MICROBIOLOGY RESEARCH ADVANCES

INFECTIOUS DISEASES

RESPONSE, RECOVERY AND TRENDS

MICROBIOLOGY RESEARCH ADVANCES

Additional books and e-books in this series can be found
on Nova's website under the Series tab.

MICROBIOLOGY RESEARCH ADVANCES

INFECTIOUS DISEASES

RESPONSE, RECOVERY AND TRENDS

PHILIPPE GEORGES
EDITOR

snova
New York

NOTICE TO THE READER

Library of Congress Cataloging-in-Publication Data

ISBN: 978-1-53616-401-5

Published by Nova Science Publishers, Inc. † New York

CONTENTS

PREFACE

An infectious disease threat is unique because of the transmissibility of diseases and the mobility of human populations. Infectious disease threats in recent years—such as Zika and Ebola outbreaks—have heightened the United States' attention to future potential threats, and raised questions about the nation's preparedness and response capabilities. Chapter 1 describes funding HHS has made available to awardees through its key preparedness and capacity-building programs—ELC, HPP, and PHEP; and these programs' performance measurement data on the awardees' infectious disease preparedness capacity.

The World Health Organization (WHO) declared the Zika virus a public health emergency of international concern in February 2016. Zika virus disease can cause adverse pregnancy and neurological outcomes. Chapter 2 examines information on what is known and not known about the epidemiology of the Zika virus, and any challenges with conducting surveillance and epidemiological studies, characteristics of different diagnostic tests authorized during the outbreak, challenges test manufacturers and users faced, and the extent to which FDA and CDC followed their own communication guidance, and the strengths and limitations of available mosquito control methods, and challenges federal agencies face supporting these efforts. Chapter 3 describes the status of funds obligated and disbursed from the Zika supplemental funding appropriated to HHS and its agencies; and how selected awardees used their Zika supplemental funding, and their experiences with applying for and managing the funding. Chapter 4 examines the status of USAID and State funding for U.S. Zika response overseas, activities supported by these funds, and implementation challenges, if any, and responses to any challenges.

The 2014-2015 Ebola outbreak in West Africa caused long-term second-order impacts, including disruptions to health systems, job loss, and food insecurity. As of September 30, 2017, of the $1.6 billion that the U.S. Agency for International Development (USAID) had obligated for the Ebola outbreak. Chapter 5 examines obligations for USAID's Ebola recovery projects, the status of USAID's implementation of these projects, and USAID's evaluation of Ebola recovery efforts. On August 1, 2018, the World Health Organization (WHO) reported a new Ebola outbreak in eastern DRC, about a week after declaring that a separate outbreak had ended in western DRC as reported in chapter 6.

Between September 2018 and May 2019, the number of African swine fever (ASF) outbreaks has rapidly increased, most notably in China, triggering economic losses in affected pork-producing countries as discussed in chapter 7.

As reported in chapter 9, Tuberculosis (TB) remains a major, and evolving, health challenge in many parts of the world and a priority for the U.S. Congress and international community.

Congress has long taken an interest in infectious disease prevention and control. According to chapter 10, the measles, mumps, and rubella (MMR) vaccine is 97% effective in preventing infection and related deaths, and routine MMR vaccination is recommended for all children.

Chapter 1 - An infectious disease threat is unique because of the transmissibility of diseases and the mobility of human populations, among other reasons. Infectious disease threats in recent years—such as Zika and Ebola outbreaks—have heightened the United States' attention to future potential threats, and raised questions about the nation's preparedness and response capabilities. A congressional report included a provision for GAO to report on the U.S. public health system's current capacity to respond to infectious disease threats. This chapter describes (1) funding HHS has made available to awardees—states and other jurisdictions—through its key preparedness and capacity-building programs—ELC, HPP, and PHEP; and (2) these programs' performance measurement data on the awardees' infectious disease preparedness capacity. To do this work, GAO analyzed HHS's data on awards provided to awardees through the three key programs using annual and supplemental appropriations, and interviewed HHS officials and non-federal stakeholders about such funding. GAO identified non-federal stakeholders representing medical and public health associations, research centers, and others through a review of relevant literature, as well as prior GAO work. GAO also reviewed the most recently available data on awardee performance on 20 measures directly related to infectious disease preparedness collectively used by the three programs. GAO categorized these 20 measures into four preparedness capacity areas.

Chapter 2 - Zika virus disease can cause adverse pregnancy and neurological outcomes. Given this ongoing threat, GAO was asked to evaluate progress made and challenges faced by federal agencies in responding to the Zika virus outbreak in the United States. GAO examined (1) information on what is known and not known about the epidemiology of the Zika virus, and any challenges with conducting surveillance and epidemiological studies, (2) characteristics of different diagnostic tests authorized during the outbreak, challenges test manufacturers and users faced, and the extent to which FDA and CDC followed their own communication guidance, and (3) the strengths and limitations of available mosquito control methods, and challenges federal agencies face supporting these efforts. GAO reviewed literature and agency documentation, and interviewed federal and state officials about the Zika virus and the U.S. response. GAO also convened an expert meeting with the assistance of the National Academy of Sciences to discuss various issues surrounding the response to the Zika virus.

Chapter 3 - Zika—a virus primarily transmitted through mosquito bites—can cause symptoms that include fever, rash, and joint and muscle pain. In pregnant women, the Zika virus can be passed to the fetus and cause severe brain defects. In response to an outbreak in the United States and its territories, Congress appropriated $932 million in September 2016 through the Zika Response and Preparedness Act to HHS and its agencies to prevent, prepare for, and respond to the Zika virus and its related health conditions, and conduct related research. The act also included a provision that GAO study the activities supported with the appropriated funds. This chapter describes (1) the status of funds obligated and disbursed from the Zika supplemental funding appropriated to HHS and its agencies; and (2) how selected awardees used their Zika supplemental funding, and their experiences with applying for and managing the funding. To do this work, GAO reviewed agency documents on Zika supplemental funding and activities, and interviewed officials from the HHS agencies and selected awardees. To select awardees, GAO identified states based on the amount of initial Zika supplemental funding they received from CDC, the Centers for Medicare & Medicaid Services, and the Health Resources and Services Administration; and selected states with the highest and lowest funding. In total, GAO selected 12 awardees: 10 states, as well as one county and one city from 2 of the 10 states. GAO provided a draft of this chapter to HHS. In response, HHS provided technical comments, which were incorporated as appropriate.

Chapter 4 - The World Health Organization (WHO) declared the Zika virus a public health emergency of international concern in February 2016. According to WHO, as of March 2017, 79 countries and territories—including 48 in the Western Hemisphere—reported evidence of ongoing Zika transmission. In April 2016, USAID and State repurposed $215 million for Zika from funds appropriated for Ebola. Subsequently, the Zika Response and Preparedness Appropriations Act, 2016, provided over $175 million in supplemental funding to USAID and State to support Zika response efforts overseas. The act also included a provision for GAO to review the status of USAID and State actions to respond to Zika. In March 2019, the Centers for Disease Control and Prevention downgraded its international travel warning for Zika. This chapter examines (1) the status of USAID and State funding for U.S. Zika response overseas, (2) activities supported by these funds, and (3) implementation challenges, if any, and responses to any challenges. GAO reviewed information from U.S. agencies and met with U.S. and host country officials in Washington, D.C. GAO also conducted fieldwork in a nongeneralizable sample of countries in Latin America and the Caribbean where agencies implemented key response activities.

Chapter 5 - The 2014-2015 Ebola outbreak in West Africa caused long-term second-order impacts, including disruptions to health systems, job loss, and food insecurity. Congress appropriated about $2.5 billion for USAID and the Department of State (State), in part, for international efforts to prevent, prepare for, and respond to an Ebola outbreak and mandated that the agencies report to congressional committees on the use of the funds. As of September 2017, USAID had allocated almost all of the appropriated Ebola funds. In 2016, USAID contracted for an evaluation of Ebola recovery activities. The fiscal year 2015 appropriations act included a provision for GAO to conduct oversight of USAID and State activities supported with funds from the Ebola response and preparedness appropriations. GAO's 2016 report (GAO-17-35) focused on USAID and State funding for Ebola response and preparedness. This chapter examines (1) obligations for USAID's Ebola recovery projects, (2) the status of USAID's implementation of these projects, and (3) USAID's evaluation of Ebola recovery efforts. GAO analyzed USAID funding data as of September 30, 2017, which are the latest data provided to Congress, reviewed project documents and evaluation plans, interviewed agency officials, and conducted fieldwork in Guinea, Liberia, and Sierra Leone.

Chapter 6 - For years, Congress has provided funds to prevent, detect, and respond to infectious disease threats, including those with pandemic potential like Ebola. In regular appropriations, since FY2014 Congress has annually provided $72.5 million to the U.S. Agency for International Development (USAID) for such efforts. From FY2015 to FY2017, Congress appropriated annually $55.1 million to the U.S. Centers for Disease Control and Prevention (CDC); in FY2018, it provided $108.2 million, including an authority to spend $50 million over three years for global health security efforts. In FY2015, Congress also provided over $5 billion in emergency funds for domestic and global efforts to contain the 2014-2015 West Africa Ebola outbreak (P.L. 113-235). Some of those unspent funds were used to contain a 2018 outbreak in western Democratic Republic of Congo (DRC) and are being used to fight the ongoing outbreak. On August 1, 2018, the World Health Organization (WHO) reported a new Ebola outbreak in eastern DRC, about one week after declaring that a separate outbreak had ended in western DRC. The ongoing Ebola outbreak—the 10th to be documented in DRC—is the largest in the country's history and has continued to spread. It is occurring in North Kivu and Ituri provinces, where a protracted conflict has caused a long-running humanitarian crisis: as of mid-2018, 4.3 million people were in need of humanitarian aid. In addition to classic public health response tools (surveillance, contact tracing, isolation, and safe burials), health workers (HWs) are using an investigational vaccine to counter the spread of disease. Unpredictable armed conflict and intermittent community resistance to these efforts are hindering all aspects of outbreak control. As of February 4, 2019, WHO reported 785 confirmed and probable Ebola cases in Ituri and North Kivu, including 484 deaths. Observers are concerned that the outbreak could spread to Goma, the capital of North Kivu, a city of over 1 million people that is also an operational hub for the United

Nations (U.N.) peacekeeping mission and international relief efforts in DRC, as well as to neighboring countries. While Uganda (which borders the most affected areas in DRC) has prior experience in Ebola control, Rwanda and Burundi do not. South Sudan's current minimal state capacity and protracted armed conflict suggest a coordinated disease control response would be highly challenging.

Chapter 7 - Between September 2018 and May 2019, the number of African swine fever (ASF) outbreaks has rapidly increased, most notably in China, triggering economic losses in affected pork-producing countries. Since September 2018, the World Organization for Animal Health (OIE)—an intergovernmental organization coordinating, supporting, and promoting animal health and disease control—has reported that over 2.8 million hogs have been culled globally due to ASF. Many industry observers believe that the actual number of culled animals is much higher. The extent of ASF outbreaks is expected to affect international trade in pork and feedstuffs. The U.S. Department of Agriculture's (USDA) Animal and Plant Health Inspection Service (APHIS) is monitoring the global spread of ASF and has developed plans to prevent ASF introduction into the United States.

Chapter 8 - Tuberculosis (TB) remains a major, and evolving, health challenge in many parts of the world and a priority for the U.S. Congress and international community. The U.S. government is one of the largest donors to global TB control efforts. The 116th Congress may consider future funding needs for TB control, particularly for vaccine research and disease surveillance and detection through strengthening health care infrastructure.

Chapter 9 - Congress has long taken an interest in infectious disease prevention and control. Measles is a highly contagious virus that is transmitted through droplets emitted from an infected person when coughing and sneezing. The virus can live for up to two hours in the airspace or on a surface where an infected person coughed or sneezed. Other people can contract the disease if they breathe contaminated air or touch their eyes, nose, or mouth after touching a contaminated surface. Up to 90% of those in the proximity of an infected person who are not immune to the disease will be infected. Symptoms usually include high fever, rash, runny nose, and ear infections. Measles can also cause hearing loss, blindness, encephalitis (an infection that causes brain swelling), severe diarrhea, and severe respiratory infections such as pneumonia. The U.S. Centers for Disease Control and Prevention (CDC) estimates that up to two of every 1,000 children infected with measles will die.

In: Infectious Diseases
Editor: Philippe Georges
ISBN: 978-1-53616-401-5

Chapter 1

INFECTIOUS DISEASE THREATS: FUNDING AND PERFORMANCE OF KEY PREPAREDNESS AND CAPACITY-BUILDING PROGRAMS*

United States Government Accountability Office

ABBREVIATIONS

ASPR	Office of the Assistant Secretary for Preparedness and Response
CDC	Centers for Disease Control and Prevention
ELC	Epidemiology and Laboratory Capacity for Infectious Diseases
HHS	Department of Health and Human Services
HPP	Hospital Preparedness Program
NOFO	notice of funding opportunity
PHEF	Public Health Emergency Fund
PHEP	Public Health Emergency Preparedness

WHY GAO DID THIS STUDY

An infectious disease threat is unique because of the transmissibility of diseases and the mobility of human populations, among other reasons. Infectious disease threats in

* This is an edited, reformatted and augmented version of United States Government Accountability Office; Report to Congressional Requesters, Publication No. GAO-18-362, dated May 2018.

recent years—such as Zika and Ebola outbreaks—have heightened the United States' attention to future potential threats, and raised questions about the nation's preparedness and response capabilities.

A congressional report included a provision for GAO to report on the U.S. public health system's current capacity to respond to infectious disease threats. This chapter describes (1) funding HHS has made available to awardees—states and other jurisdictions—through its key preparedness and capacity-building programs—ELC, HPP, and PHEP; and (2) these programs' performance measurement data on the awardees' infectious disease preparedness capacity.

To do this work, GAO analyzed HHS's data on awards provided to awardees through the three key programs using annual and supplemental appropriations, and interviewed HHS officials and non-federal stakeholders about such funding. GAO identified non-federal stakeholders representing medical and public health associations, research centers, and others through a review of relevant literature, as well as prior GAO work. GAO also reviewed the most recently available data on awardee performance on 20 measures directly related to infectious disease preparedness collectively used by the three programs. GAO categorized these 20 measures into four preparedness capacity areas.

WHAT GAO FOUND

The Department of Health and Human Services (HHS) has three key preparedness and capacity-building programs—Epidemiology and Laboratory Capacity for Infectious Diseases (ELC), the Hospital Preparedness Program (HPP), and Public Health Emergency Preparedness (PHEP). These three programs awarded about $21.2 billion to states and other jurisdictions from 2002 through 2017 to carry out public health preparedness and response efforts, including those related to infectious diseases, natural disasters, or terrorist events. Of this amount, $18.4 billion were awards funded from annual appropriations. The remaining was funded from supplemental appropriations to respond to specific infectious disease threats, including Zika, Ebola, and H1N1 pandemic influenza. HHS officials and non-federal stakeholders told GAO that supplemental appropriations were important for supporting necessary surges in capacity, but the timing of additional awards can limit response.

HHS's three key preparedness and capacity-building programs measure performance in four areas that directly relate to infectious disease preparedness capacity—electronic lab reporting, epidemiology capacity, laboratory capacity, and responder protection. The majority of awardees (states and other jurisdictions) met targets for all nine measures in the responder protection area, which measures activities related to safety and coordination for responders. However, awardee performance in the other three areas was mixed.

- *Electronic lab reporting.* One of two measures was met in this area. This area relates to the sending of laboratory reports to public health agencies via electronic means (as opposed to traditional, paper reports).
- *Epidemiology capacity.* One of three measures was met in this area. This area relates to awardees' ability to identify and respond to infectious disease outbreaks.
- *Laboratory capacity.* Five of six measures were met in this area. This area relates to both laboratory testing of certain pathogens, and communication between laboratories and other public entities.

HHS reviewed a copy of this chapter and provided technical comments, which GAO incorporated as appropriate.

HHS's Three Key Preparedness and Capacity-Building Programs: ELC, HPP, and PHEP

Program	Purpose of awards provided to states and other jurisdictions
Epidemiology and Laboratory Capacity for Infectious Diseases (ELC)	Supports epidemiologists, surveillance systems, and laboratory facilities to build state and local capacity to combat domestic infectious disease threats.
Hospital Preparedness Program (HPP)	Improves medical surge capacity by enhancing community and health system preparedness for various public health threats, including infectious disease threats.
Public Health Emergency Preparedness (PHEP)	Strengthens state and local public health departments' ability to prepare for a variety of public health threats, including infectious disease threats.

Source: GAO summary of the Department of Health and Human Services' (HHS) program information. | GAO-18-362

May 24, 2018

The Honorable Roy Blunt
Chairman

The Honorable Patty Murray
Ranking Member
Subcommittee on Labor, Health and Human Services, Education, and Related Agencies
Committee on Appropriations
United States Senate

The Honorable Tom Cole
Chairman

The Honorable Rosa DeLauro
Ranking Member
Subcommittee on Labor, Health and Human Services, Education, and Related Agencies
Committee on Appropriations
House of Representatives

An infectious disease threat is unique because of the transmissibility of diseases, the universal susceptibility of the world's population to pathogens that have not previously circulated, and the mobility of human populations. Infectious disease threats in recent years—such as Zika, Ebola, and H1N1 pandemic influenza—have heightened the United States' attention to future potential infectious disease threats and raised questions about the nation's preparedness and response capabilities. The Department of Health and Human Services (HHS) is the lead federal agency for public health and medical preparedness for, and response to, infectious disease threats. HHS provides funding to states, localities, territories, and freely associated states to aid capacity building and preparedness for infectious disease threats and other public health threats, such as natural disasters or terrorist events, through three key programs: (1) Epidemiology and Laboratory Capacity for Infectious Diseases (ELC), (2) the Hospital Preparedness Program (HPP), and (3) Public Health Emergency Preparedness (PHEP). The Centers for Disease Control and Prevention (CDC) administers ELC and PHEP, while the HHS Office of the Assistant Secretary for Preparedness and Response (ASPR) administers HPP. These three key programs routinely monitor select aspects of state and local preparedness capacity through certain performance measures.[1]

State and local governments typically lead the domestic response to an infectious disease threat. If a threat is severe enough that state and local response capabilities—including those supported by ELC, HPP, and PHEP—are overwhelmed, state and local governments become reliant on additional support from the federal government. For example, during recent infectious disease threats, HHS received supplemental appropriations to respond to Zika in 2016, Ebola in 2014, and H1N1 pandemic influenza in 2009.[2] These recent threats have generated discussions about states' and other

---

[1] Throughout this chapter, we use the term "preparedness capacity" to refer to preparedness activities, such as identifying and coordinating with partners involved in a response, as well as capacity-building activities that are critical to a response, such as laboratory services and public health surveillance.

[2] A supplemental appropriation is an act appropriating funds in addition to those already provided in an annual appropriation act. Supplemental appropriations provide additional budget authority usually in cases where the need for funds is considered too urgent to be postponed until enactment of the next regular annual appropriation bill. For Zika supplemental appropriations to HHS, see the Zika Response and Preparedness Act, Pub. L. No. 114-223, div. B tit. I, 130 Stat. 857, 901. For Ebola supplemental appropriations to HHS, see the Consolidated and Further Continuing Appropriations Act, 2015, Pub. L. No. 113-235, div. G, tit. VI., 128 Stat. 2130, 2520. For H1N1 pandemic influenza supplemental appropriations to HHS see the Supplemental Appropriations Act, 2009, Pub. L. No. 111-32, tit. VIII, 123 Stat. 1859, 1884.

jurisdictions' preparedness and response capacity, as well as federal funding to support such capacity.

A Senate Report accompanying the 2017 Consolidated Appropriations Act included a provision for GAO to study the U.S. public health system's capacity to respond to infectious disease threats.[3] This chapter describes

1. the funding that HHS has made available to awardees—states and other jurisdictions—through the three key programs that aid states' infectious disease preparedness capacity, and
2. these programs' performance measurement data on the awardees' infectious disease preparedness capacity.

To describe the funding that HHS has made available to awardees through the three key preparedness and capacity-building programs, we obtained data from ASPR and CDC on the amount of awards that the agencies made through ELC, HPP, and PHEP to states and other jurisdictions in the form of cooperative agreements from fiscal years 2002 through 2017.[4] We analyzed these data to determine the amount of awards made by CDC (through ELC and PHEP) and ASPR (through HPP) with funding from annual appropriations, as well as awards made with funding from supplemental appropriations provided to respond to specific infectious disease threats. We assessed the reliability of the award data we obtained by comparing these data to data in published reports, such as agency budget justifications; following up with agency officials regarding any discrepancies in the data; and gathering information from agencies on the internal checks they use when maintaining their data. Based on these steps, we determined that the data were reliable for our reporting purposes. We also reviewed documentation and interviewed ASPR and CDC officials, as well as non- federal stakeholders, to gather information on how awards to states and other jurisdictions have aided responses to recent infectious disease threats (Zika, Ebola, and H1N1 pandemic influenza). We identified the non-federal stakeholders to interview by reviewing relevant literature on infectious disease preparedness and response funding, as well as our prior work.[5] We selected and interviewed 10 non-federal stakeholders representing medical associations,

[3] See Pub. L. No. 115-31, § 4, 131 Stat. 135, 137; 163 Cong. Rec. H3949 (Daily ed. May 3, 2017); S. Rep. No. 114-274, at 80 (2016).

[4] For purposes of this chapter, we use the term "award," which could also be referred to as an obligation—a definite commitment by a federal entity that creates a legal liability to make payments immediately or in the future. A cooperative agreement is a legal instrument used to provide financial support when substantial interaction is expected between a federal agency and a state, local government, or other recipient carrying out the funded activity.

[5] See, for example, GAO, *Emerging Infections Diseases: Actions Needed to Address the Challenges of Responding to Zika Virus Disease Outbreaks*, GAO-17-445 (Washington, D.C.: May 23, 2017); *National Preparedness: Improvements Needed for Measuring Awardee Performance in Meeting Medical and Public Health Preparedness Goals,* GAO-13-278 (Washington, D.C.: Mar. 22, 2013); and *Influenza Pandemic: Lessons Learned from the H1N1 Pandemic Should Be Incorporated into Future Planning*, GAO-11-632 (Washington, D.C.: June 27, 2011).

public health associations, academic research centers, and organizations with emergency preparedness and response experience. The perspectives from non-federal stakeholders presented in our findings are those that the stakeholders generally agreed on, and when available, we present alternative stakeholder perspectives. While we attempted to gather similar information from all non-federal stakeholders, there were cases in which all stakeholders did not provide a perspective on each issue presented. The views of the 10 non-federal stakeholders are not generalizable beyond these stakeholders; however, they provide insights on how federal funding has aided the response to certain infectious disease threats.

To describe the three key programs' performance measurement data on awardees' infectious disease preparedness capacity, we obtained and reviewed data from ASPR and CDC on awardee performance. Specifically, we reviewed data for a total of 20 performance measures: 8 measures from ELC, 5 measures from HPP, and 7 measures from PHEP. For each measure, we reviewed the most recently available, agency-validated data (from 2015 to 2017, depending on the measure). The 20 measures we reviewed are a subset of measures used by the three programs that directly relate to infectious disease preparedness capacity. HPP and PHEP are programs that support "all-hazards" preparedness capacity, meaning they help states and other jurisdictions build capacities to respond to a range of public health threats, including, but not limited to, infectious diseases. Although many of the "all hazards" performance measures used by the programs could indirectly relate to infectious disease preparedness capacity, our review focused on those measures directly related to infectious disease preparedness capacity, as we determined through consultation with ASPR and CDC officials.[6]

Through our review of agency performance measure documentation and interviews with agency officials, we determined that the 20 performance measures fell into four areas of preparedness capacity: (1) electronic lab reporting, (2) epidemiology capacity, (3) laboratory capacity, and (4) responder protection. For our analysis, we grouped the performance measures into these four areas, with consultation from ASPR and CDC officials. In general, the majority of awardees reported data for each of the 20 measures in our review. Reasons for not reporting data included a measure not applying to the awardee or the awardee did not conduct an exercise necessary to determine their performance on a measure.[7] We calculated the percentage of awardees that achieved a

---

[6] An example of a measure that indirectly relates to infectious disease preparedness capacity is the PHEP measure that asks if public health officials have procedures in place to manage volunteers supporting a public health or medical incident. Centers for Disease Control and Prevention, *Public Health Emergency Preparedness Cooperative Agreement Budget Period 1 Performance Measure Specifications and Implementation Guidance, July 1, 2017 – June 30, 2018* (Washington, D.C.).

[7] A measure did not apply to an awardee when the measure referred to an entity, such as an Ebola treatment center, that did not exist within the awardee's jurisdiction. An Ebola treatment center is a hospital that is prepared to provide comprehensive care to people diagnosed with Ebola virus disease for the duration of a patient's illness, as designated by states and localities with CDC input. Awardees that were provided less funding, such as localities and U.S. territories, may not have been required to report data on certain measures, according to CDC officials.

performance target for each measure based on the number of awardees that reported data on the measure and to which the measure applied.

To assess the reliability of the performance measure data, we reviewed agency documentation, such as performance measure implementation guidance provided to awardees; interviewed knowledgeable ASPR and CDC officials about their data systems and data validation processes; and performed checks of the data for consistency and completeness. Based on these steps, we determined that the data for the 20 performance measures included in our review were sufficiently reliable for our reporting purposes. One limitation of performance measure data is that these data are self-reported by the awardees. ASPR and CDC officials conduct data checks to mitigate this limitation, such as looking for outliers in the data and conducting validation calls with awardees.

We conducted this performance audit from June 2017 to May 2018 in accordance with generally accepted government auditing standards. Those standards require that we plan and perform the audit to obtain sufficient, appropriate evidence to provide a reasonable basis for our findings and conclusions based on our audit objectives. We believe that the evidence obtained provides a reasonable basis for our findings and conclusions based on our audit objectives.

BACKGROUND

ELC, HPP, and PHEP are the three key HHS programs through which the department provides annual awards to states and other jurisdictions to aid capacity building and preparedness for public health threats, including infectious disease threats, natural disasters, or terrorist events. ELC was established in 1995 and currently has 64 awardees—all 50 states, 6 localities, and 8 territories and freely associated states.[8] HPP and PHEP were established in 2002 and currently have 62 awardees—all 50 states, 4 localities, and 8 territories and freely associated states.[9] ASPR and CDC provide awards through the three programs using cooperative agreements.

ELC, HPP, and PHEP Goals and Activities

Federal support through ELC, HPP, and PHEP helps states and other jurisdictions build and strengthen their abilities to effectively respond to public health threats before

---

[8] ELC's 64 awardees are the 50 states; 6 localities, which are Chicago, the District of Columbia, Houston, Los Angeles County, New York City, and Philadelphia; and 8 territories and freely associated states—American Samoa, Federated States of Micronesia, Guam, Marshall Islands, Northern Mariana Islands, Palau, Puerto Rico, and the U.S. Virgin Islands. See 42 U.S.C. § 247d-3a (authorizing awards made by ELC).

[9] HPP's and PHEP's 62 awardees are the same as the ELC awardees with the exception of 2 localities, Houston and Philadelphia. See 42 U.S.C. §§ 247d-3a, 247-3b (authorizing awards made by HPP and PHEP).

they occur. While ELC primarily supports public health infectious disease prevention and control capacity, HPP and PHEP are programs that support "all-hazards" preparedness capacity, meaning they help build capacities to respond to a range of public health threats, including infectious diseases, natural disasters, or terrorist events. According to ASPR and CDC documentation, each program has a distinct goal:

- ELC's goal is to support capacity building to combat domestic infectious disease threats. The program funds epidemiologists and activities that support surveillance systems, modernize laboratory facilities, and develop integrated information networks at local and state levels, among other disease detection and response activities. Two primary classes of ELC funding include (1) flexible, non-disease- specific funding (generally referred to as "cross-cutting" funding) to address high-priority needs related to epidemiology, laboratory, and health information systems; and (2) disease-specific, categorical funding that targets specific infectious diseases and other related public health threats, including antimicrobial-resistant bacteria, arboviral and tickborne diseases (e.g., Lyme, West Nile, Zika), foodborne disease and illnesses, healthcare-associated infections, influenza, and waterborne diseases.[10]
- HPP's goal is to improve patient outcomes and medical surge capacity by enhancing community and health care system preparedness for health consequences of various public health threats, including infectious disease threats. The program funds the development of health care coalitions—networks of health care entities and response organizations that can provide medical services, resources, or support during a public health threat. Working through these coalitions, HPP funds activities such as establishing electronic coordination and situational awareness systems to track available hospital beds and other resources, engaging with other responders through interoperable communications systems, maintaining or enhancing medical caches to protect health care workers and patients during a response, and developing and improving preparedness plans through regional exercises.[11]
- PHEP's goal is to develop effective public health emergency management and response programs nationwide. PHEP strengthens the capabilities of state, local, and territorial public health departments to prepare for, and respond to, evolving public health threats, including infectious disease threats. Activities funded include developing and exercising plans to receive, store, distribute, and dispense life-saving medicines and emergency medical supplies to the public during a

---

[10] Arbovirus, or arthropod-borne virus, refers to a virus that is transmitted via arthropods, such as mosquitoes and ticks. Other diseases in this category include chikungunya, dengue fever, Rocky Mountain spotted fever, and tularemia.

[11] A medical cache is a storage of medical supplies and medications that can be deployed in an emergency.

response to a public health threat, and coordinating emergency operations activities during a public health response to limit the health effects of life-threatening emergencies. PHEP funding also supports building epidemiological surveillance systems and laboratory capability for detecting, testing, and identifying harmful pathogens and reporting results to CDC, and conducting drills and exercises to test response capabilities.

Funding for ELC, HPP, and PHEP Awards

Awards to states and other jurisdictions through ELC, HPP, and PHEP are generally funded from annual appropriations.[12] Specifically,

- ELC awards are funded by annual appropriations to CDC, as well as amounts made available to the Prevention and Public Health Fund;[13]
- HPP awards are funded by annual appropriations to the Public Health and Social Services Emergency Fund;[14] and
- PHEP awards are funded by annual appropriations to CDC.

In addition, ASPR and CDC have, at times, provided awards to states and other jurisdictions through these programs in response to specific infectious disease threats with funding from supplemental appropriations provided by Congress to HHS. Supplemental appropriations provide budget authority for government activities, in addition to funding provided in annual appropriations or continuing resolutions.[15]

---

[12] When regular annual appropriations are not completed before the beginning of the fiscal year, funding may be provided by continuing resolutions for the full year, up to a specified date, or until regular appropriations are enacted. ELC awards are determined by a competitive technical and objective review process. HPP and PHEP annual awards are based on a formula that includes a base amount for each awardee plus population-based funding.

[13] Section 4002 of the Patient Protection and Affordable Care Act established the Prevention and Public Health Fund in 2010 to "provide for expanded and sustained national investment in prevention and public health programs to improve health and help restrain the rate of growth in private and public health care costs," and made appropriations to the fund for fiscal year 2010 and each year thereafter. Pub. L. No. 111-148, §§ 4002,10401(b), 124 Stat. 119, 541, 974 (2010) (codified as amended at 42 U.S.C. § 300u-11). Since 2010, CDC has used Prevention and Public Health Fund resources to fund ELC awards for "cross-cutting" activities, as well as other public health programs and activities. For information on activities funded by Prevention and Public Health Fund in fiscal years 2010 and 2011, see GAO, *Prevention and Public Health Fund: Activities Funded in Fiscal Years 2010 and 2011*, GAO-12-788 (Washington, D.C.: Sept. 13, 2012).

[14] The Public Health and Social Services Emergency Fund is an HHS budget account that funds authorized ASPR and other HHS office operations and activities to support the nation's ability to prepare for, respond to, and recover from the health consequences of naturally occurring and manmade threats.

[15] Budget authority authorizes an agency to enter into financial obligations that will result in outlays of federal government funds.

ELC, HPP, and PHEP Performance Measures

ELC, HPP, and PHEP awardees must fulfill certain application, financial, and reporting requirements as part of the terms of the programs' cooperative agreements. As part of these reporting requirements, awardees are required to report on performance measures, which can number 35 or more across all three programs.[16] For example, PHEP awardees must report on the percentage of volunteers that were deployed for an exercise or actual public health threat within a determined time frame, and HPP awardees are subject to several measures to assess the extent to which they have appropriate preparedness and response plans in place. Reporting on performance measures helps the agencies gauge awardees' progress on discrete activities related to preparedness capacity, as well as to determine where additional technical assistance and other resources to support awardees are needed. Further, agency officials stated that performance measures can have targets that are intended to continuously challenge awardees to meet high standards. The 20 performance measures included in this chapter (i.e., those that are directly related to infectious disease preparedness capacity) constitute a subset of the programs' measures. We reported in March 2013 that many other performance measures used by HPP and PHEP did not have targets and recommended that HHS develop targets for such measures.[17] We also recommended that HPP and PHEP performance measures remain consistent over time. Since our 2013 report, PHEP's measures have generally remained consistent in recent years, but some of these measures lack targets. HPP implemented new measures for the 2017 to 2022 project period that are not consistent with those from prior years. As of February 2018, more than half of these new measures lacked targets. ASPR officials told us that they expect measures to change over time to allow HPP to adapt to evolving public health threats, and agency guidance notes that targets may be set at a later date after establishing awardees' baseline scores.

---

[16] See Centers for Disease Control and Prevention, *Public Health Emergency Preparedness Cooperative Agreement Budget Period 1 Performance Measure Specifications and Implementation Guidance, July 1, 2017–June 30, 2018* (Atlanta, Ga.); *Instructions for Preparing Annual Performance Report/Continuation Application: Epidemiology and Laboratory Capacity for Infectious Diseases, Funding Opportunity Announcement Number: CK14-140104PPHF17* (Atlanta, Ga.); and *Epidemiology and Laboratory Capacity for Infectious Diseases Cooperative Agreement Performance Measures Guidance for Domestic Ebola Supplement, Project Period March 31, 2015 to March 30, 2018, Version 5* (Atlanta, Ga.: September 2017). See also Office of the Assistant Secretary for Preparedness and Response, *2017–2022 Hospital Preparedness Program Performance Measures Implementation Guidance* (Washington, D.C.); and *Hospital Preparedness Program Measure Manual: Implementation Guidance for Ebola Preparedness Measures* (Washington, D.C.: July 2015).

[17] See GAO-13-278.

HHS Awarded $21.2 Billion to States through Key Programs; Stakeholders Stated that Available Funding Assisted Capacity Surges, but They Also Cited Challenges

HHS's Three Key Programs Awarded $21.2 Billion to States and Other Jurisdictions from Fiscal Years 2002 through 2017; Supplemental Awards Played a Large Role in Certain Years

From fiscal years 2002 through 2017, a total of about $21.2 billion was awarded by ASPR and CDC to states and other jurisdictions through ELC, HPP, and PHEP to carry out public health preparedness and response efforts, including those related to infectious diseases, natural disasters, or terrorist events.[18] The vast majority of this amount—about 86 percent, or $18.4 billion—was provided from annual appropriations. The amount of awards from annual appropriations was mostly made by CDC through PHEP, which totaled about $11.4 billion over the time period. The amount of awards made by ASPR through HPP and by CDC through ELC totaled about $5.6 billion and $1.5 billion, respectively.

The combined amount of awards provided through the three programs' annual appropriations has generally decreased, from about $1.4 billion in fiscal year 2003 (which was when the total awards were at the highest level) to about $1.0 billion in fiscal year 2017, though funding trends between the three programs have varied over time. Specifically, the amount of awards provided through ELC from annual appropriations almost doubled, from about $0.1 billion in fiscal year 2002 to about $0.2 billion in fiscal year 2017. The amount of awards provided through HPP and PHEP from annual appropriations generally decreased, though the amount of awards has remained relatively constant in recent years. Overall, from its high in fiscal year 2003 to fiscal year 2017, HPP award amounts decreased about 54 percent. PHEP award amounts decreased about 33 percent from its high in fiscal year 2002 to fiscal year 2017. (See Figure 1.)

In addition, from fiscal years 2002 through 2017, a total of about $2.9 billion in awards has been made through the three programs from supplemental appropriations, and these awards have been a large percentage of the total award amounts provided in certain years.[19] For example, award amounts provided through ELC from supplemental appropriations in fiscal years 2015 through 2017 to respond to Ebola and Zika ranged between about 30 and 50 percent of the total award amounts during those years. (See Figure 2.)

Similarly, in fiscal years 2015 through 2017, awards were provided through HPP from supplemental appropriations to respond to Ebola, and in fiscal year 2015 these

---

[18] The nominal value of awards is presented in this chapter. Due to rounding, certain award amounts presented in this section may not sum to total award amounts reported.

[19] This amount includes about $0.3 billion through ELC, $0.4 billion through HPP, and $2.2 billion in awards through PHEP.

awards made up a large percentage of awards provided through HPP. Specifically, these award amounts totaled approximately $0.2 billion in 2015, which was about 44 percent of the total award amounts (about $0.4 billion) provided through HPP in that year. (See Figure 3.)

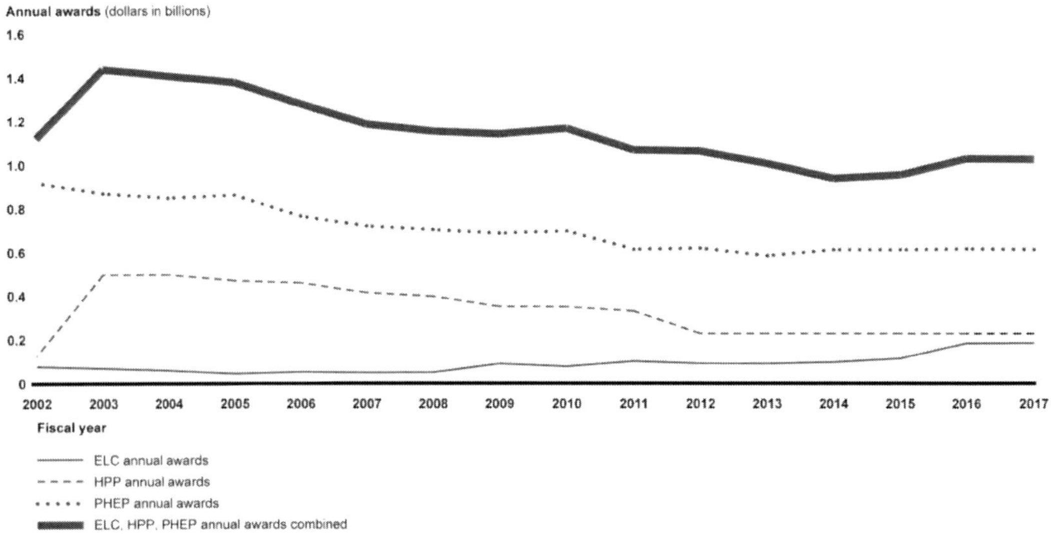

Source: GAO analysis of Office of the Assistant Secretary for Preparedness and Response and Centers for Disease Control and Prevention awards data. | GAO-18-362

Note: The Department of Health and Human Services (HHS) provides funding to states, localities, territories, and freely associated states to aid capacity building and preparedness for public health threats, including infectious disease threats, natural disasters, or terrorist events through three key programs: Epidemiology and Laboratory Capacity for Infectious Diseases (ELC), the Hospital Preparedness Program (HPP), and Public Health Emergency Preparedness (PHEP). This figure includes data on annual awards to states and other jurisdictions provided through these three programs with funding from annual appropriations to address preparedness for public health threats that include, but are not limited to, infectious disease threats.

Figure 1. Awards Provided to States and Other Jurisdictions through Three Key HHS Preparedness and Capacity-Building Programs, Annual Appropriations, Fiscal Years 2002-2017.

Awards from supplemental appropriations were also provided through PHEP in certain years, including in fiscal years 2009 and 2010 to respond to H1N1 pandemic influenza. The fiscal year 2009 award amounts for H1N1 pandemic influenza totaled close to $1.4 billion—66 percent of the total award amounts provided through PHEP in that year (about $2 billion). (See Figure 4.)

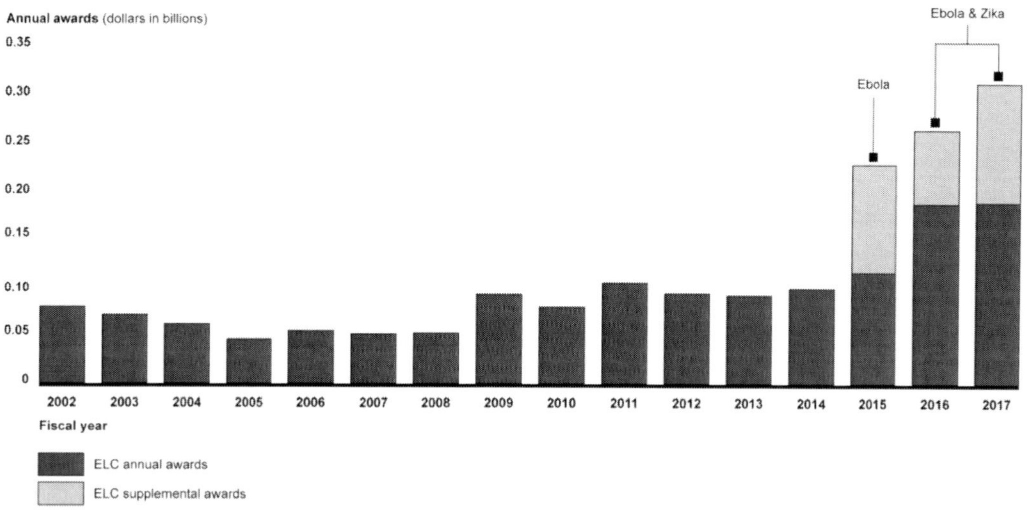

Source: Gao analysis of Centers for Disease Control and Prevention (CDC) awards data. | GAO-18-362

Note: Awards provided to respond to Zika in fiscal year 2016 were provided using funding that CDC reprogrammed away from other programs prior to supplemental appropriations being enacted. In this figure, these awards are included as awards provided from supplemental appropriations.

Figure 2. Awards Provided through Epidemiology and Laboratory Capacity for Infectious Diseases (ELC), Annual and Supplemental Appropriations, Fiscal Years 2002-2017.

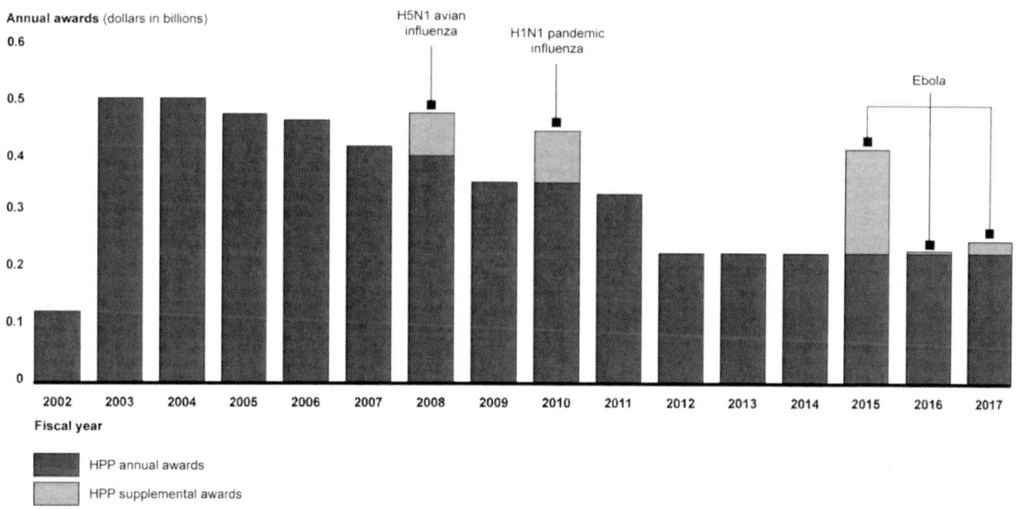

Source: GAO analysis of Office of the Assistant Secretary for Preparedness and Response awards data. | GAO-18-362

Figure 3. Awards Provided through the Hospital Preparedness Program (HPP), Annual and Supplemental Appropriations, Fiscal Years 2002-2017.

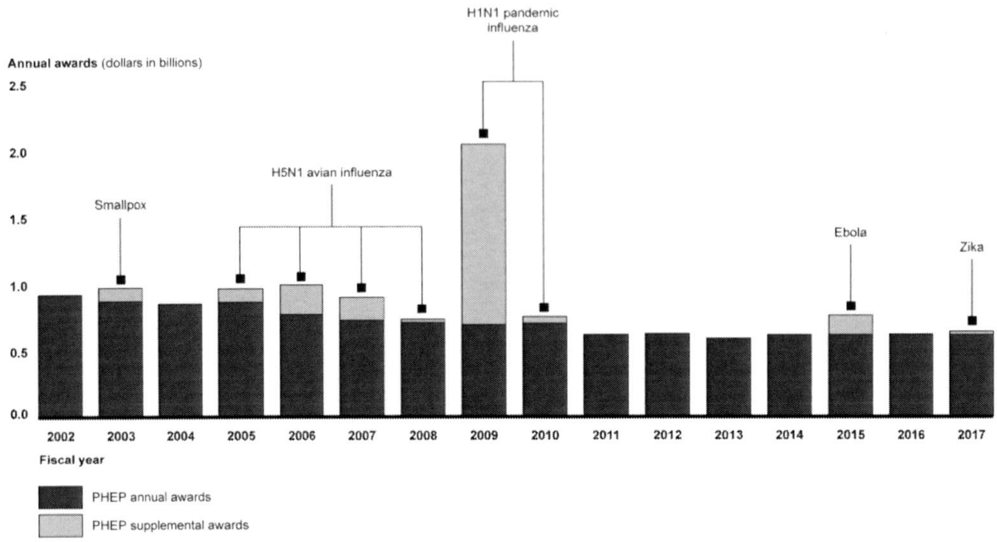

Source: GAO analysis of Centers for Disease Control and Prevention awards data. | GAO-18-362

Note: Awards provided to PHEP awardees from supplemental appropriations in fiscal years 2009 and 2010 to respond to H1N1 pandemic influenza were made through a separate granting mechanism— the Public Health Emergency Response Grant for H1N1 Influenza Pandemic. Awards provided to PHEP awardees from supplemental appropriations in fiscal year 2017 to respond to Zika were made through a separate granting mechanism—the Public Health Preparedness and Response Cooperative Agreement for All-Hazards Public Health Emergencies.

Figure 4. Awards Provided through Public Health Emergency Preparedness (PHEP), Annual and Supplemental Appropriations, Fiscal Years 2002-2017.

Stakeholders Reported that Available Funding Assisted Surges in Capacity during Recent Infectious Disease Threats; Timing of Awards Can Limit Preparedness and Response Activities

According ASPR and CDC officials, as well as most non-federal stakeholders we interviewed, awards provided through HHS's three key preparedness and capacity-building programs with supplemental appropriations were important for allowing health care systems—which include state and local public health departments, laboratories, and hospitals—to make necessary surges in capacity or take other actions, such as creating plans and training staff, to respond to infectious disease threats.[20] For example, one stakeholder told us that during the Zika threat, awards provided through ELC from supplemental appropriations allowed public health laboratories to hire additional staff and purchase laboratory testing equipment needed to conduct the high volume of Zika tests. We previously reported that awards from supplemental appropriations helped states and

[20] A health care system's ability to "surge" is the ability to have the staff and resources in place to adequately care for increased numbers of affected individuals or individuals with unusual or highly specialized needs.

local jurisdictions respond to the H1N1 pandemic influenza in 2009 and 2010.[21] For example, we found that Vermont used its award to purchase lab equipment and hire 10 temporary employees to enter vaccination data into the state's vaccine registry. We also found that Nebraska used its award to contract with nurses to administer the H1N1 influenza vaccine at mass vaccination clinics. As another example, the Association of State and Territorial Health Officials reported that the awards from supplemental appropriations provided states with resources necessary to respond to the H1N1 pandemic influenza by providing funds to support increased public health workforce capacity in surveillance and immunization.[22]

ASPR and CDC officials told us that awards provided through ELC, HPP, and PHEP are intended to establish and strengthen emergency preparedness and capacity building. Awards from annual appropriations may not fully support the need for surge capacity that states and other jurisdictions require in order to respond to an infectious disease threat, according to the officials. CDC officials said that the general decrease in PHEP awards from annual appropriations to state and local public health departments over time has limited state and local preparedness capacity. This, in turn, has increased the importance of awards from supplemental appropriations to respond to infectious disease threats. Agency officials cited a survey by the National Association of County and City Health Officials, which reported that there was a 12 percent rise in the number of local health departments that reported a decrease in their preparedness staff from 2015 levels to 2016 levels, with 34 percent reporting decreased levels in staff since 2015.[23]

Although the awards from supplemental appropriations have allowed state and local public health departments, laboratories, and hospitals to surge during a threat, most non-federal stakeholders, as well as ASPR and CDC officials, said that the timing of these awards can result in challenges to carrying out preparedness and response activities during infectious disease threats. For example, two stakeholders said that state and local public health departments' routine activities or personnel hires can be delayed while resources are used to respond to an infectious disease threat. Two stakeholders also said that PHEP awardees were affected by CDC's reprogramming of a portion of the PHEP awards from annual appropriations away from awardees to fund Zika response activities prior to the availability of supplemental appropriations.[24] According to one of these

---

[21] See GAO-11-632.

[22] See Association of State and Territorial Health Officials, *Assessing Policy Barriers to Effective Public Health Response in the H1N1Influenza Pandemic* (Arlington, Va.: June 2010), 25.

[23] In June 2016, the National Association of County and City Health Officials conducted a survey of 871 local health departments across the country. Data for the assessment were self-reported, and had a response rate of 53 percent (458 local health departments). National Association of County and City Health Officials, *The Public Health Emergency Preparedness Landscape: Findings from the 2016 Preparedness Profile Assessment* (Washington, D.C.: June 2017).

[24] The term reprogramming refers to shifting funds within an appropriation or fund account to use them for purposes other than those contemplated at the time of appropriation. In February 2016, prior to supplemental appropriations being enacted, CDC reprogrammed $44.25 million in annual appropriations away from PHEP awardees and used these funds for other activities to aid the Zika response. In September 2016, Zika supplemental funding was appropriated by the Zika Response and Preparedness Act. This funding allowed for

stakeholders, the routine PHEP preparedness activities that awardees had planned were delayed or were not fully operational until the amounts of the reprogrammed awards were returned as new awards to the PHEP awardees. According to an April 2016 survey of PHEP awardees conducted by the National Association of County and City Health Officials and other organizations, about 72 percent of responding jurisdictions reported that ongoing preparedness program areas (e.g., surveillance, epidemiological activities, and laboratory services) were likely to be affected by the reprogramming.[25]

ASPR and CDC officials also told us that it can take up to 4 months to disseminate awards through the existing programs, once supplemental appropriations are enacted. ASPR and CDC officials said that although the process for administering funds through ELC, HPP, and PHEP is familiar to states and other jurisdictions, these cooperative agreement programs do not allow for rapid dissemination of funds, because the agencies must follow their cooperative agreement administrative requirements and protocols. For example, before awarding funds from supplemental appropriations, the agencies have to create and provide notice of funding opportunities (NOFO) that jurisdictions have to apply to and be approved for before funds can be disseminated. For example, CDC officials stated that the process to get awards from supplemental appropriations to ELC awardees took about 4 months for the Ebola response and about 3 months for Zika.

In October 2017, CDC issued a new NOFO that is intended to shorten the amount of time it takes the agency to disseminate funding to respond to public health threats. This NOFO establishes a list of awardees, with existing emergency preparedness and response capacity, that are pre- approved for funding by CDC when a public health threat occurs, including infectious disease threats. According to CDC officials, any CDC program, including ELC and PHEP, could use this funding mechanism. The NOFO requires that awardees have administrative structures and plans in place to receive funding, as well as plans to respond to a public health threat. According to CDC officials, awards could potentially be provided within 2 weeks to pre-approved awardees after supplemental appropriations are enacted, as opposed to months under the current cooperative agreement programs. According to officials, all of the 64 ELC and PHEP awardees have applied to the NOFO and have been deemed eligible.[26]

---

the restoration of $44 million back to PHEP so that the program could reinstate the remaining awards. According to CDC officials, the agency restored the remaining $0.25 million from its operating budget so that the full amount of the funding—$44.25 million—was eventually provided to the PHEP awardees.

25 The majority of jurisdictions also reported that vector control, contractual services, supplies, and staffing levels were likely to be affected. The survey was fielded between April 8, 2016, and April 15, 2016, to all 62 PHEP awardees. The survey was completed by representatives from 61 jurisdictions for a total response rate of 98.4 percent. National Association of County and City Health Officials, the Association of State and Territorial Health Officials, Council of State and Territorial Epidemiologists, and the Association of Public Health Laboratories, *Impact of the Redirection of Public Health Emergency Preparedness (PHEP) Funding from State and Local Health Departments to Support National Zika Response* (Washington, D.C.: May 2016).

26 The NOFO was open to all 64 ELC and PHEP awardees, as well as five tribes, which CDC defines as federally or state recognized American Indian or Alaska Native tribal governments serving a population of at least 50,000 members. According to CDC officials, no tribes had applied to the NOFO. Agency officials told us that they

As of February 2018, the agency had begun notifying these awardees that they are on CDC's pre-approved list for funding in the case of a future public health threat. The NOFO does not apply to ASPR programs, including HPP, and ASPR officials told us that the agency does not have plans to develop a similar opportunity for ASPR programs.[27]

ASPR and CDC officials, as well as all non-federal stakeholders, also noted that a funding mechanism to fund rapid response activities when additional support is needed would be beneficial and could help address timing challenges. Such a mechanism could include the use of the existing Public Health Emergency Fund (PHEF) or a new emergency response fund specific to infectious disease.[28] The availability of any such fund for immediate use would be subject to available appropriations. According to CDC officials and most non-federal stakeholders we interviewed, such a mechanism could allow HHS to provide additional funds to state and other jurisdictions for a rapid response to infectious disease threats while the department waits for any supplemental appropriations to be enacted by Congress. While one non-federal stakeholder stated that PHEF, with available funding, could be a viable funding mechanism for funding infectious disease threats, the stakeholder cautioned against the use of such a fund without having clear definitions as to when it should be used. The stakeholder stated that there should be ongoing investments at all levels of government for preparedness and capacity-building activities, and that PHEF or another type of emergency fund should not be used to make-up for a lack in those investments. A few other stakeholders also commented that they would not want an emergency fund to be a substitute to providing ongoing funding to preparedness and capacity-building programs, such as ELC, HPP, and PHEP. (See app. I for six factors that the non-federal stakeholders said may be considered for an emergency response fund, whether using an existing fund like PHEF or creating a new fund.)

---

were contacting the tribes to ensure they were aware of the opportunity. They also said that the application process for the NOFO will be reopened at a later date, and eligible tribes will have the opportunity to apply.

[27] According to CDC and ASPR officials, the agencies are in the process of shifting the responsibility for HPP grants management—which includes administration of the HPP cooperative agreements—from CDC to ASPR. While ASPR has had programmatic management responsibility for HPP, CDC has had grants management responsibility for HPP (in addition to its programmatic management and grants management responsibilities for ELC and PHEP). Officials told us that this change will begin in July 2019, and that moving the HPP grants management to ASPR will allow more staff to oversee the HPP administrative process, which could aid the timeliness of awards provided from supplemental appropriations.

[28] PHEF, established in 1983, is available to the Secretary of Health and Human Services to respond to a public health emergency, including infectious disease threats. See Pub. L. No.98-49, 97 Stat. 245 (1983) (codified as amended at 42 U.S.C. § 247d). A Congressional Research Service report issued in 2009 indicated that the fund had not received an appropriation since Congress reauthorized it in 2000. Congressional Research Service, *Public Health and Medical Response to Disasters: Federal Authority and Funding*, RL33579 (Washington, D.C.: Apr. 29, 2009). According to HHS's 2016 budget justification estimates, PHEF has no balance.

Majority of Awardees Met Targets for All Responder Protection Measures, but Performance Was Mixed Across Other Areas

Table 1. Performance Measures Used by HHS's Three Key Preparedness and Capacity-Building Programs, by Preparedness Capacity Area

Program	Performance measure	Preparedness capacity area[a]			
		Electronic lab reporting	Epidemiology capacity	Laboratory capacity	Responder protection
ELC	Percentage of laboratory reports received electronically.	√	-	-	-
	Number of new electronic lab reporting feeds established.	√	-	-	-
	Investigated reported outbreaks.	-	√	-	-
	Laboratory test turnaround time completed within established time frame.	-	-	√	-
	Laboratories have designated a biosafety officer.	-	-	-	√
	Laboratories have conducted risk assessments and mitigated risks.[b]	-	-	-	√
	Laboratories have a biosafety plan in place that has been reviewed and communicated.	-	-	-	√
	Standard operating procedure in place to perform risk assessments for laboratories.	-	-	-	√
HPP	Ebola treatment centers can access personal protective equipment.[c]	-	-	-	√
	Assessment hospitals can access personal protective equipment.[d]	-	-	-	√
	Frontline facilities can receive information on personal protective equipment from their health care coalition.[e]	-	-	-	√
	Emergency medical services agencies that are required to participate in awardee's concept of operations are engaged in the process of developing an operational plan for the state.[f]	-	-	-	√
	Health care coalitions that participate in an advisory group that makes recommendations on the prevention of health care-associated infections.	-	-	-	√
PHEP	Percentage of required disease reports received on time.	-	√	-	-
	Percentage of required disease reports for which initial control measures were initiated on time.[g]	-	√	-	-
	Completed emergency contact drill one on time.[h]	-	-	√	-
	Completed emergency contact drill two on time.[h]	-	-	√	-
	Proportion of laboratory response network-biological proficiency tests passed.[i]	-	-	√	-

Program	Performance measure	Preparedness capacity area[a]			
		Electronic lab reporting	Epidemiology capacity	Laboratory capacity	Responder protection
PHEP	Submitted subtyping results from E. coli samples to a national database.[j]	-	-	√	-
	Submitted subtyping results from E. coli samples to a national database.[j]	-	-	√	-
Total number of measures in each area		**2**	**3**	**6**	**9**

Legend: √ = Performance measure included in preparedness capacity area. - = Performance measure not included in preparedness capacity area.

Source: GAO analysis of Office of the Assistance Secretary for Preparedness and Response (ASPR) and the Centers for Disease Control and Prevention (CDC) performance measurement information. | GAO-18-362

Note: The Department of Health and Human Services (HHS) provides funding to states, localities, territories, and freely associated states to aid capacity building and preparedness for public health threats, including infectious disease threats, natural disasters, or terrorist events, through three key programs: Epidemiology and Laboratory Capacity for Infectious Diseases (ELC), the Hospital Preparedness Program (HPP), and Public Health Emergency Preparedness (PHEP). This table shows the performance measures used in these key programs that are directly related to infectious disease preparedness capacity, as we determined through consultation with ASPR and CDC officials.

[a] We categorized the 20 performance measures in this table into four preparedness capacity areas. While the agencies have not categorized the performance measures, ASPR and CDC officials agreed with our categorization of the performance measures into these areas.

[b] Risk assessments involve identifying potential hazards, assessing risks associated with those hazards, and establishing precautions and standard procedures to minimize exposure to those risks.

[c] Ebola treatment centers are hospitals that are prepared to provide comprehensive care to people diagnosed with Ebola virus disease for the duration of a patient's illness, as designated by states and localities with CDC input after conducting site visits.

[d] Ebola assessment hospitals are those that are prepared to receive and isolate a patient with potential Ebola virus disease, as designated by the state.

[e] Most U.S. acute care facilities that are equipped for emergency care (such as hospital-based emergency departments, urgent care clinics, and critical access hospitals) are frontline facilities.

[f] A concept of operations is an overview of the processes and steps for an effective system or operation, such as a response to an infectious disease outbreak.

[g] Initial control measures vary by disease. Some examples of control measures include identification of potentially exposed individuals, investigation into the causes of an infectious disease threat after it is identified, and immunization.

[h] Drill one is time to complete notification between CDC, on-call laboratorian, on-call epidemiologist, and then back to CDC; drill two is the reverse direction: time to complete notification between CDC, on-call epidemiologist, on-call laboratorian, and then back to CDC.

[I] The laboratory response network-biological is a group of state, local, and other public health laboratories that provides routine and specialized laboratory testing to quickly respond to public health threats.

[j] Subtyping procedures can identify certain attributes of bacteria to distinguish between bacteria of the same species. Subtyping can be used to predict the severity and transmissibility of a certain strain of bacteria, such as E. coli or Listeria monocytogenes.

The 20 performance measures we reviewed for HHS's three key preparedness and capacity-building programs (ELC, HPP, and PHEP) fell into four preparedness capacity areas: electronic lab reporting, epidemiology capacity, laboratory capacity, and responder protection.[29] The majority of awardees (states and other jurisdictions) that reported on performance measures in the responder protection area met all performance targets in this

[29] The 20 performance measures included in our review directly relate to infectious disease preparedness capacity. While the agencies have not categorized the performance measures, ASPR and CDC officials agreed with our categorization of the performance measures in the four areas.

area. However, awardee performance in the other three preparedness capacity areas was mixed.

ELC had measures in each of the four preparedness capacity areas, while PHEP had measures in two areas, and HPP's performance measures fell into one of the four preparedness capacity areas. (See Table 1.) The programs' performance measures are meant to demonstrate accountability and identify awardees' strengths, weaknesses, and areas for improvement on discrete activities related to preparedness capacity. According to CDC officials, the measures can include targets that are intended to challenge awardees to continuously meet high standards.

Of the 20 measures, we found that the majority of reporting awardees met the performance targets for 9 of the 9 measures in the responder protection area, 5 of the 6 measures in the laboratory capacity area, 1 of the 2 measures in the electronic lab reporting area, and 1 of the 3 measures in the epidemiology capacity area. These areas, and related awardee performance, are discussed in detail in the sections that follow.

Responder Protection

The responder protection performance measures apply to ELC's and HPP's Ebola awards from supplemental appropriations, and measure activities related to safety and coordination for laboratorians, hospital and emergency personnel, and other responders, including the coordination of these responders. The measures assess the extent to which awardees can safely respond in the event of a highly contagious infectious disease threat. Though these performance measures were designed specifically for Ebola, ASPR and CDC officials told us that these measures may also have some application to preparedness for other highly infectious diseases. For each of the four ELC measures in this area, the majority of ELC awardees met each target—the percentage of reporting awardees that met the target ranged from 77 to 97 percent. For each of the five HPP measures in this area, the majority of HPP awardees met each target—the percentage of reporting awardees that met the target ranged from 61 to 97 percent. (See Table 2.)

According to CDC officials, the benefits of the ELC measures in this area include promoting a culture of safety within the awardee's jurisdiction, learning new technologies and procedures that could be used during a highly contagious infectious disease outbreak, and establishing written plans and procedures to train staff on how to respond to certain risks. These measures all asked for a "yes" or "no" response, and CDC's target was for awardees to submit a "yes" to each measure.

Table 2. Awardee Performance on Responder Protection Performance Measures, by Program

Program	Performance measure	Target	Percent of reporting awardees that met target[a]
ELC	Laboratories have designated a biosafety officer.	Awardee reported "yes."	97 percent (n = 61)
	Laboratories have conducted risk assessments and mitigated risks.	Awardee reported "yes."	87 percent (n = 60)
	Laboratories have a biosafety plan in place that has been reviewed and communicated.	Awardee reported "yes."	90 percent (n = 60)
	Standard operating procedure in place to perform risk assessments for laboratories.	Awardee reported "yes."	77 percent (n = 60)
HPP	Ebola treatment centers can access personal protective equipment.	All Ebola treatment centers accessed within 10 minutes.	97 percent (n = 29)
	Assessment hospitals can access personal protective equipment.	All assessment hospitals accessed within 10 minutes.	94 percent (n = 49)
	Frontline facilities can receive information on personal protective equipment from their health care coalition.	All frontline facilities received within 8 hours.	68 percent (n = 56)
	Emergency medical services agencies that are required to participate in awardee's concept of operations are engaged in the process of developing an operational plan for the state.	All required emergency medical services agencies engaged.	85 percent (n = 55)
	Health care coalitions that participate in an advisory group that makes recommendations on the prevention of health care-associated infections.	80 percent of health care coalitions participated.	61 percent (n = 57)

Source: GAO analysis of awardee performance measurement data provided by the Office of the Assistance Secretary for Preparedness and Response (ASPR) and the Centers for Disease Control and Prevention (CDC). | GAO-18-362

Note: Data are from October 1, 2016, through March 31, 2017, for Epidemiology and Laboratory Capacity for Infectious Diseases (ELC) and from May 18, 2015, through May 17, 2016, for the Hospital Preparedness Program (HPP), according to ASPR and CDC officials. These are the most recent years for which validated data were available.

[a] The percentages in this column are based on the subsets of awardees that provided data and to which the measure applied, or (n). While almost all awardees reported data on eight of the nine measures, the exact number of awardees that provided data varied across measures. Some awardees did not report data for certain measures, because, for example, they did not conduct the exercise necessary to determine performance on a measure, or were not required to report on a measure, according to ASPR and CDC officials. For example, HPP's Ebola treatment center measure was not required of many awardees, because they did not have Ebola treatment centers within their jurisdictions.

ASPR officials stated that the HPP measures in this area related to medical facilities' ability to quickly access personal protective equipment in the case of a potentially highly contagious infectious disease. The measures also assess coordination among various health care entities to help ensure that groups, such as emergency medical services and health care advisory groups, are involved in the planning for an infectious disease threat. The majority of awardees have already met targets for each of the five performance measures in this area, even though the targets set by ASPR are 5-year targets that do not need to be achieved until 2020. While ASPR has not yet established targets for awardees to aim for every year, officials stated they are planning to establish interim targets for these performance measures in 2018, using data collected in 2016 and 2017 as a benchmark.

Laboratory Capacity

Laboratory capacity refers to both laboratory testing of certain pathogens and communication between laboratories and other public entities. ELC had one measure and PHEP had five measures in this area. Half of the reporting awardees (50 percent) met the target for ELC's only measure in this area, while a large majority of PHEP awardees met the targets for each of the five PHEP measures in this area—the percentage of reporting awardees that met the target ranged from 75 to 100 percent. (See Table 3.)

Table 3. Awardee Performance on Laboratory Capacity Performance Measures, by Program

Program	Performance measure	Target	Percent of reporting awardees that met target[a]
ELC	Laboratory test turnaround time completed within established time frame.	Varied between 2 and 65 days.	50 percent (n = 48)
PHEP	Completed emergency contact drill one on time.	Completed within 45 minutes.	96 percent (n = 51)
	Completed emergency contact drill two on time.	Completed within 45 minutes.	96 percent (n = 52)
	Proportion of laboratory response network-biological proficiency tests passed.	Failed no more than one proficiency test.	100 percent (n = 53)
	Submitted subtyping results from E. coli samples to a national database.	90 percent of samples within 4 working days.	90 percent (n = 52)
	Submitted subtyping results from Listeria monocytogenes samples to a national database.	90 percent of samples within 4 working days.	75 percent (n = 40)

Source: GAO analysis of awardee performance measurement data provided by the Centers for Disease Control and Prevention (CDC). | GAO-18-362

Note: Data are from calendar year 2015 for Epidemiology and Laboratory Capacity for Infectious Diseases (ELC); from July 1, 2016, through June 30, 2017, for Public Health Emergency Preparedness's (PHEP) two emergency contact drill measures; and from July 1, 2014, through June 30, 2015, for PHEP's other three measures, according to CDC officials. These were the most recent years for which validated data were available.

[a] The percentages in this column are based on the subset of awardees that provided data and to which the measure applied, or (n). While most awardees reported data for these measures, the exact number of awardees that provided data varied across measures. According to CDC officials, some awardees did not report data for certain measures, because, for example, they did not perform the necessary testing to determine performance on a measure, or were not required to report on a measure, as was the case for some localities and U.S. territories.

CDC officials stated that the ELC measure in this area—turnaround time for laboratory tests—allows awardees to choose diseases for which they would like to focus on to improve the timeliness of their laboratory testing. Targets for this measure were set by the awardee and varied from 2 to 62 days. Certain circumstances may make it more difficult for an awardee to meet the target, such as implementing complex laboratory procedures, according to CDC officials. Performance varied widely among awardees that missed the target; for example, several awardees missed their selected target by one or two days, while others missed the target by a week or more.

PHEP's two emergency contact drill measures in this area assess whether there is effective contact between on-call epidemiologists and laboratorians, which relates to how quickly they can respond during a public health threat, such as an infectious disease outbreak. The other three PHEP measures are important, because they ensure that laboratories have the capability to detect and report potentially deadly diseases. CDC established the targets for all five of these measures.

Electronic Lab Reporting

Electronic lab reporting involves sending clinical and laboratory reports to public health agencies via electronic means (as opposed to traditional paper reports). ELC had two measures in this area. The majority of reporting ELC awardees (58 percent) met the performance target for one of the two ELC performance measures in this area (establishing two or more electronic lab reporting feeds), while 16 percent met the target for the other measure (increasing the percentage of laboratory reports received electronically by at least 10 percentage points).[30] (See Table 4.)

Table 4. Awardee Performance on Electronic Lab Reporting Performance Measures

Program	Performance measure	Target	Percent of reporting awardees that met target[a]
ELC	Percentage of laboratory reports received electronically.	Increased at least 10 percentage points.	16 percent (n = 19)
	Number of new electronic lab reporting feeds established.	Two or more.	58 percent (n = 19)

Source: GAO analysis of awardee performance measurement data provided by the Centers for Disease Control and Prevention (CDC). | GAO-18-362

Note: Data are from calendar year 2016 for the two Epidemiology and Laboratory Capacity for Infectious Diseases' (ELC) measures in this area, according to CDC officials. These are the most recent years for which validated data were available.

[a] The percentages in this column are based on the subsets of awardees that provided data and to which the measure applied, or (n). The two measures in this table did not apply to the majority of awardees, because these measures were only required of awardees that did not receive at least 75 percent of their laboratory reports electronically.

According to CDC officials, using electronic lab reporting instead of paper reports results in timelier, more complete, and more accurate reports. ELC applies these measures to awardees that have not already reached the program threshold of reporting at

[30] Electronic lab reporting feeds are direct data lines that electronically load laboratory results from a laboratory's data system to another data system, such as a public health department's data system.

least 75 percent of their laboratory reports electronically. CDC officials stated that the process of submitting reports via electronic lab reporting requires significant technical expertise and repeated communication between the laboratories, hospitals, and the state's public health department. CDC-established targets measure whether or not awardees are increasing their volume of reports received via electronic lab reporting each year. Awardees who have not met ELC's reporting threshold may struggle with electronic lab reporting for several reasons, such as difficultly hiring or maintaining skilled personnel to advance electronic lab reporting or implementing electronic reporting in low volume laboratories, according to CDC officials. The performance of the ELC awardees that did not meet the electronic lab reporting target varied widely. For example, over 20 percent of awardees submitted a smaller proportion of laboratory reports electronically in 2016 than they did in 2015, while other awardees came close to meeting the target (a 10 percent increase in electronic reports).

Epidemiology Capacity

Epidemiology capacity refers to identifying and responding to infectious disease outbreaks.[31] ELC had one measure in this area, and PHEP had two. The majority of reporting ELC awardees (84 percent) met the established target for ELC's measure; however, few PHEP awardees met the targets of the two PHEP measures in this area—the percentage of reporting awardees that met the target ranged from 10 to 12 percent. (See Table 5.)

ELC's measure in this area—the percent of total outbreaks investigated— is meant to assess the extent to which state public health agencies can effectively respond, prevent, and control infectious disease outbreaks. The measure indicates the proportion of outbreaks that were investigated by each awardee for reportable diseases compared to the total number of outbreaks, with the CDC-established target of investigating 100 percent of outbreaks, according to CDC officials.

The two PHEP measures in this area are key to being able to initiate timely investigations and limit the spread of disease. CDC officials stated that the nature of a disease may make it difficult for an awardee to meet the performance targets. For example, the source of foodborne diseases can be particularly difficult to track in order to implement control measures, especially when contamination may have originated outside of the United States. While few PHEP awardees met the targets for submitting all disease reports and implementing all initial control measures on time, awardee performance varied by disease. For example, among the awardees that had cases of disease, only 15

[31] CDC defines disease outbreak as the occurrence of cases of disease in excess of what would normally be expected in a defined community, geographical area, or season. In some situations, a single case of disease may qualify as an outbreak. Awardees are also permitted to use their own definitions of what constitutes an outbreak when reporting performance measure data, according to CDC officials.

percent of disease reports were received on time and 17 percent of initial control measures were implemented on time for E. coli, but both targets were met 77 percent of the time for measles.

Table 5. Awardee Performance on Epidemiology Capacity Performance Measures, by Program

Program	Performance measure	Target	Percent of reporting awardees that met target[a]
ELC	Investigated reported outbreaks.	All reported outbreaks investigated.	84 percent (n = 61)
PHEP	Percentage of required disease reports received on time.	Disease reports received on time across all diseases.[b]	Across all six diseases combined: 10 percent (n = 52)[c] • Botulism: 63 percent • Tularemia: 50 percent • E. coli: 15 percent • Hepatitis A: 28 percent • Measles: 77 percent • Meningococcal: 30 percent
	Percentage of disease reports for which required initial control measures were initiated on time.	Initial control measures implemented on time across all diseases.[b]	Across all six diseases combined: 12 percent (n = 52)[d] • Botulism: 69 percent • Tularemia: 54 percent • E. coli: 17 percent • Hepatitis A: 36 percent • Measles: 77 percent • Meningococcal: 62 percent

Source: GAO analysis of awardee performance measurement data provided by the Centers for Disease Control and Prevention (CDC). | GAO-18-362

Note: Data are from calendar year 2015 for Epidemiology and Laboratory Capacity for Infectious Diseases (ELC) and from July 1, 2015, through June 30, 2016, for Public Health Emergency Preparedness (PHEP), according to CDC officials. This is the most recent year for which validated data were available.

[a] The percentages in this column are based on the subsets of awardees that provided data and to which the measure applied, or (n). While almost all awardees reported data for these measures, the exact number of awardees that provided data varied across measures. Some awardees did not report data for a measure, because, for example, the awardee was not required to report on a measure, as was the case for some localities and U.S. territories.

[b] This target is not indicated in CDC's performance measurement guidance to PHEP awardees. Rather, it is an expectation that CDC has for the awardees, according to CDC officials.

[c] CDC officials stated that awardees determine their own reporting time frames for each of the six diseases that are required to be reported, and CDC expects each awardee to report all required diseases within those time frames. We have provided the percent of reporting awardees that met this expectation as it applies to all six diseases combined, as well as by each of the six diseases individually. Reporting time frames for what is considered "on time" vary by awardee but are from immediately to within 1 week, depending on the disease, according to CDC officials.

[d] CDC officials stated that CDC determines the initial control measure time frames for each of the six diseases that are required to be reported, and CDC expects each awardee to implement all required initial control measures within those time frames. We have provided the percent of reporting awardees that met this expectation as it applies to all six diseases combined, as well as by each of the six diseases individually. The time frames for what is considered "on time" vary by disease and are from within 24 hours to 1 week, according to CDC officials.

Agency Comments

We provided a draft of this chapter to the Secretary of Health and Human Services for comment. HHS provided technical comments, which we incorporated as appropriate.

We are sending copies of this chapter to the appropriate congressional committees, the Secretary of Health and Human Services, and other interested parties.

Marcia Crosse
Director, Health Care

APPENDIX I: NON-FEDERAL STAKEHOLDERS' VIEWS ON FACTORS TO CONSIDER FOR AN EMERGENCY RESPONSE FUND

Table 6. Six Factors That May Be Considered for an Emergency Response Fund, According to Non-Federal Stakeholders

Factor	Stakeholder discussion
Who determines when to use an emergency fund	Most of the non-federal stakeholders stated that it would be beneficial if the Secretary of Health and Human Services were authorized to determine when to use an emergency fund. Two stakeholders explained that it would be beneficial for the Secretary to make the determination, because the Department of Health and Human Services (HHS) is in charge of the public health response in the case of emergencies. Further, one of these stakeholders said that the Secretary can consult with, and benefit from, the technical and scientific knowledge of the Centers for Disease Control and Prevention (CDC) when making the decision. One stakeholder said that it would be beneficial for the use of such a fund to be determined by the CDC Director, because the agency has the expertise to dealing with public health threats. One stakeholder commented that a benefit of the existing Public Health Emergency Fund (PHEF) is that its use is determined by the Secretary of Health and Human Services.[a]
	One non-federal stakeholder stated that it could be beneficial for use of the fund to be determined at the White House level because a cross-agency response is often required.
What factors would trigger the use of an emergency fund	A few non-federal stakeholders said that no one specific factor, or set of factors, could be used to determine when to trigger the use of an emergency fund. For example, one stakeholder provided the example that the factors for Zika and Ebola were very disparate, and both outbreaks started abroad with little mortality in the United States; however, according to the stakeholder, it would have been appropriate to use an emergency fund for both. Further, two other stakeholders commented that while factors such as morbidity and mortality rates are important, these rates might not be fully known before it is appropriate to take emergency action to stop an infectious disease threat. As a result of the varying
	factors, a few stakeholders commented it would be important to consult with subject matter experts—including the Secretary of Health and Human Services and other public health professionals, such as those within CDC—to determine if and when to trigger the use of an emergency fund.
	A few non-federal stakeholders also said that the capacity of the state and local response entities and whether their resources have been depleted are considerations for determining when to use an emergency fund. For example, two stakeholders told us that those with authority over a fund need to be in communication with the state and local public health departments, and use of an emergency fund could be considered when state and local capacities are overwhelmed.
Methods to determine the amount of available funding	While a few non-federal stakeholders supported the idea of maintaining a set amount in an emergency fund, there was no consensus on how that amount should be calculated. Two stakeholders liked the idea of using a formula that included data on past infectious disease response spending as a basis for determining the amount to maintain in an emergency fund, though two other stakeholders agreed that past events (and their costs) do not determine future events.
	A few non-federal stakeholders commented that it was important that any appropriations to an emergency fund supplement, but not supplant, regular annual appropriations that support preparedness and capacity- building programs. This is the case for funds appropriated to PHEF. 42 U.S.C. § 247d(c).

Factor	Stakeholder discussion
Activities to fund with an emergency fund	A few non-federal stakeholders stressed that an emergency fund could be reserved for activities that need immediate action. For an infectious disease threat, a few non-federal stakeholders mentioned a variety of activities that could be funded with an emergency fund—including state and local public health laboratory operations and surveillance, risk communications, mass dispensing of medical countermeasures, and other activities—to provide additional surge capacity, some of which may be unpredictable.[b] Because of the unpredictability of the next big infectious disease threat, a few stakeholders said that it would be beneficial for an emergency fund to be flexible in terms of the activities it is allowed to fund.
	A few non-federal stakeholders commented that it would be most beneficial for an emergency fund to be used for defined, short-term needs over long-term public health threats, such as the opioid epidemic. For example, one stakeholder stated that while PHEF could be used to support the initial response to any public health threat, it would not be beneficial for it to support any long-term or ongoing response efforts. Long-term public health threats, such as the opioid epidemic, could rapidly deplete the fund without making a difference in the threat itself, according to the stakeholder.
Accountability for use of an emergency fund	Most non-federal stakeholders generally agreed that it would be beneficial to have reporting requirements attached to an emergency fund, which include financial accountability measures, and a few of these stakeholders commented that such requirements are already in place for existing preparedness and capacity-building programs, as this is a part of good governance.[c]
	A few non-federal stakeholders also said that requiring an after action report following the emergency would be beneficial.
Whether an emergency fund would be specific to infectious disease threats	One non-federal stakeholder told us that it would be beneficial to have a fund specific to infectious disease threats, while half of the non-federal stakeholders we interviewed did not agree with having an emergency fund limited to infectious disease threats. One of these stakeholders commented that an emergency fund is needed to surge quickly for any type of public health threat—including bioterrorism and radio-nuclear threats—and that often the same core resources are needed to respond to infectious disease threats, as well as these other types of threats.
	A few other stakeholders stated that there is not a consensus on how broad or narrow a fund should be. One of these stakeholders said that although there is not consensus, besides hurricanes, the last three big public health threats were infectious disease threats, so it would make sense to start with that type of event. A fund limited to infectious disease threats could be put it in place, used, evaluated, and then analyzed over time to determine if it should be expanded to other public health threats.

Source: GAO summary of information received from non-federal stakeholders interviewed. | GAO-18-362

[a] PHEF, established in 1983, is available to the Secretary of Health and Human Services to respond to a public health emergency, including infectious disease threats. See Pub. L. No.98-49, 97 Stat. 245 (1983) (codified as amended at 42 U.S.C. § 247d). A Congressional Research Service report issued in 2009 indicated that the fund had not received an appropriation since Congress reauthorized it in 2000. Congressional Research Service, *The Public Health and Medical Response to Disasters: Federal Authority and Funding, RL33579* (Washington, D.C.: Apr. 29, 2009). According to HHS's 2016 budget justification estimates, PHEF has no balance.

[b] A health care system's ability to "surge" is the ability to have the staff and resources in place to adequately care for increased numbers of affected individuals or individuals with unusual or highly specialized needs.

[c] We previously reported on the application, financial, and reporting requirements that awardees must adhere to as part of the terms of the cooperative agreements of two programs that support preparedness capacity—the Hospital Preparedness Program and Public Health Emergency Preparedness. These include adhering to the HHS Office of Assistant Secretary for Preparedness and Response and CDC guidelines for the appropriate use of cooperative agreement funds, undergoing biennial financial audits of their cooperative agreement funds, and submitting midyear and end-of-year progress reports and periodic financial reports. For more detailed information, see GAO, *National Preparedness: Improvements Needed for Measuring Awardee Performance in Meeting Medical and Public Health Preparedness Goals*, GAO-13-278 (Washington, D.C.: Mar. 22, 2013).

Ten non-federal stakeholders told us that a mechanism to fund rapid response to an infectious disease threat could be beneficial during infectious disease threats. Such a mechanism could include the use of the existing Public Health Emergency Fund or a new emergency response fund specific to infectious disease.

The availability of any such fund for immediate use would be subject to available appropriations. Stakeholders reported six factors that may be considered for a new emergency response fund. The table below summarizes the information from stakeholders regarding the factors.

In: Infectious Diseases
Editor: Philippe Georges
ISBN: 978-1-53616-401-5

Chapter 2

EMERGING INFECTIOUS DISEASES: ACTIONS NEEDED TO ADDRESS THE CHALLENGES OF RESPONDING TO ZIKA VIRUS DISEASE OUTBREAKS*

United States Government Accountability Office

ABBREVIATIONS

AMCA	American Mosquito Control Association
APHL	Association of Public Health Laboratories
ASPR	Assistant Secretary for Preparedness and Response
ASTHO	Association of State and Territorial Health Officials
BARDA	Biomedical Advanced Research and Development Authority
BSL	biological safety level
Bti	*Bacillus thuringiensis israelensis*
CDC	Centers for Disease Control and Prevention
CLIA	Clinical Laboratory Improvement Amendments
CSTE	Council of State and Territorial Epidemiologists
DOD	Department of Defense
EPA	Environmental Protection Agency
EUA	Emergency Use Authorization
FDA	Food and Drug Administration

* This is an edited, reformatted and augmented version of United States Government Accountability Office; Report to Congressional Requesters, Publication No. GAO-17-445, dated May 2017.

FIFRA	Federal Insecticide, Fungicide, and Rodenticide Act
HHS	Department of Health and Human Services
IgG	immunoglobulin G
IgM	immunoglobulin M
IMM	integrated mosquito management
IVM	integrated vector management
MAC-ELISA	IgM antibody capture enzyme-linked immunosorbent assay
MMWR	Morbidity and Mortality Weekly Report
NACCHO	National Association of County and City Health Officials
NIAID	National Institute of Allergy and Infectious Diseases
NIH	National Institutes of Health
NNDSS	National Notifiable Diseases Surveillance System
NPDES	National Pollution Discharge Elimination System
NSTC	National Science and Technology Council
OSTP	Office of Science and Technology Policy
PAHO	Pan American Health Organization
PRNT	plaque reduction neutralization test
RNA	ribonucleic acid
RT-PCR	reverse transcriptase-polymerase chain reaction
SARS	severe acute respiratory syndrome
SVAZE	Sistema de Vigilancia Activa de Zika en Embarazos
WHO	World Health Organization
ZAPSS	Zika Active Pregnancy Surveillance System
ZIP	Zika in Infants and Pregnancy

WHY GAO DID THIS STUDY

Zika virus disease can cause adverse pregnancy and neurological outcomes. Given this ongoing threat, GAO was asked to evaluate progress made and challenges faced by federal agencies in responding to the Zika virus outbreak in the United States.

GAO examined (1) information on what is known and not known about the epidemiology of the Zika virus, and any challenges with conducting surveillance and epidemiological studies, (2) characteristics of different diagnostic tests authorized during the outbreak, challenges test manufacturers and users faced, and the extent to which FDA and CDC followed their own communication guidance, and (3) the strengths and limitations of available mosquito control methods, and challenges federal agencies face supporting these efforts.

GAO reviewed literature and agency documentation, and interviewed federal and state officials about the Zika virus and the U.S. response. GAO also convened an expert meeting with the assistance of the National Academy of Sciences to discuss various issues surrounding the response to the Zika virus.

WHAT GAO RECOMMENDS

GAO is making five recommendations to FDA and CDC, including that CDC establish a transparent process for providing test manufacturers access to diagnostic tests and FDA and CDC provide information to help ensure that users of diagnostic tests can compare performance. Agencies agreed with four recommendations but raised some concerns with the fifth. GAO has addressed these concerns in the report.

WHAT GAO FOUND

Since Zika virus disease was a newly emerging disease threat in the United States, and relatively little was known about the Zika virus prior to the 2016 U.S. outbreak, the Centers for Disease Control and Prevention (CDC), and the states were not fully equipped with needed information and resources at the beginning of the outbreak. This presented several challenges for Zika virus disease surveillance and research efforts, such as challenges related to establishing a national definition for reporting cases. Knowledge about Zika virus epidemiology has increased in the past year, including information about Zika virus disease incidence and distribution of cases, and its associated adverse health outcomes. Most of the 5,197 Zika virus disease cases reported by April 5, 2017 in the United States were associated with travel from affected areas outside the continental United States. Only two states had disease cases of local, mosquito- borne transmission—216 were in Florida and 6 in Texas. While much has been learned about the epidemiology of the Zika virus, many unknowns remain, including the actual number of infections and the full spectrum of outcomes.

The 16 Zika virus diagnostic tests authorized during the outbreak varied in their performance and operational characteristics. For example, they varied in their ability to detect the virus and provide accurate results. In developing the diagnostic tests, manufacturers faced challenges in several areas, including access to clinical samples and other authorized diagnostic tests for comparison purposes. Users of the tests also encountered challenges, including determining the most accurate test to use, and obtaining equipment needed to conduct the tests. Some manufacturers raised concerns about the difficulty in developing diagnostic tests that met the Food and Drug Administration's (FDA) requirements for Emergency Use Authorization and some users expressed concerns about selecting tests amongst those authorized. GAO also determined that CDC and FDA did not follow some of their guidance in communicating with users of diagnostic tests, including providing clear information that would have enabled users to more easily compare performance across different tests.

Mosquito control programs in the United States are implemented at state and local levels and are critical to mitigating the risks associated with the Zika virus. Control methods include applying pesticides, reducing available water sources for breeding, and using personal protection. Each method has its strengths and limitations. For example, some control methods are more effective at reducing mosquito populations while others help prevent individuals from mosquito bites. Similarly, each method has some limitations, for example, there is varied public opposition to the use of certain pesticides. CDC supports state and local mosquito control activities primarily by providing guidance on mosquito control methods and funding to support certain mosquito control efforts. Challenges federal agencies faced in supporting these activities include sustaining staff expertise in mosquito control during periods when there are no outbreaks, funding constraints, and effectively communicating information about the geographical distribution of mosquitoes that transmit the Zika virus.

May 23, 2017

The Honorable Greg Walden
Chairman

The Honorable Frank Pallone, Jr.
Ranking Member
Committee on Energy and Commerce
House of Representatives

The Honorable Tim Murphy
Chairman

The Honorable Diana DeGette
Ranking Member
Subcommittee on Oversight and Investigations
Committee on Energy and Commerce
House of Representatives

The Honorable Fred Upton
House of Representatives

Emerging infectious diseases such as Zika virus disease constitute an ongoing threat to the health of people in the United States and around the world. Many advances in medical research and treatments were made in the past century, but infectious diseases have been nevertheless a leading cause of death worldwide (they account for one of every five deaths). Additionally, infectious diseases impose a heavy societal and economic burden on individuals, families, communities, and countries.

Infectious diseases are a continuous threat because of (1) emergence— at times rapid—of new infectious diseases; (2) reemergence of previously known infectious diseases; and (3) persistence of intractable infectious diseases.

Changes in human demographics, behavior, and land use—among other factors—bring people into closer and more frequent contact with pathogens and contribute to infectious disease emergence. This may involve exposure to animal carriers of disease and increased opportunities for pathogens to jump between animal and human reservoirs. In addition to Zika virus, other examples of emerging infectious diseases include Ebola virus disease, severe acute respiratory syndrome (SARS), influenza, dengue, and chikungunya, among others. The Zika virus attracted attention from health officials in the United States and abroad after geographic and time-period similarities between reported cases of Zika virus infection and adverse health outcomes, especially in newborns, were reported in Brazil in 2015—a pattern that was also observed during a Zika virus outbreak in French Polynesia in 2014.

As shown in Figure 1, the Zika virus is primarily transmitted to humans by infected mosquitoes but can also be transmitted from mother-to-child during pregnancy or around the time of birth, or from person to person through sexual contact or blood transfusion.[1] The virus can cause signs and symptoms that include fever, rash, conjunctivitis ("pink eye" where the eyes appear red or pink), and joint and muscle pain, although most people with Zika virus infection have only mild or no symptoms. Disease surveillance and epidemiological studies have established that Zika virus infection in a pregnant woman can cause birth defects in newborns and is also associated with increased cases of nervous system illnesses in infected adults.[2]

---

[1] Centers for Disease Control and Prevention. "Clinical Guidance for Healthcare Providers for Prevention of Sexual Transmission of Zika Virus," accessed February 21, 2017. https://www.cdc.gov/zika/hc-providers/clinical-guidance/sexualtransmission.html.

[2] Surveillance is the systematic and continuous collection, analysis, and interpretation of data, closely integrated with the timely and coherent dissemination and assessment of the results by those who have the right to know so that action can be taken. See Miquel Porta ed., *A Dictionary of Epidemiology*, 6th ed. (New York: Oxford University Press, 2014), 274. Epidemiologic studies determine the extent and distribution of the disease in a population, its causes and factors, modes of transmission, natural history, and developing preventive strategies or interventions. See Dona Schneider and David E. Lilienfeld, *Lilienfeld's Foundations of Epidemiology*, 4th ed. (New York: Oxford University Press, 2015).

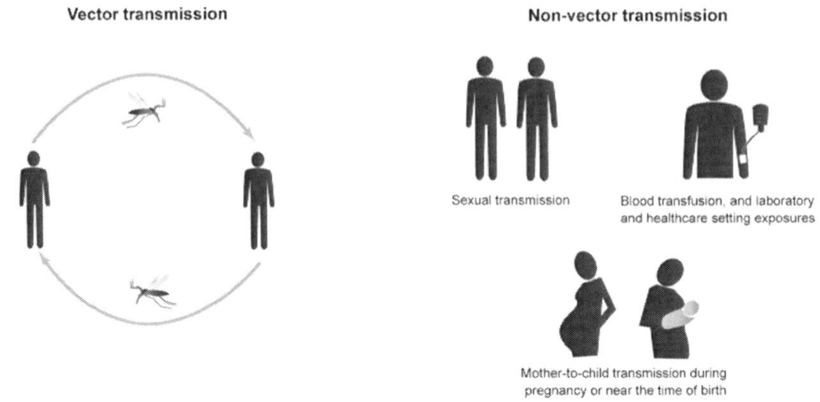

Source: GAO analysis of Centers for Disease Control and Prevention information. | GAO-17-445.

Figure 1. Zika Virus Can Be Transmitted by Mosquitoes (Vectors) and in Other Ways.

Because of concern about the threat and emergence of Zika virus disease in the United States, you asked us to review a number of issues related to the Zika virus and the U.S. response to the outbreak. This chapter (1) provides information on what is known and not known about the epidemiology of the Zika virus and determine the challenges, if any, in conducting surveillance and epidemiological studies, (2) determines the characteristics of different Zika virus diagnostic tests and any challenges manufacturers and users faced, and the extent to which the Centers for Disease Control and Prevention (CDC) and Food and Drug Administration (FDA) followed their own communication guidance during the U.S. outbreak, and (3) identifies available mosquito control methods, describes their strengths and weaknesses, and identifies any challenges federal agencies and others face in assisting mosquito control efforts.[3]

To conduct this work, we reviewed relevant documentation, such as FDA's guidance to manufacturers, product labels, and agencies' reports on epidemiology of the Zika virus. We also interviewed officials from key federal agencies and departments responding to the domestic Zika virus outbreak, including the Department of Defense (DOD), Environmental Protection Agency (EPA), and Department of Health and Human Services (HHS) including CDC, FDA and National Institutes of Health (NIH).

We also convened, with the assistance of the National Academy of Sciences, a 2-day meeting with 16 experts knowledgeable about the Zika virus to discuss issues related to the outbreak. These experts represented academia, the federal government, state government, and industry and combined expertise in epidemiology, diagnostic testing, and mosquito control.

To assess the Zika virus outbreak in terms of epidemiology, diagnostic tests, and mosquito control, we selected two cities for site visits in the continental United States based on their reported Zika virus cases at the time of our site visit selection: New York

[3] In this chapter, users of diagnostic tests include laboratory personnel, health care providers, and others in the medical and scientific communities.

City, New York, which had the largest number of cases acquired from travel outside the United States, and Miami, Florida. Florida was the only state with local mosquito-borne transmission at the time of our site selection.[4] For both site visits, we interviewed and collected information from officials in the city and state public health departments.

To provide information on what is known about Zika virus epidemiology and the challenges in conducting surveillance and epidemiological studies, we reviewed surveillance case count data from CDC and data reported jointly by the Pan American Health Organization (PAHO) and the World Health Organization (WHO). We reviewed peer-reviewed journal articles, agency documents, and reports about Zika virus infection and associated health outcomes. We interviewed federal and selected state and city officials about challenges in Zika virus surveillance and epidemiology, including initial response efforts. We also interviewed representatives from key public health organizations, including the Association of State and Territorial Health Officials (ASTHO), Council of State and Territorial Epidemiologists (CSTE), National Association of County and City Health Officials (NACCHO), and PAHO.[5]

To determine the characteristics of different Zika virus diagnostic tests, we reviewed and compared the product labels, letters of authorization, and factsheets for healthcare providers and patients for each test posted on the FDA website in April 2017. To determine the strengths and limitations of different diagnostic tests and the challenges associated with Zika virus diagnostic testing, research, development, and regulatory approval, we interviewed several manufacturers of Zika diagnostic tests. We also interviewed officials at selected public health laboratories and asked officials at selected federal laboratories about the strengths and limitations of different diagnostic tests. We compared the information that we gathered from our interviews and agency documents to *Standards for Internal Control in the Federal Government*.[6]

To determine whether CDC and FDA followed their own communication guidance, we compared information collected from agency interviews, our expert meeting, scientific professional societies, and relevant agencies' documents to internal agency guidance documents, such as FDA's transparency initiative information.[7]

---

[4] We did not visit Puerto Rico or other U.S. territories with laboratory-confirmed Zika virus disease cases; however, Puerto Rican scientists participated in our expert group meeting.

[5] ASTHO is a national nonprofit organization representing public health agencies and their employees in the United States and its territories, including the District of Columbia. CSTE is a professional organization of public health epidemiologists from every U.S. state and territory as well as Canada and Great Britain. NACCHO is an association of nearly 3,000 local health departments across the United States. PAHO provides technical cooperation and facilitates partnerships to improve health and quality of life, is the specialized health agency of the Inter-American System, and serves as the Regional Office for the Americas of WHO.

[6] GAO, *Standards for Internal Control in the Federal Government*, GAO-14-704G (Washington, D.C.: September 2014).

[7] Department of Health and Human Services, Food and Drug Administration Transparency Task Force, *FDA Transparency Initiative: Improving Transparency to Regulated Industry* (Washington, D.C.: FDA, January 2011), and Department of Health and Human Services, Food and Drug Administration, *FDA Transparency Initiative: Increasing Public Access to FDA's Compliance and Enforcement Data* (Washington, D.C.: HHS, April 2014).

To identify available mosquito control methods and their strengths and limitations, we reviewed agency documents and peer-reviewed literature and interviewed experts and officials from eight mosquito control entities.[8]

To assess the challenges federal agencies face in assisting mosquito control efforts in the United States, we interviewed federal agency officials from CDC, EPA, and FDA as well as experts in the federal government, academia, state and local governments, and experts from our meeting. (More information on our objectives, scope, and methodology is in appendix II).

We conducted this performance audit from June 2016 to May 2017 in accordance with generally accepted government auditing standards. Those standards require that we plan and perform the audit to obtain sufficient, appropriate evidence to provide a reasonable basis for our findings and conclusions based on our audit objectives. We believe that the evidence obtained provides a reasonable basis for our findings and conclusions based on our audit objectives.

BACKGROUND

Zika Virus: An Overview

The Zika virus is related to dengue, yellow fever, West Nile, and Japanese encephalitis viruses, among others.[9] The virus was first identified in the Zika Forest in Uganda, Africa in 1947, from where it moved east, causing only sporadic human disease until 2007. The first documented outbreak of Zika virus disease was reported in Yap State, Federated States of Micronesia, in 2007 and subsequent outbreaks occurred in Southeast Asia and the Western Pacific.[10] Some researchers have suggested that several combined factors contributed to the current outbreak and that travel was a major factor.[11] Figure 2 illustrates the spread of the Zika virus over time.

In February 2016, a WHO emergency committee on the Zika virus noted a strong association in time and place between Zika virus infection and a rise in detected cases of congenital malformations and neurological complications, suspecting a causal relationship.

---

[8] We selected a nongeneralizable sample of mosquito control entities. More information about our selection methods is in appendix II.

[9] Zika virus is a member of the genus Flavivirus which is made up of positive, single- stranded, enveloped ribonucleic acid (RNA) viruses found in arthropods (primarily ticks and mosquitoes) and can occasionally infect humans and other vertebrates.

[10] Robert S. Lanciotti and others, "Genetic and Serologic Properties of Zika Virus Associated with an Epidemic, Yap State, Micronesia, 2007," *Emerging Infectious Diseases*, vol. 14, no. 8 (2008): 1232–39.

[11] Gretchen Vogel, Jon Cohen, and Martin Enserink. "Zika Virus: Your Questions Answered." *Science*, January 29, 2016. http://www.sciencemag.org/news/2016/01/zika-virus-your-questions-answered.

WHO declared that the recent cluster of microcephaly cases and other neurological disorders, including Guillain-Barré syndrome, reported in Brazil and following a similar cluster in French Polynesia in 2013, constituted a Public Health Emergency of International Concern which required urgent and coordinated research.[12] The Secretary of Health and Human Services also designated the Zika virus a public health emergency in Puerto Rico in August 2016.[13]

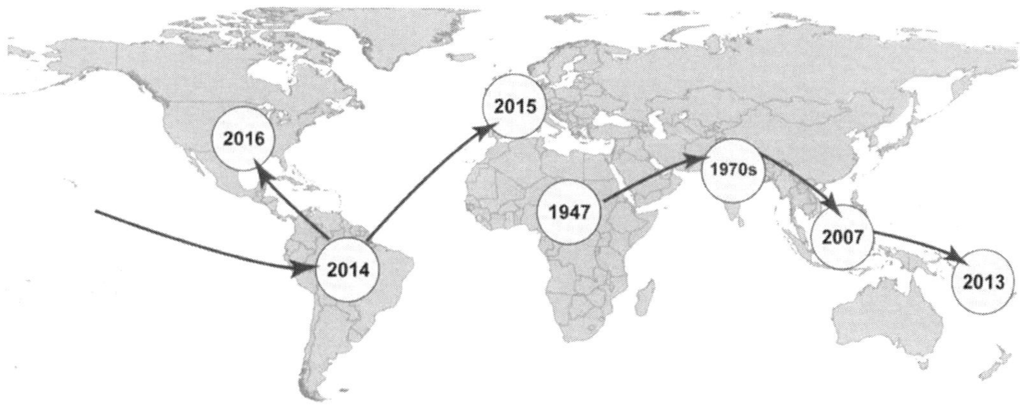

Source: GAO analysis of World Health Organization Information. | GAO-18-445.

Figure 2. Spread of the Zika Virus Around the World, 1947-2016.

Microcephaly is a rare nervous system disorder that causes a baby's head to be smaller than expected and not fully developed, which can lead to impaired thought processes, delayed motor function, and other adverse outcomes. Guillain-Barré syndrome is a rare disorder in which the body's immune system attacks the nervous system outside the brain and spinal cord, causing muscle weakness and, in some cases paralysis, although most people recover.

Currently available Zika virus prevention methods include various mosquito control and control methods, guidance on safe sex practices if a person has or is suspected of having Zika virus or has traveled to an area with high rates of local transmission, and guidance for travel to areas affected by Zika virus. Although at present no vaccine has been approved by the FDA to prevent Zika virus disease, several vaccines are in different development phases.

[12] In November 2016, WHO declared a Public Health Emergency of International Concern after research demonstrated the link between Zika virus infection and microcephaly; WHO's Emergency Committee on Zika virus determined that a robust technical mechanism is required to manage the global response. However, the Zika virus and associated health outcomes remain a significant public health challenge.

[13] The public health emergency declaration is a tool the federal government used to provide additional support to Puerto Rico's government to respond to the Zika outbreak and to grant access to certain federal funds. The last time HHS declared a public health emergency was in 2012, after Superstorm Sandy struck the eastern coast of the United States.

Zika Virus Surveillance Overview

The Zika virus was added to the list of nationally notifiable diseases in February 2016. CDC collects data on new cases of notifiable diseases through its National Notifiable Diseases Surveillance System (NNDSS), by encouraging states and territories to report laboratory-confirmed cases.[14] Arthropod-borne viruses (also called arboviruses) are also reported in a surveillance system that is specific to arboviral diseases, called ArboNET.[15] Reporting nationally notifiable diseases, including the Zika virus, from states and territories to CDC is voluntary. States and territories rely on healthcare providers or laboratories to report cases to their local, state, or territorial health departments according to the laws or regulations within their jurisdictions. A surveillance case definition is a set of uniform criteria used to define a disease for public health surveillance, with the purpose of enabling public health officials to classify and count cases consistently across reporting jurisdictions.[16]

Key terms related to epidemiology

Emerging Infections: Infectious disease that is newly recognized; one that has been recognized before but is newly appearing in a different population or geographic area than previously affected; one that is newly affecting many more individuals; and/or one that has developed new attributes (e.g., resistance or virulence).

Epidemiology: The study of the occurrence and distribution of health-related events, states, and processes in specified populations, including the study of the determinants influencing such processes and the application of this knowledge to control relevant health problems.

Incidence: The number of new cases of a disease in a defined population within a specified time.

Incidence rate: The rate at which new events occur in a population expressed as the number of new cases divided by the population at risk in a defined time period.

Outbreak: An epidemic limited to a localized increase in the incidence of a disease as in a village, town, or closed institution.

Surveillance: Systematic and continuous collection, analysis, and interpretation of data, closely integrated with the timely and coherent dissemination of the results and assessment to those who have the right to know so that action can be taken.

Source: Miquel Porta (ed.), *A Dictionary of Epidemiology*, 6th ed. (New York: Oxford University Press, 2014). | GAO-17-445.

CSTE—a professional organization of member states and territories representing public health epidemiologists—recommends that state health departments report cases of

[14] NNDSS enables public health officials at local, state, territorial, federal, and international levels to voluntarily share notifiable disease-related health information and allows public health officials to use this information to monitor, control, and prevent the occurrence and spread of those diseases. The Zika virus was declared a nationally notifiable condition for surveillance reporting in the United States with the Office of Management and Budget approval of a revision to the system, which authorized CDC to receive case notifications of the Zika virus.

[15] Arboviruses are any of a group of viruses that are transmitted by mosquitoes, ticks, or other arthropods (an animal such as an insect or spider).

[16] Surveillance case definitions are not intended to be used by healthcare providers for making a clinical diagnosis or determining how to meet an individual patient's health needs.

selected diseases to CDC's NNDSS, in accordance with CSTE's position statements that establish case definitions and are reviewed by CDC. The CSTE Zika virus interim case definition position statement was published in February 2016 and revised in June 2016. By April 2017, all states with the exception of Alaska, and three U.S. territories reported Zika virus cases to CDC through the ArboNET system, according to CDC's reports.

To understand more about Zika virus infection, CDC established the U.S. Zika Pregnancy Registry and is collaborating with state, tribal, local, and territorial health departments to collect information about pregnancy and infant outcomes following laboratory evidence of possible Zika virus infection during pregnancy. According to CDC, the data collected through this registry will be used to update recommendations for clinical care, to plan for services for pregnant women and families affected by Zika virus, and to improve prevention of Zika virus infection during pregnancy.[17] The Puerto Rico Department of Health and CDC developed the Zika Active Pregnancy Surveillance System (ZAPSS)/Sistema de Vigilancia Activa de Zika en Embarazos (SVAZE) to evaluate the association between possible Zika virus infection during pregnancy and adverse outcomes during pregnancy, birth, and early childhood up to 3 years of age.[18] Pregnant women in Puerto Rico with laboratory evidence of possible Zika virus infection (positive or equivocal test results, regardless of whether they have symptoms) and prenatally or perinatally exposed infants born to these women will be actively monitored.[19] According to CDC, this information has been used to inform best practices in care for women infected with Zika virus during pregnancy and their infants. CDC compiles data from the aforementioned systems to regularly update its website information regarding case counts and its Morbidity and Mortality Weekly Report (MMWR) of notifiable diseases.[20]

Diagnostic Tests for the Zika Virus

Accurate diagnostic tests have a key role in patient management and the control of most infectious diseases. Good quality diagnostic tests that are fit for purpose and can provide accurate results can help in reducing the burden of infectious diseases. The choice of which diagnostic test to use can depend on several factors, such as: which tests are approved for use by regulatory authorities, which tests are available for use at the

---

[17] Centers for Disease Control and Prevention, "U.S. Zika Pregnancy Registry," accessed April 5, 2017, https://www.cdc.gov/zika/reporting/registry.html.

[18] Centers for Disease Control and Prevention, "Zika Active Pregnancy Surveillance System (ZAPSS)/Sistema de Vigilancia Activa de Zika en Embarazos (SVAZE)," accessed April 5, 2017. https://www.cdc.gov/zika/reporting/zapss.html.

[19] According to HHS officials, it is important to note that pregnant women have been included in the registries regardless of symptoms from the initiation of these registries because it was recognized at the onset that surveillance of asymptomatic pregnant women was important.

[20] CDC issues annual summaries for notifiable diseases a few months into the following year, once the data have been finalized.

patient's health care location, and the physician's decision on which of the available tests he or she judges might be useful in clinical decision making. Zika virus diagnostic testing is now performed in federal, state, and commercial laboratories.

HHS, through FDA, oversees the safety and effectiveness of diagnostic tests, which are regulated as medical devices sold in the United States.[21] FDA can authorize the use of unapproved medical products, including diagnostic tests or an unapproved use of approved medical products for certain emergencies.[22] Under an Emergency Use Authorization (EUA), these medical products can be used in emergencies under certain conditions, when there are no adequate, approved, and available alternatives. An EUA for a specific diagnostic test is intended to be temporary and only remains in effect for the duration of the declared emergency unless it is revoked, for example because of issues with the diagnostic test.

Before FDA may issue a EUA, the Secretary of Health and Human Services must declare that circumstances exist justifying the authorization (see Figure 3).[23] In appropriate circumstances, an HHS EUA declaration may support issuance of more than one EUA. For example, based on an HHS EUA declaration that circumstances exist to justify the authorization of emergency use of diagnostics for a specified biological agent, FDA may authorize emergency use for multiple diagnostic tests to meet the need, provided that each EUA meets the statutory criteria for issuance.[24] The FDA website

---

[21] Diagnostic testing devices are called *in vitro* diagnostic products. 21 C.F.R. § 809.3. FDA regulates *in vitro* diagnostic products using a risk-based framework by classifying each device into one of three categories (Classes I-III). The class number determines the level of regulation and the appropriate premarket process required for that diagnostic test to establish a reasonable assurance of safety and effectiveness. See 21 U.S.C. § 360c.

[22] The Emergency Use Authorization (EUA) authority allows FDA to help strengthen the nation's public health protections against chemical, biological, radiological, or nuclear (CBRN) threats by facilitating the availability and use of medical countermeasures needed during public health emergencies. Under section 564 of the Federal Food, Drug, and Cosmetic Act, as amended, the FDA Commissioner may allow unapproved medical products or unapproved uses of approved medical products to be used in an emergency to diagnose, treat, or prevent serious or life-threatening diseases or conditions caused by CBRN threat agents when there are no adequate, approved, and available alternatives.

[23] This declaration must be based on one of the following four actions: (1) a determination by the Secretary of Homeland Security that there is a domestic emergency, or a significant potential for a domestic emergency, involving a heightened risk of attack with a CBRN agent(s), (2) a determination by the Secretary of Defense that there is a military emergency, or a significant potential for a military emergency, involving a heightened risk to United States military forces of attack with a CBRN agent(s), (3) a determination by the Secretary of Health and Human Services that there is a public health emergency, or a significant potential for a public health emergency, that affects, or has a significant potential to affect, national security or the health and security of United States citizens living abroad, and that involves a CBRN agent or agents, or a disease or condition that may be attributable to such agent(s), or (4) the identification by the Secretary of Homeland Security of a material threat that is sufficient to affect national security or the health and security of United States citizens living abroad. After the Secretary of Health and Human Services issues an EUA declaration based on one of these four determinations, and after consulting (to the extent feasible and appropriate given the applicable circumstances) with the Assistant Secretary for Preparedness and Response (ASPR), the Director of the NIH, and the Director of CDC, the Commissioner may authorize the emergency use of an unapproved product or an unapproved use of an approved product, provided that other statutory criteria are met. 21 U.S.C. § 360bbb-3(b).

[24] Food and Drug Administration, "Emergency Use Authorization of Medical Products and Related Authorities: Guidance for Industry and Other Stakeholders," accessed April 21, 2017, https://www.fda.gov/RegulatoryInformation/Guidances/ucm125127.htm.

includes a current list of available diagnostic tests and associated letters of authorization, fact sheets, and product labels. The letter of authorization includes the criteria for issuance, the scope of the authorization, waiver of certain requirements, and conditions and duration of authorization. Fact sheets are available for public health providers and for patients. Product labels include the intended use, procedures for conducting the test, and performance characteristics, among others.

HHS determined that the Zika virus posed a significant potential for a public health emergency affecting national security and declared in February 2016 that circumstances justified EUA of Zika virus diagnostic tests.[25] FDA's analytical and clinical evaluation of an EUA for a medical product is limited in comparison to the extensive evaluation required for premarket notification (also called a 510(k) review) or premarket approval.[26]

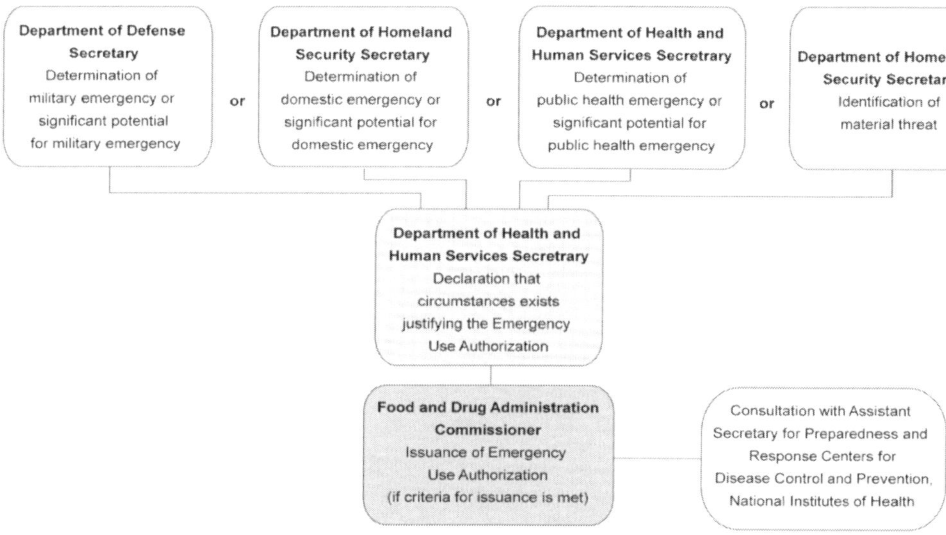

Source: GAO analysis of FDA information. | GAO-17-445.

Figure 3. Prerequisites for Issuing an Emergency Use Authorization for Medical Products.

Laboratory developed tests, on the other hand, are intended for clinical use, not for commercial sale and distribution, and are designed, manufactured and used within a single laboratory or laboratory network. FDA has generally not enforced premarket review and other applicable FDA requirements for laboratory developed tests because such tests are relatively simple and generally available on a limited basis. However, according to an expert from out meeting, laboratory developed tests have increased in technical and analytical complexity.

---

[25] See 21 U.S.C. § 360bbb-3(b)(1)(C).

[26] The premarket notification, or 510(k), process allows developers to demonstrate to FDA that the medical device seeking approval is substantially equivalent to a device already legally on the market. 21 C.F.R. Part 807. Premarket approval is the more stringent approach for new devices, requiring developers to provide scientific evidence, typically clinical data, showing that the device is safe and effective. 21 C.F.R. Part 814.

FDA has authorized under EUA two different types of diagnostic tests for the Zika virus—molecular and serologic. Molecular tests are used to detect genetic material in samples of bodily fluids, such as serum and urine. Serologic tests are diagnostic tests that detect antibodies against the Zika virus in the blood. CDC manufactured and received authorization for both types of tests, one called Trioplex (molecular) and the other, Immunoglobulin M Antibody Capture enzyme linked immunosorbent assay, called MAC-ELISA (serological). Trioplex is a real time reverse transcription polymerase chain reaction test (real time RT-PCR) and the MAC-ELISA is used to detect antibodies created against the Zika virus.[27]

Mosquito Control Efforts

Because Zika virus disease cannot yet be prevented by drugs or vaccines, mosquito control is critical in mitigating risks associated with this disease. According to a CDC webpage, Zika virus is transmitted to people mainly through the bite of infected *Aedes aegypti* or possibly *Aedes albopictus* mosquitoes, which an article in a CDC journal reports are present in the United States and widely distributed globally[28] Figure 4 shows the potential range of the *Aedes aegypti* and *Aedes albopictus* mosquitoes in the United States. The *Aedes aegypti* mosquitoes are reportedly the primary mosquito spreading Zika virus in the Americas, while the *Aedes albopictus* mosquitoes share many of the same traits as *Aedes aegypti*.[29]

A female mosquito that bites someone with Zika virus of sufficient titer can obtain the virus, allow it to multiply within it, and enter its salivary gland such that subsequent humans bitten by this mosquito can potentially be infected with the Zika virus.[30] According to experts, the *Aedes aegypti* mosquitoes are primarily daytime biters and can bite multiple human hosts in succession. According to the CDC, mosquito control measures that reduce the number of potentially infectious mosquitoes can help reduce the spread of the Zika virus.

---

[27] Reverse transcription polymerase chain reaction (RT-PCR) is a technique to amplify genetic material that uses a reverse transcriptase enzyme to convert ribonucleic acid (RNA) to deoxyonucleic acid (DNA). ELISA is a technique designed for detecting and quantifying substances such as antibodies. Antibodies are made by the body in response to antigens such as viruses.

[28] Anna R. Plourde and Evan M. Bloch, "A Literature Review of Zika Virus," *Emerging Infectious Diseases*, Vol. 22 No. 7 (2016); and Centers for Disease Control and Prevention, Transmission and Risks, accessed May 15, 2017, https://www.cdc.gov/zika/transmission/index.html.

[29] Edward B. Hayes, "Zika Virus outside Africa," *Emerging Infectious Diseases,* vol.15, no. 9 (2009): 1347–50; and National Science and Technology Council, *A Strategy for Integrating Best Practices with New Science to Prevent Disease Transmission by Aedes Mosquito Vectors*, (Washington, D.C.: December, 2016).

[30] According to the National Science and Technology Council (NSTC), male mosquitoes are needed to fertilize mosquito eggs but do not bite humans or transmit diseases such as the Zika virus. One scientific study reported that an infected *Aedes aegypti*, but not *Aedes albopictus*, mosquito can transmit the Zika virus to some of its progeny. Saravanan Thangamani and others, "Vertical Transmission of Zika Virus in *Aedes aegypti* Mosquitoes," *American Journal of Tropical Medicine and Hygiene,* vol. 95, no. 5 (November 2016): 1169–73.

Mosquito control in the United States is implemented and overseen at the state and local levels, by entities such as mosquito control districts and health agencies.[31] CDC, using sources such as the American Mosquito Control Association, identified over 900 entities in the United States that perform mosquito control; however, not all geographic areas within the United States are covered by a mosquito control entity. Federal agencies support such control entities with funding and subject matter experts and may regulate some control methods such as pesticides.

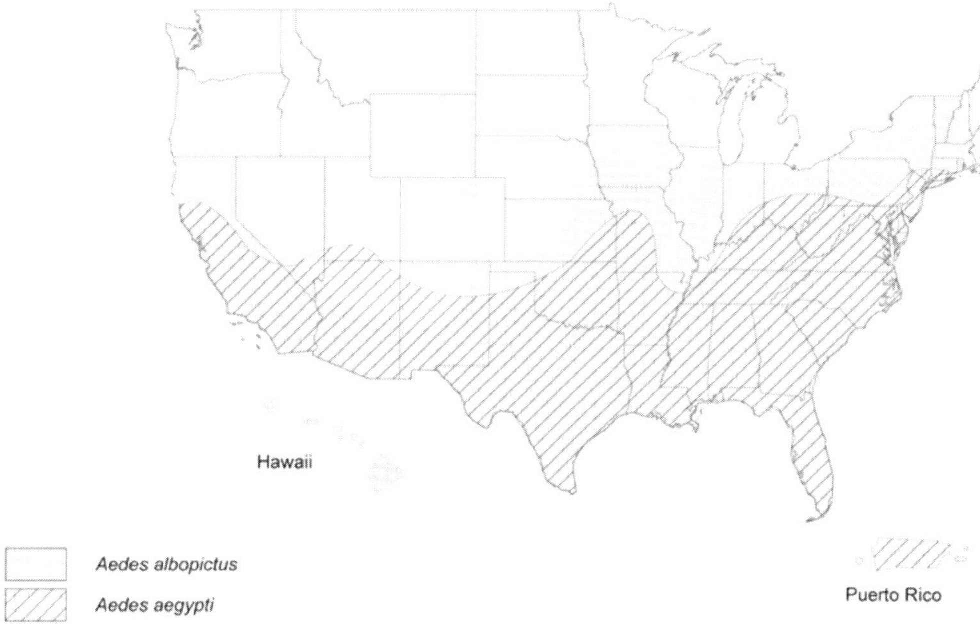

Source: GAO, adapted from CDC. | GAO-17-445.

Figure 4. Potential U.S. Range of *Aedes aegypti* and *Aedes albopictus* Mosquitoes.

HHS is the lead federal agency for public health and medical response to disease outbreaks and it leverages national public health and medical resources to prepare for and respond to disease outbreaks. For a Zika virus response, HHS coordinates activities across federal agencies to prevent and reduce Zika virus disease transmission and detect Zika virus disease and infection in communities where it may emerge. It would provide clinical guidance for diagnosis and case management. Table 1 shows the role of federal agencies and other agencies with respect to Zika virus disease in the United States.

[31] Mosquito control districts are established to provide only one or limited number of designated services, in this case mosquito control, and have sufficient administrative and fiscal autonomy to qualify as independent governments.

Federal Agency Roles in a Zika Virus Outbreak Response

Table 1. Federal agency roles in addressing Zika virus disease: Diagnostics, epidemiology, and mosquito control

Agency	Activity
Environmental Protection Agency (EPA)	• the lead agency for pesticide registrations and pesticide usage information; and • focuses on appropriate pesticide use, including technical assistance on wide-area spraying, residential treatments, review of health and safety data in the registration process, including data relating to the efficacy of pesticides used against mosquitoes carrying disease.
U.S. Department of Health and Human Services	
Assistant Secretary for Preparedness and Response (ASPR)	• focuses on preparedness planning and response; building federal emergency medical operational capabilities; countermeasures research, advance development, and procurement; and grants to strengthen the capabilities of hospitals and health care systems in public health emergencies and medical disasters; • provides federal support, including medical professionals through ASPR's National Disaster Medical System, to augment state and local capabilities during an emergency or disaster; • coordinates and aligns key HHS preparedness and response activities within the Department to maximize the use of available resources; and • supports collaboration and information sharing between public health and medical partners in the U.S. government.
Biomedical Advanced Research and Development Authority (BARDA)	• collaborates with partners from the Public Health Emergency Medical Countermeasures Enterprise to address medical countermeasure needs for the Zika response domestically and globally;[a] • helps in the transition of medical countermeasure candidates from early development to advanced research and development and then to FDA approval; • develops four strategic goals to address medical countermeasure needs for the Zika response through new vaccines, rapid diagnostics, screening tests for donated blood and virus inactivation in blood products; and • assists medical countermeasure developers.
Centers for Disease Control and Prevention (CDC)	• command center for monitoring and coordinating the emergency response to Zika, bringing together CDC scientists with expertise in arboviruses like Zika, reproductive health, emerging infections during pregnancy, birth defects, developmental disabilities, and travel health; • supports public health investigations and surveillance; • develops diagnostic tests for Zika and conducts studies on the link between Zika and health outcomes; • monitors and reports pregnancy and birth defect cases of Zika; • provides clinical guidance and education to state and local health officials, pregnant women and families and healthcare providers; • supports state and local health departments in improving access to clinical services for maternal child health populations and children with special needs; • conducts surveillance to identify potential mosquito habitats and provides funding for mosquito control; • supports Zika virus readiness and response capacity in states and territories where mosquito populations are known to transmit the Zika virus, with a priority focus on areas with ongoing Zika transmission; and

Agency	Activity
Centers for Disease Control and Prevention (CDC)	• technical lead for coordinating international public health and medical assistance, including sharing laboratory and clinical samples of biological material and responding to requests for coordinating international deployment of HHS public health and medical personnel and medical countermeasures.
Food and Drug Administration (FDA)	• facilitates development of diagnostic tests by providing manufacturers Emergency Use Authorization review templates that outline FDA's current recommendations for analytical and clinical validation studies needed to support an EUA submission; • works with manufacturers to support their diagnostic development programs, helping ensure that their tests are properly validated before being used to inform patient care;
	• with EPA, reviews innovative strategies to help suppress the population of virus-carrying mosquitoes and mitigate the threat of vector-borne epidemics; • engages with commercial and government developers, including the National Institute of Allergy and Infectious Diseases (NIAID) and BARDA, to advance the development of investigational vaccines for Zika virus; and • monitors for fraudulent products and false product claims related to the Zika virus and acts to protect consumers.
National Institutes of Health (NIH)	• works with its partners in government, academia, and the pharmaceutical and biotechnology industries to better understand the Zika virus, the disease it causes, and ways to combat it by supporting investigators through research grants and contracts; and • conducts and supports research in areas such as the natural history of the disease, basic research on the Zika virus, how it causes disease (or pathogenesis), and the consequences of Zika virus infection on pregnant women and infants, diagnostic testing to rapidly determine if someone is or has been infected with Zika and to distinguish from other flaviviruses, and vector biology, as well as treatments and vaccines.

Source: GAO analysis based on information supplied by agencies listed above. | GAO-17-445.

[a]The Public Health Emergency Medical Countermeasures Enterprise coordinates federal efforts to enhance responses to chemical, biological, radiological, and nuclear threats and preparedness for emerging infectious diseases from a medical countermeasures perspective across federal departments and agencies.

Challenges to Gathering New Information About Zika Virus Epidemiology

Surveillance and research during the recent Zika virus outbreaks in the United States and abroad have established new information about the epidemiology of Zika virus. Since the Zika virus was a newly emerging infectious disease threat in the United States, and relatively little was known about the virus prior to 2016, CDC and the states were not fully equipped with information and resources needed for a rapid response at the outset of the recent outbreaks. This presented surveillance and research challenges in addressing the Zika virus knowledge gaps.

What Is Known About the Epidemiology of Zika Virus

Knowledge about Zika virus epidemiology has increased in the past year, including information about Zika virus disease incidence and distribution of cases and its associated adverse health outcomes.

Zika Virus Cases Reported in the U.S. States and Territories

Between January 1, 2015 and April 5, 2017, reported Zika virus disease cases numbered 5,197 in the United States.[32] Florida and New York had the largest number of reported cases, followed by California and Texas.[33]

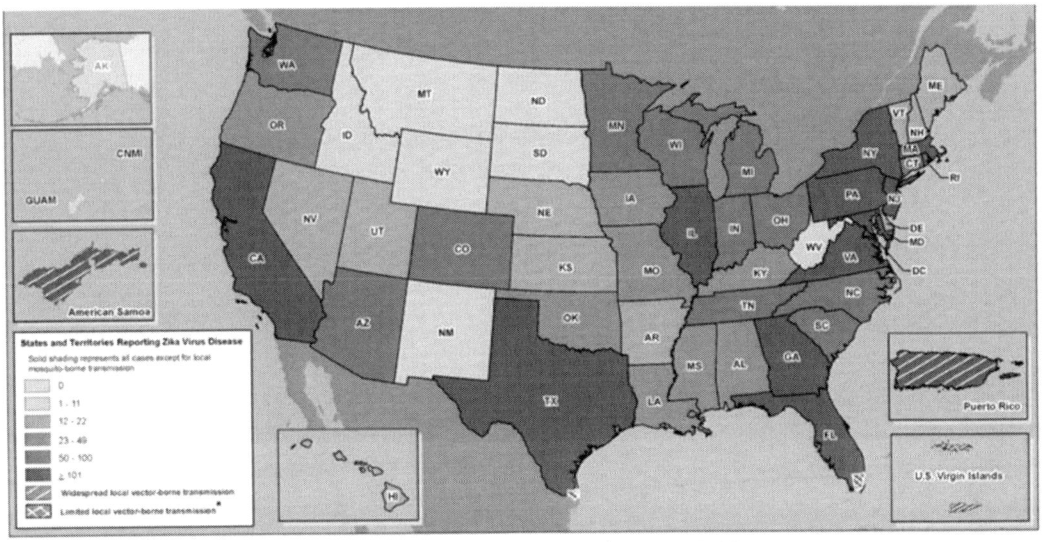

Source: Centers for Disease Control and Prevention (CDC). | GAO-17-445.

Figure 5. Laboratory-Confirmed Zika Virus Disease Cases That States and Territories Reported to ArboNET, April 5, 2017.

With the exception of Alaska, every state and three territories reported at least one Zika virus disease case by April 5, 2017. (See Figure 5.) Ten states reported more than 100 cases each. Ninety-four percent of all cases in U.S. states and the District of Columbia were travel-associated. According to a CDC analysis of reported cases between January 1, 2016 and July 31, 2016 in U.S. states and the District of Columbia, 66 percent of the 2,354 travel-related cases were associated with travel to countries and territories in the Caribbean, followed by Central America (18 percent), South America (10 percent), North America (5 percent), and Southeast Asia and the Pacific Islands (<1 percent).

---

[32] "Zika virus disease" case definition includes only cases that meet both laboratory and clinical (symptoms) criteria. (see appendix IV for detailed case definitions for Zika virus surveillance.) CDC provides provisional disease case counts from Zika virus reports from U.S. states and territories. It classifies these data as provisional until a few months into the next year.

[33] Number of reported cases: Florida (N=1,116), New York (N=1,016), California (N=438), Texas (N=320).

According to CDC, the first identified occurrence of local (mosquito-borne) areas of transmission and the first identified outbreak of mosquito-borne Zika virus infection in the continental United States occurred in Florida in Miami-Dade and Broward counties during June–August, 2016.[34] This led to the designation of red zones for those areas and guidance for people living in or traveling to those areas.[35] Texas is the only other state that has since reported locally-acquired cases. As of April 5, 2017, 216 of the total reported cases in Florida and 6 of the total cases in Texas were locally-acquired. Seventy-four reported cases in U.S. states and the District of Columbia were acquired through other routes, including maternal-fetal transmission, person-to-person through sexual transmission, and laboratory transmission.[36]

At 36,504 reported cases, the U.S. territories had about seven times the number of cases as U.S. states, and most of these cases were presumed to have been acquired through local mosquito-borne transmission; only 143 cases reported in the U.S. territories were among travelers returning to territories from other affected areas.[37] CDC reports that with local transmission in the territories, it is not possible to determine whether infection was caused by mosquito-borne or sexual transmission.

In addition to routinely updating cumulative Zika virus disease case counts on its Zika webpage, CDC periodically publishes Zika case demographic and other information in its MMWR. For example, 63 percent of the 2,382 Zika virus disease cases reported between January 1, 2016 and July 31, 2016 in U.S. states and the District of Columbia were female, and the same percentage was reported in an analysis of Puerto Rico cases between November 1, 2015 and October 20, 2016.[38] CDC noted that the higher proportion of women with symptomatic disease could be because of care-seeking behavior, differential exposure to mosquitoes or other risks, or testing of pregnant women increased.

The median age of reported Zika virus disease cases was 39 years in U.S. states and the District of Columbia. Preliminary CDC analysis indicated that reported cases in U.S. states typically were among older persons compared to cases in U.S. territories. According to CDC, the age difference observed in this preliminary analysis was most likely due to differences in the traveler population versus the general population. The majority of cases in U.S. states were travel-associated, while most cases in U.S. territories

---

[34] A. Likos. "Local Mosquito-Borne Transmission of Zika Virus—Miami-Dade and Broward Counties, Florida, June–August 2016," *Morbidity and Mortality Weekly Report,* vol. 65, no. 38 (September 30, 2016):1032—38.

[35] See CDC guidance at https://www.cdc.gov/zika/intheus/florida-update.html (accessed May 14, 2017) for more details.

[36] Other routes include sexual transmission (N=45), mother-to-child (congenital) infection (N=27), laboratory transmission (N=1), and person-to-person through an unknown route (N=1).

[37] Number of reported cases: American Samoa (N=132), Puerto Rico (N=35,375), U.S. Virgin Islands (N=997).

[38] William L. Walker and others, Zika Virus Disease Cases—50 States and the District of Columbia, January 1–July 31, 2016," *Morbidity and Mortality Weekly Report*, vol. 65, no. 36 (September 16, 2016): 983–86; Matthew Lozier and others, Incidence of Zika Virus Disease by Age and Sex—Puerto Rico, November 1, 2015–October 20, 2016, *Morbidity and Mortality Weekly Report*, vol. 65, no. 44 (November 11, 2016): 1219–23.

were acquired through presumed local mosquito-borne transmission, according to a CDC Zika case count update report.

Zika Virus Infection Can Cause Microcephaly and Other Adverse Health Outcomes

In a paper published in May 2016, CDC authors applied criteria for causality in a review of available data and concluded that a causal relationship exists between prenatal Zika virus infection and microcephaly and other serious brain abnormalities.[39] In September 2016, a WHO Zika causality statement concluded that the most likely explanation of available evidence from outbreaks of Zika virus infection and clusters of microcephaly is that Zika virus infection during pregnancy is a cause of congenital brain abnormalities including microcephaly.[40] Other studies have sought to estimate the risk of adverse health outcomes to pregnant women infected with Zika virus. For example, a CDC study estimated that the risk of microcephaly from Zika virus infection in the first trimester in Brazil was between about 100 to 1300 cases per 10,000 births, compared to an estimated baseline risk of 2 to 12 cases per 10,000 births.[41] According to CDC and WHO, microcephaly is just one of a range of birth defects that could be related to Zika virus infection.[42]

WHO reported that by January 18, 2017, 29 countries or territories had reported microcephaly and other central nervous system malformations that were potentially associated with Zika virus infection.[43] In the United States, the U.S. Zika Pregnancy Registry publicly reports about twice a month the total number of pregnant women with laboratory evidence of possible Zika virus infection who were reported to the registry. The March 28, 2017 update included 1,716 pregnant women in U.S. states and the District of Columbia with laboratory evidence of possible Zika virus infection. Of 1,311 completed pregnancies as of March 28, 2017 with laboratory evidence of Zika virus infection in U.S. states and the District of Columbia, there were 56 live born infants reported to have birth defects and 7 pregnancy losses with birth defects. As of March 28, 2017, 3,461 pregnant women with laboratory evidence of Zika virus infection in U.S.

---

[39] Sonja A. Rasmussen and others, "Zika Virus and Birth Defects—Reviewing the Evidence for Causality," *New England Journal of Medicine,* 374 (May 19, 2016): 1981–87.

[40] World Health Organization (WHO) *Zika Causality Statement*. accessed May 3, 2017, http://www.who.int/emergencies/zika-virus/causality/en/.

[41] Michael A. Johansson and others, "Zika and the Risk of Microcephaly," *New England Journal of Medicine*, 375 (2016): 1–4. The estimates of risk due to infection during the first trimester of pregnancy ranged from 0.88 percent with a 95 percent credible interval of 0.80 to 0.97 percent when assuming an 80 percent overall Zika virus infection rate and 100 percent over-reporting of microcephaly cases, to 13.2 percent with a 95 percent credible interval of 12.0 to 14.4 percent when assuming a 10 percent Zika virus infection rate and no over-reporting. A credible interval means that the measure of interest lies with 95 percent probability in the interval.

[42] Centers for Disease Control and Prevention (CDC), "Key Messages—Zika Virus Disease," accessed April 21, 2017, https://www.cdc.gov/zika/pdfs/zika-key-messages.pdf; World Health Organization (WHO) Zika Causality Statement, accessed May 3, 2017, http://www.who.int/emergencies/zika-virus/causality/en/.

[43] World Health Organization (WHO), *Situation Report: Zika Virus Microcephaly Guillian- Barré Syndrome 20 January 2017 Data as of 18 January 2017*, accessed April 12, 2017, http://www.who.int/emergencies/zika-virus/situation-report/20-january-2017/en.

territories were reported to the U.S. Zika Pregnancy Registry or to the Zika Active Pregnancy Surveillance System for Puerto Rico. CDC noted in this update that Puerto Rico was not using the same case inclusion criteria, and CDC was not reporting numbers for adverse pregnancy outcomes in the territories at that time. A CDC report in April 2017 provided data on the impact of Zika virus on pregnant women and babies for 2016, including that 44 states reported cases of pregnant women with evidence of Zika virus infection and most were travel-associated, and about 1 in 10 pregnant women with confirmed Zika virus had a fetus or baby with birth defects.[44]

As of January 18, 2017, 21 countries or territories had reported an increase in the incidence of Guillain-Barré syndrome or laboratory confirmation of a Zika virus infection among Guillain-Barré syndrome cases.[45] CDC also reported that its own research suggested a strong association between Guillain-Barré syndrome and Zika virus, but also noted that only a small proportion of persons with a recent Zika virus infection got Guillain-Barré syndrome.[46] CDC reported that of 56 suspected cases of Guillain-Barré syndrome with onset of neurologic signs identified between January 1 and July 31, 2016 in Puerto Rico, 20 patients had no evidence of Zika virus infection, compared to 34 patients who had evidence of Zika virus or flavivirus infection.[47]

What Is Not Known about the Epidemiology of Zika Virus

While much has been learned about the epidemiology of Zika virus, many unknowns remain, including

- the total number of infections;
- the biological mechanisms, risks, reasons for geographic differences, and full spectrum of outcomes associated with maternal-fetal transmission;
- the presence and duration of the virus in different bodily fluids;
- the role of prior Zika virus infections or exposure to other related flaviviruses; and
- the full spectrum of outcomes of Zika virus infection.

---

[44] Centers for Disease Control and Prevention, "Vital Signs April 2017", accessed May 17, 2017, https://www.cdc.gov/vitalsigns/pdf/2017-04-vitalsigns.pdf.

[45] World Health Organization, *Situation Report: Zika Virus Microcephaly Guillain-Barré Syndrome 20 January 2017 Data as of 18 January 2017*, accessed April 12, 2017, http://www.who.int/emergencies/zika-virus/situation-report/20-january-2017/en/.

[46] Centers for Disease Control and Prevention, "Key Messages—Zika Virus Disease," accessed April 21, 2017, https://www.cdc.gov/zika/pdfs/zika-key-messages.pdf.

[47] Two of the 56 patients were pending test results. Of the 34 patients with evidence of Zika virus or flavivirus infection, 26 had confirmed or presumptive Zika virus infection, and 8 had presumptive flavivirus infection. Whether an infection is classified as confirmed or presumptive depends on the laboratory evidence. Emilio Dirlikov and others. "Guillain- Barré Syndrome During Ongoing Zika Virus Transmission — Puerto Rico, January 1–July 31, 2016," *Morbidity and Mortality Weekly Report*, vol. 65, no. 34 (September 2, 2016): 910-914.

The Total Number of Infections Is Not Known

Zika virus case counts obtained from the national disease surveillance system underestimate the total number of Zika virus infections over a specified time period, for reasons including that an infected person

- may not seek medical care because they have only mild or no symptoms, or other reasons,
- may not be diagnosed because of limitations in Zika virus diagnostic testing, and
- surveillance reporting can be incomplete for a variety of reasons.

First, the ArboNET surveillance system captures only reported Zika virus disease and infection cases. As such, the case counts does not capture the suspected high proportion of infected people who are asymptomatic and may not seek care and get a diagnosis of Zika virus infection. One study estimated that about 18 percent of Zika-infected persons will have clinical symptoms of the infection.[48] CDC and WHO have reported that about 80 percent of people who have Zika virus infection won't have any symptoms.

Findings from a May 2017 study in Puerto Rico also suggested there is a high rate of asymptomatic people infected with Zika virus who are not diagnosed. The study applied results from a blood donor population that was screened for Zika virus to estimate the number of Zika infections in the population of Puerto Rico and estimated that there were over 450,000 Zika virus infections in Puerto Rico over approximately four months in mid-2016.[49] In comparison, 35,375 disease cases were reported in Puerto Rico from January 1, 2015 through April 5, 2017, according to a CDC Zika virus disease case count update report. The Puerto Rico blood donor study authors concluded that results from blood donation screening during arboviral outbreaks can supplement routine clinical and surveillance data for improved targeting of prevention efforts.

Second, limitations in Zika virus diagnostic testing can also affect the accuracy of the number of Zika virus cases reported in disease surveillance due to inaccurate laboratory test results. Some Zika diagnostic tests can determine that a recent flavivirus infection has occurred, which may or may not be caused by Zika virus. This is because the antibodies produced in response to flavivirus infection (Zika, dengue, West Nile, yellow fever) are cross-reactive and may produce a positive result in a test for any of these viruses. This is of particular concern in areas where there has been co-circulation of flaviruses, such as dengue virus in Puerto Rico. The ability of the test to detect the virus also depends on the

---

[48] Mark R. Duffy and others, "Zika Virus Outbreak on Yap Island, Federated States of Micronesia," *New England Journal of Medicine,* vol. 360 (2009): 2536–43. This study estimated that about 18 percent of infected persons have a clinical illness with a 95 percent confidence interval range of 10 to 27 percent.

[49] Michelle S. Chevalier and others, "Use of Blood Donor Screening Data to Estimate Zika Virus Incidence, Puerto Rico, April–August 2016," *Emerging Infectious Diseases,* vol. 23, no. 5 (2017). The estimated number of incident Zika virus infections in Puerto Rico between April 3–August 12, 2016 was 469,321 with a 95 percent confidence interval of 401,477 to 559,126, based on screening of 21,468 blood donors.

type of test used, when it is used, and the type of specimen collected. CDC recommends additional criteria and testing strategies for pregnant women for definitive diagnoses. The different types of Zika virus diagnostic tests, their challenges, and testing strategies for mitigating these challenges are discussed later in this chapter.

Third, according to CDC documentation, notifiable disease reporting is likely incomplete, and the completeness varies depending upon the disease and the reporting state or territory. Factors that can influence completeness of reporting include the availability of diagnostic facilities; control measures in effect, public awareness of a specific disease, the state and local health officials responsible for disease control and public health surveillance, changes in methods for public health surveillance, or introduction of new diagnostics tests or other diseases. However, CDC documentation states that it has undertaken efforts to educate providers on Zika virus infection and provided guidance for screening and testing.

The Biological Mechanisms, Risks, and Reasons for Geographic Differences in Outcomes Associated with Maternal-Fetal Transmission Are Unclear

The mechanisms of causality between Zika virus infection and microcephaly are not well-understood.[50] According to a recent CDC Zika virus key messages document published on its website, questions also remain regarding the timing, risk, and full spectrum of adverse pregnancy outcomes as a result of Zika virus infection.[51] Adding to the complexity, microcephaly is also caused by other environmental and genetic factors, including infections such as rubella during pregnancy, maternal exposure to toxic chemicals such as heavy metals or smoking, injuries to the developing brain, genetic abnormalities such as Down syndrome, and severe malnutrition during fetal life.

The reasons for differences in the reported incidence of microcephaly and other birth defects between geographic areas with Zika virus outbreaks are also not well-understood. For example, in Brazil in 2015, municipalities with high reports (defined as greater than 20 cases per 10,000 municipalities) of confirmed cases (per 10,000 live births) of newborns and children with changes in growth related to Zika virus infection and other infectious etiologies were concentrated in the Northeast region, although there was wider dispersion in other regions in 2016.[52]

There is also wide variation in reported microcephaly cases relative to Zika virus cases in different countries. Using case data from PAHO, we found a wide variation among countries in the ratio of number of reported cases of birth defects associated with Zika virus infection to the total number of confirmed locally-acquired and travel-

---

[50] Jin-Na Wang and Feng Ling, "Zika Virus Infection and Microcephaly: Evidence for a Causal Link," *International Journal of Environmental Research and Public Health,* vol. 13, no. 1031 (October 2016).

[51] Centers for Disease Control and Prevention, "Key Messages—Zika Virus Disease," accessed April 21, 2017, https://www.cdc.gov/ZIKA/PDFS/ZIKA-KEY-MESSAGES.PDF.

[52] Pan American Health Organization / World Health Organization. *Zika - Epidemiological Report Brazil.* (Washington, D.C.: 2017).

associated cases of Zika virus as of March 9, 2017 (Table 2). For example, there were about 55 Zika virus cases for every birth defect case in Brazil, whereas in Colombia there are about 77 Zika virus cases for every birth defect case.

Table 2. Zika virus cases and birth defects associated with the Zika virus reported in the Americas, 2015–2017, as of March 9, 2017

Zika virus cases				
Country	**Confirmed locally acquired**	**Travel-associated**	**Confirmed birth defects**[a]	**Ratio of birth defects to Zika virus cases**[b]
Brazil	130,840	0	2,386	1:55
Colombia	9,802	0	128	1:77
Dominican Republic	345	0	54	1:6
United States	222	4,813	52	1:97
Guatemala	890	0	37	1:24
Martinique	21	0	22	1:1
French Guiana	483	10	17	1:29
Guadeloupe	382	0	14	1:27
Bolivia	192	4	14	1:14
Puerto Rico	39,339	137	12	1:3290
All other PAHO member countries	22,984	758	31	1:766

Source: GAO analysis of data from the Pan American Health Organization (PAHO). I GAO-17-445.

Note: PAHO refers to travel-associated cases as "imported" cases and to locally acquired cases using the epidemiologic term "autochtonous" cases.

[a]Congenital syndrome associated with the Zika virus infection.

[b]Ratio of confirmed congenital syndrome (birth defects) cases associated with Zika virus to the total confirmed and imported Zika virus cases. Ratios in epidemiology can be used when there is not necessarily a relationship between the numerator and denominator, whereas in a proportion, the numerator is always part of the denominator. Proportions are not appropriate for this table because the mothers of the infants with confirmed congenital syndrome may or may not be included in the confirmed Zika virus case counts, as these do not have the same inclusion criteria.

According to literature we reviewed, some possible reasons for these variations include differences in mosquito prevention and family planning practices, environmental factors, population differences, and surveillance system differences (including case definitions).

The Presence and Duration of the Virus in Different Bodily Fluids Is Not Well-Understood

It is not well-understood how long the Zika virus can remain in different bodily fluids or how long it can be transmitted to other people. CDC reports that Zika can remain in semen longer than in other bodily fluids, including vaginal fluids, urine, and blood. One case report study found that Zika virus was detectable in semen at 69 days after symptom onset,[53] and another study reported a maximum duration of Zika virus genetic material in semen of 125 days after symptom onset.[54]

The Role of Prior Zika Virus Infections or Exposure to Other Related Flaviviruses is Not Clear

The role of previous Zika virus infections or related flaviviruses such as dengue virus is unclear. According to WHO, it is not known whether Zika virus presence in a population over time results in widespread or low-level immune protection or possibly no protection.[55] The cross-reactivity between Zika virus and related flaviviruses has not been established, although some studies are beginning to address this gap. For example, a study published in December 2016 suggests that preexisting dengue virus immunity may enhance Zika virus infection and lead to greater disease severity.[56] Another study published in April 2017 found evidence that antibodies against related flaviviruses such as dengue and West Nile can cross-react with Zika virus and could increase disease severity.[57]

The Full Spectrum of Outcomes of Zika Virus Infection is Not Known

The full spectrum of outcomes from maternal-fetal transmission is not known. A paper published by CDC authors identified research gaps that need rapid and systematic assessment, including a complete understanding of the frequency and full spectrum of clinical outcomes resulting from fetal Zika virus infection and of the environmental factors that influence emergence.[58] Another review paper noted that with causality between Zika virus infection and adverse pregnancy outcomes having been established, the critical research issues can turn to understanding the full spectrum of outcomes and quantifying the relative and absolute risks among infants who are born to women who were infected at different times during pregnancy, and identifying factors that modify the risk of an adverse pregnancy or birth outcome, such as coinfection with another virus, preexisting immune response to another flavivirus, genetic background of the mother or fetus, and severity of infection.[59]

The associations between Zika virus infection and Guillain-Barré syndrome are also unclear. It has been reported that the most likely explanation of an association is that Zika

---

[53] Marta Arsuaga and others, "Probable Sexual Transmission of Zika Virus from a Vasectomized Man," *Lancet Infectious Diseases,* vol. 16 (2016):1107.

[54] Gabriela Paz-Bailey and others, "Persistence of Zika virus in Bodily Fluids – Preliminary Report," *The New England Journal of Medicine,* (2017): 1-9.

[55] World Health Organization, "Emergencies: One Year into the Zika Outbreak: How an Obscure Disease Became a Global Health Emergency," accessed April 26, 2017, http://www.who.int/emergencies/zika-virus/articles/one-year-outbreak/en/.

[56] Lauren M. Paul and others, "Dengue Virus Antibodies Enhance Zika Virus Infection," *Clinical & Translational Immunology,* vol. 5, no. 12 (2016).

[57] Susana V. Bardina and others, "Enhancement of Zika Virus Pathogenesis by Preexisting Antiflavivirus Immunity," *Science,* vol. 356, no. 6334 (2017): 175-80.

[58] Lyle Petersen and others, "Zika Virus", *The New England Journal of Medicine*, vol. 374 (2016): 1552-63.

[59] Sonja A. Rasmussen and others, "Zika Virus and Birth Defects," 1981–87.

virus infection can trigger Guillain-Barré syndrome.[60] According to CDC documentation, CDC collaborates with state and local health departments to investigate possibly unusually large numbers or clusters of Guillain-Barré syndrome cases, and Puerto Rico has a surveillance system for Guillain-Barré syndrome.

Three Key Challenges to Zika Virus Surveillance

CDC, CSTE, and state and local public health agencies faced several challenges in implementing surveillance for Zika virus and its associated health outcomes. These challenges involved establishing early case definitions, timely communication of critical information, and interoperability between surveillance databases.

Establishing Case Definitions Challenged the Collection of Consistent and Timely Information

We identified several challenges related to establishing case definitions for Zika virus infection and disease surveillance. According to CDC officials, typically, the process for adding a new disease to the national notifiable disease list is that the CSTE votes during its annual meetings whether to add the disease. If approved, the disease is usually made notifiable the following January. According to CDC officials, this allows time to plan and prepare for implementation, including the information technology aspects of reporting the disease. However, because of the emergent nature and emergency response needed for Zika virus, CSTE released an interim case definition in February 2016 so that Zika virus disease would become immediately notifiable.

These interim definitions included only laboratory diagnosed cases in persons who also reported certain clinical criteria. CDC officials and representatives from public health organizations told us that as more was learned about Zika virus, including the need to capture asymptomatic cases, the interim case definitions were revised. CSTE approved the revised case definitions position statement in June 2016, which included laboratory confirmed, asymptomatic cases (Zika virus infection) and some revisions related to laboratory diagnostic testing.

These changes presented some challenges, according to some public health officials and organizational representatives we interviewed. CDC and CSTE officials told us that because there were two case definitions approved during the year, changes had to be made to the reporting system twice, and all cases classified according to the first definition had to be reclassified based on the new definition, which takes time.[61] CDC officials also told us that another challenge is that jurisdictions use different systems and

---

[60] World Health Organization. *Guillain–Barré Syndrome Fact sheet, updated October 2016*, accessed April 26, 2017, http://www.who.int/mediacentre/factsheets/guillain-barre-syndrome/en/.

[61] According to CDC, CSTE recommended that all jurisdictions reclassify all previously reported 2016 Zika virus disease and congenital infection cases according to the new case definitions from June 2016.

have different capacities related to surveillance and informatics expertise, which required a lot of resources from CDC and others to assist these jurisdictions.

CDC officials noted that it takes time for states to reclassify their older cases. CDC designates Zika virus cumulative case counts as provisional on its Zika virus case counts website.[62] CDC officials told us that cases can be added or removed as new information becomes available, and that due to lags in investigation, testing, and reporting, newly reported cases often occurred weeks or even months earlier than the reported date.

Experts at our meeting and public health officials at selected sites emphasized the importance of educating health care providers, including on testing and reporting guidelines. For instance, an official from one of the selected sites stated that "a well-informed clinician is the best reporting tool." HHS officials told us that CDC engaged frequently with key professional organizations such as the American College of Obstetricians and Gynecologists to provide updated information; however gaps remain among providers who do not access up-to-date information provided on the CDC or professional organization websites.

Information Dissemination and Communication Were Not Always Timely

Public health officials from a selected site and representatives of public health organizations had some positive things to say regarding the assistance that federal agencies, or more specifically CDC, provided in responding to the Zika virus outbreaks. For example, officials from one selected site told us that a lot of guidance was coming out rapidly from CDC, and in general the guidance was very helpful and made providers more comfortable in patient care. Representatives from a public health organization told us that they viewed the U.S. government's response to Zika as much stronger and more organized, forward leaning, inclusive, and transparent than it was for response to some earlier diseases, especially recognizing the many unknowns about Zika virus. Representatives from another public health organization told us that CDC demonstrated flexibility in its willingness to make modifications to Zika virus reporting based on feedback from states.

Nonetheless, we identified some challenges regarding the communication of guidance from CDC early in Zika virus surveillance implementation. For example, officials from one selected site told us that they were sometimes not able to get guidance consistently because entities within CDC did not talk with each other, and that CDC could not come to a quick conclusion about who to include in the Zika virus case definition. Representatives from a public health organization told us that they were sometimes not informed of changes in Zika-related information before learning about a change from a CDC media release, but that this had improved compared to 5 or 10 years ago.

---

[62] See CDC Zika virus case counts website at: https://www.cdc.gov/zika/geo/united-states.html, accessed April 10, 2017.

However, according to HHS officials, CDC frequently uses media outlets to disseminate important information to reach a broad audience. CDC also provided updated guidance for diagnosis and clinical practice, including several clinical guidelines and health alert network messages.[63]

Public health officials in selected sites also told us that earlier in the Zika virus response, challenges resulted from officials from different CDC units needing to establish communication channels that had not existed before the Zika virus outbreak. Officials from one selected site told us about difficulty in communication and the importance of agency-wide communication and partnerships, and relationships that can make things happen faster. Officials from this site also told us that communication across different units improved over time. CDC officials similarly told us that many people were involved across CDC, including from birth defects and reproductive health, and arboviral diseases units, and that rarely were so many different people involved in a response effort.

The Interoperability of Surveillance Databases Was Lacking

There are separate systems for Zika virus cases and associated health outcomes surveillance that collect different information but also some of the same information, and these systems are not electronically linked. Officials from selected sites and representatives from a public health organization told us that having several different surveillance systems that were not interoperable was a challenge. Representatives we interviewed from one public health organization noted that states took issue with having to report data to the pregnancy registry that they already reported to other registries. Officials from one site we visited told us that there were questions as to whether different tracking systems are necessary, and that it is a challenge that they have different requirements. In another selected site, officials told us it is challenging when changes need to be made in the system because there's no cross-communication in the data.

However, HHS officials told us that surveillance systems for infectious diseases and surveillance of pregnancies and pregnancy outcomes and birth defects serve very different purposes and are also tailored to each jurisdiction's needs. HHS officials also noted that the different and complementary surveillance systems serve equally important, yet very different critical needs during public health emergencies.

Two Key Challenges in Conducting Epidemiological Zika Virus Research

We identified two key challenges for Zika virus epidemiological research: study designs needed for establishing association and causality challenged linking Zika virus

[63] Health alert messages are disseminated through CDC's Health Alert Network, which is CDC's primary method of sharing cleared information about urgent public health incidents with public information officers; federal, state, territorial, and local public health practitioners; clinicians; and public health laboratories.

and associated health outcomes, and insufficient data and lack of developed models challenged prediction of the spread of the virus.

Establishing Association and Causality between Zika Virus Infection and Adverse Health Outcomes Faced Study Design Challenges

We identified challenges in linking the Zika virus with associated health outcomes. CDC was able to report pregnancy outcomes of women who were infected with or are suspected to have been infected with Zika virus and reported to the pregnancy registries. According to HHS officials, combining this prospective monitoring of pregnant women with retrospective birth defect surveillance allows for a comprehensive picture of pregnancy outcomes and has already provided critical information to inform the public health response to Zika virus. However, because the Zika pregnancy registry only includes pregnant women who have laboratory evidence of Zika virus infection, there is no control group of pregnant women without Zika virus in the pregnancy registry.

According to HHS officials, studies that prospectively follow an identified group of people over time to monitor for both disease and outcomes are needed. WHO also noted that cohort studies of the populations currently at risk are needed to determine both absolute and relative risks of a Zika- affected pregnancy, the role of co-factors and effect modifiers, and to determine whether there is a specific congenital Zika virus syndrome.

NIH recently launched such a study–Zika in Infants and Pregnancy (ZIP)–that aims to enroll as many as 10,000 pregnant women at up to 15 sites in Puerto Rico and abroad in order to study the outcomes of pregnant women who test positive for the Zika virus as well as those who test negative and their infants.[64] The researchers plan to compare birth outcomes between mothers who were infected with Zika virus and those who were not, documenting the frequency of microcephaly and other adverse health outcomes. The study will also evaluate how the timing of infection affects pregnancy outcomes and the role that environmental influences, social determinants and other infections, such as dengue fever, may have on the health of the study participants and their newborns.

However, there are challenges in conducting prospective cohort studies such as the ZIP study. These studies can take years before complete results are available and published in peer-reviewed journals. For example, the ZIP study start date was June 2016, and the estimated study completion date is June 2018.[65] Prospective cohort studies that follow large numbers of individuals in multiple sites for many months or years are also generally expensive and time-consuming.

---

[64] The Zika in Infants and Pregnancy (ZIP) trial will enroll participants in their first trimester of pregnancy and follow them throughout their pregnancies to determine if they become infected with the Zika virus and, if so, the outcomes in mother and infant. The infants will be followed for at least one year after birth.

[65] See https://clinicaltrials.gov/ct2/show/study/NCT02856984, accessed May 13, 2017. According to HHS officials, to mitigate delays in using study results, NIH has planned for interim analyses to obtain and disseminate information as the ZIP study proceeds.

Predicting the Spread of the Zika Virus Was Challenged by Insufficient Data and Lack of Developed Models

Modeling and simulation studies that accurately estimate the number of disease cases in a population or predict cases of a disease can improve planning and allocating scarce public health resources.[66] According to an April 2017 Zika virus key messages report, CDC has not been able to predict how much the Zika virus will spread in the continental United States. CDC officials told us that there was no epidemiologic model that looked at both types of transmission together–sexual and mosquito-borne. In addition, there are several major assumptions that need to be made for descriptive and predictive modeling of the Zika virus, including the number of infections and the overall number of pregnant women. CDC officials told us that as of October 2016, many uncertainties remained for Zika virus modeling. The models are constantly being refined and updated.

A December 2016 report from an intergovernmental committee on infectious disease modeling noted the importance and potential of outbreak prediction and modeling to improve outbreak preparedness. The report outlined three major challenges concerning

- data- and information-sharing, including the need for timely and accurate data and information, especially at the beginning of a novel disease outbreak, when knowledge about the pathogen and data on the epidemiological situation is limited;
- outbreak model development and decision support, including a systematic effort to synthesize results across modeling efforts and support on how to use this information in outbreak response decision-making; and
- science of disease emergence, which involves the need for better understanding of the processes that drive disease emergence and transmission well enough to predict where and when diseases are likely to emerge.

Characteristics of Different Diagnostic Tests Varied, Manufacturers and Users Faced Several Challenges, and FDA and CDC Did Not Consistently Communicate Sufficient Information

Authorized diagnostic tests used for the recent Zika virus outbreak varied in their performance and operational characteristics.[67] Diagnostic test manufacturers faced

[66] Descriptive modeling tries to estimate what probably occurred or is occurring now, while predictive modeling predicts cases in the future.

[67] Performance characteristics of a test used to describe the quality of a diagnostic test result including the analysis of accuracy, precision, sensitivity, and specificity, among others. Operational characteristics include among others, the time to perform a test, its technical simplicity or ease of use, users' acceptability, and the stability of the test under user conditions.

challenges in several areas, including research and development, testing, and regulatory approval of these tests. Diagnostic test users also encountered challenges, including determining the most accurate test to use, comparing clinical performance characteristics across tests, and obtaining equipment required to conduct authorized tests. Both manufacturers and users we spoke with raised issues about the EUA process. Moreover, CDC and FDA did not consistently communicate sufficient information about Zika virus diagnostic tests that could have enabled users to more easily identify the test that could detect the smallest amount of virus in a sample.

Molecular and Serological Zika Virus Diagnostic Tests Varied in Performance and Operational Characteristics

There are currently no available diagnostic tests cleared by FDA for the detection of Zika virus. By April 12, 2017, FDA had authorized 16 diagnostic tests for the Zika virus (13 molecular tests and 3 serologic tests) under EUAs following the public health emergency declaration.

According to FDA officials, they revoked one test, and as a result, 15 diagnostic tests are currently authorized. These authorized diagnostic tests for the Zika virus vary in their performance and operational characteristics. Molecular and serologic tests have different strengths and limitations, but some of the limitations can be mitigated by using an algorithm that CDC published.[68]

Molecular Tests Varied in Their Ability to Detect Zika Virus

Authorized molecular diagnostic tests for the Zika virus varied in their performance characteristics, and some may not have been sensitive enough to detect Zika virus infection in samples that were collected when the level of virus was low, namely, towards the end of, or after, the recommended collection time post onset of symptoms. The product labels for these authorized Zika virus diagnostic tests list a variety of different performance characteristics, including: analytical sensitivity, cross-reactivity, interference, and clinical evaluation.[69] The differences between these performance characteristics are important for understanding the accuracy of the diagnostic test. For instance, the limit of detection listed on manufacturers' product labels using their own samples and protocols range from 5.9 copies/mL (less virus is needed for detection) to

---

[68] The CDC-issued algorithm is a step-by-step protocol intended to assist laboratories in combining results from multiple samples and methods to make appropriate decisions about next testing steps.

[69] Analytic sensitivity (limit of detection) is defined as the lowest concentration of virus that can be consistently detected 95 percent of the time in a defined type of specimen. Cross- reactivity is when antibodies to similar viruses react, such as dengue, leading to tests that are not specific for the Zika virus. For example, a person previously infected with another flavivirus such as dengue could be falsely identified as also having been exposed to the Zika virus (and vice versa). Clinical evaluation is a measure of a specific assay evaluated against a comparator assay with clinical samples.

42,000 copies/mL (more virus is needed for detection) (appendix V has more details on these characteristics). If a person had 1,000 copies/mL of Zika virus RNA in his or her blood stream, the test that had the lower limit of detection (5.9 copies/mL) would indicate a positive result, while the test with the higher limit of detection (42,000 copies/mL) would incorrectly indicate a negative result (called a false negative). The limit of detection is an important measure for the Zika virus, which can be present in relatively low levels in the body. It is important to note that a negative result by molecular testing should be followed by serological testing, according to CDC's guidance, in order to reduce the risk of false negative results.

FDA created Zika virus reference material for molecular tests to compare test results to ensure accuracy. We found that the limit of detection varied between different tests when performed using samples and protocols FDA provided from 100 detectable units/mL to 30,000 detectable units/mL (See appendix V). The diagnostic accuracy of a new test refers to the extent of agreement between the outcome of the new test seeking authorization and the reference standard.[70]

Key terms related to diagnostic tests

- Comparator assay: An assay used as the reference method for assessing the performance characteristics of another test method.
- FDA Reference Materials: Genetic material from two current Zika virus strains in human plasma and three controls for blind testing to establish performance testing provided by FDA.
- Limit of detection: The measure of how much virus needs to be in a sample for the assay to detect the presence of the virus.
- Operational characteristics: The time to perform the test, its technical simplicity or ease of use, user acceptability, and the stability of the test under user conditions.
- Performance characteristics: A description of quality of a diagnostic test result including the analysis of accuracy, prevision, sensitivity, and specificity, among others.
- Sensitivity: The proportion of patients with the infection (determined by the result of the reference or "gold standard" test) who have a positive result using the test under evaluation.
- Specificity: The proportion of patients without the infection (determined by the result of the reference or gold standard test) who have a negative result using the test under evaluation.
- Test: Any method for obtaining additional information regarding a patient's health status.

Source: Food and Drug Administration, Department of Health and Human Services, and Shabir Banoo and others, "Evaluation of Diagnostic Tests for Infectious Diseases: General Principles, *Nature Reviews: Microbiology* (2010): S17-S29. I GAO-17-445.

According to FDA officials, when a new test is evaluated by comparison to a nonreference standard, as with the Zika virus, one cannot directly calculate unbiased estimates of sensitivity and specificity and therefore these terms are not appropriate. Instead, estimates called positive percent agreement and negative percent agreement are

---

[70] A reference standard is the best available method for establishing the presence or absence of the target condition. The reference standard can be a single test or method or a combination of methods and techniques, including clinical follow-up, according to FDA's guidance document.

calculated and reflect the agreement of the new test with the nonreference standard.[71] According to FDA officials, a major disadvantage with agreement measures is that agreement is not a measure of "correctness." The two tests could agree; however, agreement does not indicate how good or poor test sensitivities and specificities are (for example, both tests could agree because they are both false negatives). Also, that two tests are not in agreement does not necessarily mean that the new test is inaccurate and the comparator test is correct.

Molecular Tests Varied in Ease of Use and Timeliness

The authorized molecular diagnostic tests for the Zika virus after the public health emergency declaration also varied in their operational characteristics. These molecular diagnostic tests vary in their ease of use—some require manual steps, while others have some automation. Automation potentially allows for faster and more consistent processing and fewer staff resources. The time to perform individual authorized molecular diagnostic tests for the Zika virus is around 4 hours. One manufacturer using automation can process multiple samples in 8 hours. However, all the authorized molecular tests for the Zika virus have to be performed at Clinical Laboratory Improvement Amendments (CLIA) high complexity laboratories.[72]

Strengths and Limitations of Molecular Diagnostic Tests

Molecular diagnostic tests can be designed to be more specific to a single virus and, as a result, have fewer issues with identifying the specific virus compared to serological testing. These tests detect specific virus sequences of genetic material. According to a manufacturer we interviewed, some Zika virus diagnostic molecular tests detect multiple targets, meaning a test detects multiple segments of genetic material from the Zika virus, rendering the test more accurate since it can still detect the virus even if there is an alteration in one of the segments that the test is detecting. Molecular tests can also be used to simultaneously detect other viruses such as dengue, chikungunya, and Zika (see Table 3 for strengths and limitations for both types of tests).

---

[71] According to FDA's guidance document, positive percent agreement is the proportion of non-reference standard positive subjects in whom the new test is positive and negative percent agreement is the proportion of non-reference standard negative subjects in whom the new test is negative.

[72] According to its website, the Centers for Medicare & Medicaid Services regulates all laboratory testing (except for research) performed on humans in the United States through the Clinical Laboratory Improvement Amendments (CLIA) and covers approximately 254,000 laboratory entities. The Division of Laboratory Services within the Survey and Certification Group, under the Center for Clinical Standards and Quality, is responsible for implementing the CLIA program. See https://www.cms.gov/Regulations-and-Guidance/Legislation/CLIA/index.html?redirect=/clia/, accessed April 3, 2017. Laboratories obtain a CLIA certificate that corresponds to the complexity of the testing they conduct. For tests developed by a laboratory or that have been modified from the approved manufacturer's instructions, the complexity category defaults to high complexity per the CLIA regulations.

Molecular diagnostic tests give a definitive diagnosis independent of other tests when the result is positive. To reliably detect the Zika virus, molecular diagnostic tests should be performed within two weeks after symptom onset (see Figure 6).

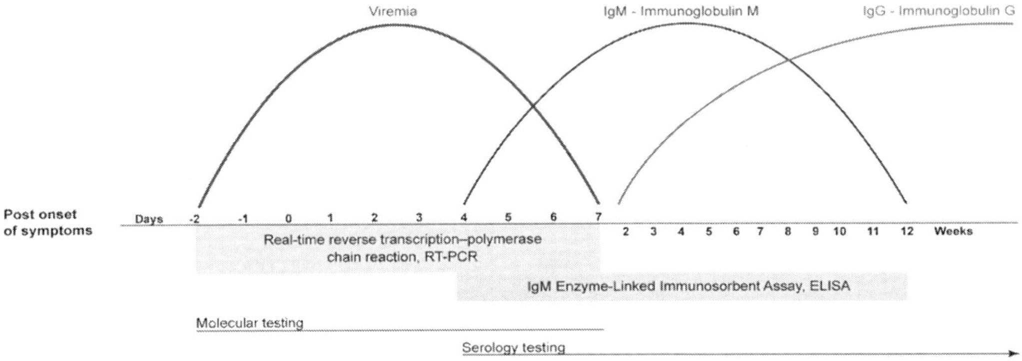

Source: GAO analysis of Centers for Disease Control and Prevention (CDC) and World Health Organization (WHO) data. | GAO-17-445.

Note: This figure is not to scale and for illustrative purposes only. According to a CDC report, viremia (presence of virus in the blood) is expected to occur from several days before onset until a week after illness onset (for the purposes of this figure, we assume that several days is at least two days and a week as seven days).

Figure 6. Zika Virus and Antibodies after Infection.

Table 3. Strengths and limitations of molecular and serologic diagnostic tests for Zika virus infection identified by Food and Drug Administration

Type of test	Strength	Limitation
Molecular	• For some devices, extraction and detection are automated, increasing the throughput • High sensitivity • High specificity: no cross-reactivity with dengue, West Nile, and yellow fever viruses • Robust and well-understood tests and formats • Range of specimen types: serum, plasma, urine, cerebral spinal fluid, amniotic fluid, whole blood	• Window of time for detection is limited • Asymptomatic pregnant women in area with active Zika transmission: not possible to determine window of time for molecular testing • Due to manufacturers design, currently authorized for Clinical Laboratory Improvement Amendments high complexity laboratories
Serologic (Immunoglobulin M)	• Covers a wider window of time (up to 12 weeks) • Can be used to detect recent exposure to the Zika virus in asymptomatic patients • High Sensitivity for primary infection but reports on the sensitivity for secondary infections are mixed	• Potential cross-reactivity with other antibodies against other flaviviruses (dengue, West Nile, yellow fever), especially in South America and Puerto Rico • Confirmatory testing required by following the CDC-issued algorithm which can include the plaque reduction neutralization test

Source: GAO analysis based on Food and Drug Administration Information I GAO-17-445.

A negative molecular test does not rule out Zika virus infection because the amount of virus in the sample could be too low to be detected at the time of molecular testing. Some scientists have expressed concern over the limit of detection of some authorized molecular diagnostic tests, which could have resulted in missed Zika virus infections by molecular testing and increase the need for serological follow-up testing; however, additional testing according to CDC guidance is intended to correct these false negative findings. An expert from our meeting stated that the sensitivity limitation of molecular testing cannot be overcome by additional testing if the molecular test is negative based on low levels of virus but before the body has developed an antibody response.

Specifically, CDC guidance specifies that negative samples from molecular tests should be sent for serology testing.

Serological Tests Varied in Their Ability to Detect Zika Virus Antibodies

Serology tests can be used to detect the Zika virus-specific IgM antibodies that typically develop during the first week of illness and persist for about 12 weeks.[73] As previously mentioned, three serological tests were authorized for the Zika virus, of which CDC manufactured one (the MAC-ELISA) and the two others were commercially manufactured. Officials at a public health laboratory we interviewed said that one of the commercially authorized tests had better specificity than the CDC MAC-ELISA when compared using 30 different samples. However, the laboratory officials found that the commercially authorized test was easier to perform but more time consuming to interpret and evaluate.

Manufacturers evaluated cross-reactivity by testing specimens from patients with antibodies to other diseases that could potentially cause false positive results. Our analysis of the data provided by manufacturers in their EUA fact sheets and labeling found that one of the commercial tests did not demonstrate any cross-reactivity when compared to other flaviviruses and to nonflaviviruses during the initial qualification testing. An expert from our meeting stated that false positives based on cross- reactivity may depend on complex mixtures of antibodies at different states of infection, so it is complicated to assess this problem in a comprehensive and definitive manner. However, data provided in the EUA fact sheets and labeling for the CDC MAC-ELISA demonstrate that this assay had significant cross reactivity to dengue virus but not to other flaviviruses. CDC did not perform experimental studies for nonflaviviruses for the CDC MAC-ELISA test, stating in the label that the scientific literature indicated that only minimal cross-reactivity is expected with antibodies against other virus families.[74]

---

[73] IgM is a basic antibody produced by the immune system created in response to an initial exposure to an antigen; in this case, the antigen is part of the Zika virus. It is the first antibody that the body makes in response to a new infection and can be found in the blood.

[74] D. A. Martin and others, "Standardization of immunoglobulin M capture enzyme-linked immunosorbent assays (MAC-ELISA) for routine diagnosis of arboviral infections." *Journal of Clinical Microbiology*, vol. 38 (2000): 1823-26.

The positive percent agreement listed on the label for one of the commercial tests is 100 percent, and for the CDC MAC-ELISA is 93.98 percent.[75] The negative percent agreement is 92.5 percent for one of the commercial tests, but the CDC MAC-ELISA does not list a negative percent agreement in the product label. One of the commercial tests also showed that there is no interference with substances normally found in serum, while the CDC MAC-ELISA test did not include this information in the product label. According to HHS officials, the three diagnostic tests use different antigens for detection of Zika virus antibodies, which may be cross-reactive with antibodies from related flaviviruses. According to HHS officials, a side-by-side comparison of the performance of these diagnostic tests has demonstrated some cross-reactivity to other flaviviruses by each assay.

Serological Tests Varied in Their Timeliness and Throughput

Of the serologic tests authorized for Zika virus diagnosis, one takes three hours and the CDC MAC-ELISA takes three days to administer. Some diagnostic users we interviewed stated that one of the commercially authorized tests was easier to use and a more efficient assay than the CDC MAC-ELISA because it is automated. According to FDA, automation decreases the time and staff required to run the samples. The CDC MAC- ELISA test takes approximately 2 to 3 days because laboratories are required to perform two overnight incubations in the laboratory to complete the test; in contrast one of the commercial tests only takes about 3 hours, in part because the plates are pre-coated. Similarly, one of the commercially authorized tests can run 28 samples per plate, while the CDC MAC-ELISA test can run 8 samples per plate.

Diagnostic users we spoke with stated that running the CDC MAC-ELISA in this format created issues with test throughput and capacity. One reason for different number of samples per plate between the tests is that the outer wells of the plates are used in one of the commercial tests and not in the CDC MAC-ELISA test. In addition, each CDC test sample was run in triplicate at the same time, decreasing the number of samples that can be run at one time.

Strengths and Limitations of Serological Diagnostic Tests

Serologic tests for IgM can diagnose a recent infection for a wider range of time (from about 7 days to up to 12 weeks after infection) compared to molecular tests, which generally detect current infections. Another strength of serologic tests is that they can be used to detect recent exposure to the Zika virus in asymptomatic patients.

---

[75] The performance of the tests was determined with 55 clinical specimens, and compared to the CDC MAC-ELISA and plaque reduction neutralization test (PRNT) or the CDC Trioplex test. For the CDC MAC-ELISA, the 93.98 positive percent agreement was determined by comparing results with the PRNT using serum submitted to CDC Fort Collins for testing from 2015 to the present with 166 samples.

One limitation of these tests is that antibodies produced against one flavivirus may be cross-reactive to other flaviviruses, so a positive Zika virus IgM result does not necessarily indicate a Zika virus infection. The reason is that related flaviviruses such as dengue, yellow fever, West Nile, and Japanese encephalitis, which can be caused by a previous natural infection or vaccination, can give a positive Zika virus IgM result by a serology test. This has proven to be an issue in South America, Central America, Mexico, and Puerto Rico, where multiple flaviviruses are circulating, according to FDA officials.

Another limitation is that positive results need to be confirmed by using the CDC algorithm, which can include the plaque reduction neutralizing testing (PRNT) that is performed only at CDC or one of CDC's designated confirmatory testing laboratories (currently there are five designated state public health laboratories, according to HHS officials).[76] The PRNT requires about six days to complete, and the logistics of specimen shipment can further extend the time, according to HHS officials. According to CDC officials, CDC typically takes three weeks to send PRNT results but reporting time may be longer during the summer. Based on our analysis of a recent FDA document, this prolonged period between getting the IgM results and the PRNT confirmatory results may have led some clinicians and patients to make family planning decisions without confirmation of Zika virus infection.

Because the PRNT measures virus-specific neutralizing antibodies to confirm infection, not only does it take more time, but it is also difficult to perform. The test requires mixing patient serum with live Zika virus to determine how effective the serum is at neutralizing the virus in cell culture.[77] However, neutralizing antibodies may still react to related viruses. According to FDA officials, the PRNT is a well-recognized, established standard laboratory technique and therefore did not have to go through FDA approval or authorization. However, as mentioned above, only a few laboratories are able to perform the PRNT for the Zika virus. According to a CDC document, PRNT is considered the "gold-standard" for confirmatory testing for Zika virus infection. An expert from our meeting stated that there can still be cross-reactivity with PRNT that confounds interpretation of the results. The five state public health laboratories that perform Zika virus PRNT have demonstrated capacity and proficiency to perform PRNT testing on their own, according to HHS officials.

Finally, according to CDC officials, neutralizing antibodies to the Zika virus develop shortly after IgM antibodies and consist primarily of IgG antibodies.[78] Serology testing could be used to detect IgG antibodies; however, the United States has no EUA test for detecting Zika virus specific IgG at this time. The associations between the Zika virus

---

[76] The plaque reduction neutralization test (PRNT) measures virus-specific neutralizing antibody titers and, according to CDC report, should be performed against various related flaviviruses to rule out false-positive ELISA results.

[77] Cell culture is the growth of microorganisms such as bacteria and yeast, or human, plant, or animal cells in the laboratory. Cell cultures may be used to diagnose infections, to test new drugs, and in research.

[78] Neutralizing antibodies reduce or destroy infectivity of an infectious agent by partial or complete destruction of the agent. Neutralizing antibodies are expected to persist for many years after flavivirus infections.

and adverse health outcomes in newborns and the ability to detect infections older than 12 weeks could be relevant to family planning and clinical care of patients, if such tests were available. However, IgG is typically highly cross-reactive to other flaviviruses and can remain elevated for years following an infection or vaccination, so it is difficult to determine when a patient has an elevated IgG if it is elevated for a recent infection, a prior flavivirus infection (possibly years earlier) or both.

Overall Limitations of Diagnostic Testing Can be Addressed Through the Use of Algorithms

As discussed above, different types of diagnostic tests for the Zika virus have different strengths and limitations. As a result, rather than a single diagnostic test being considered in isolation, multiple tests and sample types are often needed to establish a definitive laboratory diagnosis.

Table 4. Overview of diagnostic testing algorithms

Samples collected from all individuals with symptoms less than 14 days after the onset:
Serum or paired urine and serum samples with a Zika virus molecular diagnostic test, a positive result in any specimen is sufficient to diagnose Zika virus infection If Zika virus molecular results are negative, serum should be tested for the presence of Immunoglobulin M (IgM) antibodies (serology testing). Testing for dengue IgM antibodies should also be performed if the patient is pregnant or potentially exposed to dengue virus. Currently, one Emergency Use Authorization (EUA) serology test recommends that samples with a result of presumptive positive for other flavivirus have follow-up testing with a Food and Drug Administration (FDA) cleared dengue serology test.
Serum collected from individuals presenting with symptoms 14 days or more after onset:
Initial testing should be done with IgM serology test for Zika virus. For non-pregnant symptomatic patients, a reactive IgM serology test result is followed by plaque reduction neutralization test to confirm the diagnosis.
Additional criteria and testing strategies apply for pregnant women:
If a positive IgM serology test is obtained in specimens collected more than 14 days or more after onset of symptoms or potential exposure, testing with a molecular test should be performed. If the Zika molecular test results are negative, testing should proceed to plaque reduction neutralization test to test for the presence of neutralizing antibodies to Zika virus. IgM serology testing for dengue virus is recommended for symptomatic pregnant women.
Asymptomatic pregnant women meeting epidemiological criteria for testing:
Specimens collected from a pregnant woman presenting less than 14 days from exposure should be tested with molecular testing. If negative, a second serum specimen should be collected 2-12 weeks following exposure and tested by Zika virus IgM serology testing. Serum specimens collected from asymptomatic pregnant women 2-12 weeks following a potential exposure or from pregnant women without symptoms living in an area of ongoing transmission should be tested by serology testing. If reactive, molecular testing should be performed on all appropriate specimen types available. If the molecular test is negative, plaque reduction neutralization testing* should be performed for confirmation of the IgM result.

Source: Centers for Disease Control and Prevention (CDC). | GAO-17-445.

Note: For detailed information and the algorithms, information on testing infants, and links to additional guidance on testing pregnant women, see https://www.cdc.gov/zika/laboratories/lab-guidance.html.

*Plaque Reduction Neutralization Test (PRNT) is not currently routinely recommended for testing of any specimens in Puerto Rico.

The window of acute Zika virus infection is small. Viral RNA is the first thing that can be detected in an infected person in multiple specimen types. In blood, as the immune response develops and antibodies rise, levels of viral RNA decline. Zika virus diagnostic tests that have been authorized since the public health emergency declaration varied in their ability to detect the Zika virus or antibodies to Zika virus. Consequently, a test that is less sensitive may produce a false negative result, while a more sensitive test may detect the virus.

CDC provides guidance for determining the order of testing (known as testing algorithms) with different types of tests based on the strengths and limitations of the different test types, presence of symptoms, pregnancy status, and time between symptom onset or exposure and sample collection. For individuals with symptoms, the time between symptom onset and sample collection dictates test order. For pregnant women who have no symptoms but meet certain epidemiological criteria for testing, time between exposure or return from travel dictates test order. The testing order algorithms are shown in Table 4.

Manufacturers and Users Faced Several Challenges in Developing and Using Zika Diagnostic Tests

We identified five challenges that manufacturers of diagnostic tests faced related to Zika virus diagnostic testing, research, and development, and regulatory approval: (1) biological aspects of the virus and the immune response, including low levels of virus in the bodily fluids of infected patients for short periods of time and the cross-reactivity of antibodies to other flaviviruses, (2) difficulty in accessing well-characterized clinical samples, (3) getting access to EUA tests for use as a comparator assay, (4) gaining cooperation with international entities, and (5) challenges interacting with FDA during review. Challenges users of the diagnostic tests faced included: (1) requirements to purchase new specific equipment to be compliant with the EUA label on a test they wanted to use; and (2) determining the most accurate test because information in the EUA labels for some of the performance characteristics were not easily comparable. Consequently, users could not easily compare diagnostic test performance measures from product labels.

Manufacturers Faced Several Challenges Developing Diagnostic Tests

The first challenge to manufacturers developing diagnostic tests was the lack of knowledge of Zika virus biology and infections, especially at the beginning of the U.S. outbreak. The best sample type to use for molecular testing was uncertain at the beginning of the outbreak. For instance, the Zika virus had been found to be present longer in urine than in serum or plasma, but information on just how long the virus could persist in different bodily fluids was still evolving. Compared to related viruses, the Zika virus is present at low levels in bodily fluids of patients during an active infection. Manufacturers also faced challenges in identifying ways to test for antibodies, as well as unique Zika virus antigens to target due to issues with extensive cross-reactivity with other flaviviruses.[79] Information is still evolving about antigens that are unique to the Zika virus and how long the virus persists in various bodily fluids, making it difficult to develop diagnostic tests for the virus.

Second, the lack of well characterized clinical samples for diagnostic test development was identified as a major challenge for developing Zika virus diagnostic tests, according to the federal agency officials and manufacturers we interviewed, and all the experts who participated in our meeting. However, several manufacturers told us that obtaining samples for testing was difficult because of high costs, potential cross-reactivity with other flaviviruses, and an insufficient number of samples. For example, one manufacturer had to pay more than $200,000 to acquire samples from commercial vendors. According to another manufacturer we interviewed, a single clinical sample for the Zika virus can cost around $450. Manufacturers told us they requested, but were not able to obtain, samples from CDC in the early stages of the outbreak and one manufacturer stated this was because not enough samples were available. One manufacturer stated that this delayed the development of its test. According to HHS officials, to help address the lack of samples for test development, BARDA, a component of ASPR, provided characterized samples to test manufacturers, once the samples became available in midsummer 2016. However, HHS officials stated that no test manufacturer received enough samples from BARDA for the EUA testing requirements and had to acquire samples from other sources to support the EUA application.

BARDA officials told us they have worked closely with CDC and manufacturers to collect and characterize clinical samples that can be used to develop and validate diagnostic tests to detect Zika virus infection.[80] Manufacturers also had issues with clinical samples, since samples sourced from Central and South America were not well characterized, because other circulating flaviviruses could cause cross- reactivity, creating uncertainty in the outcome of a given test.

Third, FDA recommends that manufacturers perform clinical evaluation studies that compare their tests to another "comparator" assay that is laboratory developed, an in-house assay, or an EUA test. The selection and quality of the comparator assay directly affects the measurements of the test performance. A CDC document states that CDC

---

[79] Antigens are epitopes of the virus that are important to the immune response. An epitope is the part of an antigen molecule an antibody attaches itself to.

[80] BARDA provides an integrated, systematic approach to the development and purchase of the necessary vaccines, drugs, therapies, and diagnostic tools for public health medical emergencies. BARDA distributes some clinical samples to manufacturers that meet minimal criteria, including manufacturers that have contacted FDA to obtain the EUA template, which indicates interest in developing a test toward FDA clearance that might be considered for use on an EUA. It distributes to manufacturers that either have had a Zika test in development or have the ability to do so (for example, have FDA authorized serologic tests for other viruses). See table 1.

rarely has the resources needed to fully respond to public health emergencies but should provide a consistent, fair, and transparent review process for all public-private initiatives. However, according to CDC officials, they did not make their EUA test available to some commercial manufacturers for use as a comparator assay. One manufacturer we interviewed said its request to CDC for reagents to perform the Trioplex test was denied since it was a commercial manufacturer. Another manufacturer told us it attempted to purchase an EUA test from another manufacturer but was unable to because the other manufacturer refused to sell the EUA diagnostic test.

According to HHS officials, in order to obviate this challenge, FDA allows manufacturers to use laboratory developed tests as comparator tests. An expert at our meeting, stated a manufacturer had to establish their own assay because commercial manufacturers cannot purchase the Trioplex test or create it since it is unpublished.

Two of the 12 authorized molecular diagnostic test labels have CDC's Trioplex listed as their comparator assay. CDC was the first manufacturer to receive an EUA and therefore the Trioplex test was the first authorized molecular test that other tests attempting to get EUA could be compared to. According to CDC officials, diagnostic tests CDC created are distributed only to public health laboratories performing Zika virus clinical diagnoses because in the early stage of the response, CDC did not have the capacity to adequately support public health laboratories and also supply commercial manufacturers with CDC tests for performance testing. CDC officials also stated that issues with intellectual property rights, such as patents, or material transfer agreements, may prevent sharing reagents, individual components and technology. An expert from our meeting stated that this could have been overcome by publishing the test protocol with specific details about the test. However, CDC distributed its tests to four manufacturers through technology transfers, when no shortage of reagents was experienced by September 2016. CDC officials we spoke with were unclear of how the process to transfer authorized CDC tests to manufacturers originally started. *Standards for Internal Control in the Federal Government* state that agencies should document their operational processes to ensure that the organization meets its objectives. Without a clear and transparent process for distributing CDC diagnostic tests, the agency may not be able to develop the capacity of the commercial sector during an outbreak.

Fourth, interacting with international entities to obtain samples and perform testing presented some challenges. Some foreign countries have laws that must be followed when collecting samples. A manufacturer we interviewed faced import challenges trying to perform a diagnostic test in another country. One manufacturer told us it took 6 weeks for diagnostic manufacturers to ship materials to another country for testing, and the import tax was $30,000. An expert from our meeting also stated that obtaining CDC import permits was challenging.

Fifth, manufacturers had mixed opinions on the effectiveness of communication from FDA. Specifically, representatives of some manufacturers said that FDA did a good job communicating with them throughout the EUA process during the recent outbreaks while some said that communication with FDA could be improved. FDA interacts with manufacturers about potential EUA products to help ensure that manufacturers submit complete EUA applications and thereby enhances FDA's ability to review and ultimately authorize the EUA.[81] FDA stated that its review expertise is scarce, making it imperative to prioritize efforts to move the best diagnostic tests forward first (that is, the test that is most effective in addressing an unmet public health need). However, one manufacturer we interviewed stated that the longer time for communication and time to receive authorization from FDA were challenging in developing diagnostic test for Zika virus. According to FDA, the average time between pre-EUA, a time when FDA begins review of fact sheets and other documentation before the submission and EUA submission is 87.6 days, with a range of 14 to 178 days for Zika diagnostic tests. The average time once an application was submitted to the authorization date was 7.4 days, with a range of 1 to 26 days. A manufacturer suggested an improvement would be to shorten the time to respond to inquiries.

FDA developed templates for molecular and serology diagnostic tests and sent them to manufacturers in order to support obtaining an EUA. According to FDA officials, templates provided transparency in terms of the studies required for a successful EUA submission and streamlined submission for the manufacturers. FDA officials stated that updates to studies were communicated to manufacturers as new information became available during the Zika outbreak, including by direct communication with manufacturers and through FDA's webpages. As new information on Zika virus became available, FDA instituted changes to the EUA to ensure that manufacturers were demonstrating adequate performance for their diagnostic tests. However, some manufacturers requested greater clarity. Some manufacturers we interviewed stated that FDA changed its requirements for authorization throughout the process. HHS officials stated that they had to incorporate new information about the Zika virus into their review process as it became available throughout the outbreak, consequently changing the required amount of analytical and clinical data requested from manufacturers before they could make EUA authorizations.

Diagnostic Test Users Faced Challenges Acquiring Equipment and Determining the Most Accurate Test

Zika virus diagnostic test users we interviewed faced challenges because they had to purchase new equipment to be compliant with the EUA label on a test they wanted to use. It was difficult to determine the most accurate test because information on the EUA

---

[81] As of March 2017, FDA had 133 inquiries to request the EUA templates or information on where to source clinical samples. According to FDA officials, 71 of the 133 queries required extensive feedback and interactive communications and resulted in 45 pre-EUA submissions and 16 complete EUA submissions.

labels of the performance characteristics of tests were not comparable or not available on the CDC website.

First, although CDC officials stated that all states had at least one public health laboratory that had the equipment to run the CDC MAC-ELISA test, representatives from several laboratories we interviewed stated that they had to acquire new equipment to be able to perform a certain EUA diagnostic test. For instance, implementation of serological testing within another federal laboratory was delayed because additional equipment was needed to perform the authorized test. CDC officials stated that the agency is working to expand diagnostic testing capacity within both public health and commercial laboratories in the United States.

Second, diagnostic test users also faced challenges in determining the most accurate test because information on the labels was not easily comparable. An FDA document states that the agency should share information that is up-to-date, understandable, and easily accessible so diagnostic test users has some basis for choosing medical products to purchase and use.[82] Moreover, according to this document, posting compilation or analysis of data can benefit users since all users may not have the ability or resources to independently analyze raw data.[83] By comparing the diagnostic test labels, we found that the labels had units listed differently for key performance characteristics, data had to be extracted from each product insert, and some of the information could not be readily compared with other data. We also found that performance characteristics are listed on the diagnostic test labels, but it is not available in a consolidated format.

According to FDA officials, the agency began collecting information using FDA Reference Materials because different manufacturers were using different samples and potentially different methods to determine the limit of detection of their tests.[84] Using common samples across manufacturers allowed FDA to directly compare the limits of detection across different molecular diagnostic tests. However, the FDA Reference Materials were available only after certain diagnostic tests were already authorized under EUA. Therefore, those diagnostic test labels did not initially list the limit of detection using the FDA Reference Materials until their labels were updated.

FDA officials stated that if manufacturers had not previously performed the limit of detection using the FDA Reference Materials, they would need to perform those tests and provide results to FDA. This would allow users to compare limits of detection for tests that were performed using the same samples and procedures. FDA officials stated that they were waiting to receive all the results from all the manufacturers with an authorized diagnostic test before considering consolidating information about performance characteristics, since this information was already publically available in the updated product labels of the individual tests. All authorized molecular test manufacturers had

[82] Food and Drug Administration, Transparency Initiative.
[83] Food and Drug Administration, Transparency Initiative.
[84] FDA Reference Materials were made available to all test manufacturers, free of charge, provided that they demonstrated the feasibility of their assay, according to FDA officials.

submitted limit of detection data using the FDA Reference Materials to FDA by March 6, 2017.

Until limit of detection data have been extracted and summarized from all the diagnostic test labels, it may be difficult and time-consuming for users to compare the performance characteristics and results of diagnostic tests. By waiting until FDA has all the information before compiling information about performance characteristics, it will be time-consuming for users to compare the limit of detection across the authorized molecular diagnostic tests.[85] This will become especially important with the mosquito season approaching and public health laboratories making decisions about which tests to use.

Another challenge users faced was related to the lack of information on comparator assays. An FDA document recommends that there should be a clear description of all methods used and how and what data were collected when performing comparison testing, including a description of the comparator assay "nonreference standard."[86] Experts at our meeting agreed that identifying the comparator assay would make it easier to compare the risks and benefits of different Zika virus diagnostic tests.[87] The selection and quality of the comparator assay directly affects the legitimacy of the comparison of the test performance.[88] When we compared product labels for different molecular tests, we found that 6 of 12 product labels did not identify the comparator assay and that the comparator assay could fall into one of three types: (1) another EUA test, (2) a laboratory developed test, or (3) an in-house assay (see appendix V).

FDA officials stated that the comparator assay for authorized diagnostic tests can be either another authorized test or a validated reference method and manufacturers are allowed to decide if they will identify the comparator assay. However, the manufacturers are not required to do so. According to FDA officials, comparison studies for EUA diagnostic tests are based on a relatively low number of clinical specimens, and the levels of viral RNA in a number of specimens can be low. In addition, FDA officials stated that these two factors preclude definitive conclusions regarding the comparative performance of devices, and FDA staff are concerned that studies using comparator assays in labeling may be used to make inappropriate claims and could be misinterpreted by end users. The use of FDA Reference Material allows for a more rigorous analysis of the comparative sensitivities of the assays from the various manufacturers, according to FDA officials.

---

[85] For example, three diagnostic tests have the same limit of detection listed for serum (1000 detectable units/mL) using the FDA Reference Materials and have three different limit of detections listed on their product labels when manufacturers use their own samples and protocols (721 copies/mL or 0.05 tissue culture infectious dose /mL, 30 copies/mL and 250 RNA copies/mL).

[86] Food and Drug Administration, *Guidance for Industry and FDA Staff: Statistical Guidance on Reporting Results from Studies Evaluating Diagnostic Tests* (Washington, D.C.: March 13, 2007).

[87] A comparator assay is used as the reference method for assessing the performance characteristics of another test method.

[88] Shabir Banoo and others, "Evaluation of Diagnostic Tests for Infectious Diseases: General Principles", *Nature Reviews: Microbiology* (2010): S17-S29.

However, without knowing the identity of the comparator assay, it is more difficult for users to compare performance characteristics across different diagnostic tests and determine the most appropriate test to use. According to an expert at our meeting, this information would be helpful for laboratories in determining what test to use in the face of multiple approved tests. Although the criteria for procuring diagnostic tests can vary, for most laboratories the paramount focus is on test performance.

Standards for Internal Control in the Federal Government state that agencies are to communicate quality information externally through reporting lines so that external parties can help an entity achieve its objectives and address related risks.[89]

Issues with Centers for Disease Control and Prevention (CDC) molecular diagnostic test sensitivity	
A CDC scientist (who later became a whistleblower) alleged that the Emergency Operation Center at CDC endangered public health when it failed to disclose that an emergency use authorized CDC test used to detect Zika virus—called the Trioplex Real-time RT-PCR assay (Trioplex)—was substantially less sensitive than another CDC laboratory developed test (Singleplex). After raising concern about the test's sensitivity, an Office of Special Counsel (OSC) investigation was conducted. OSC encouraged CDC to promote scientific debate on this issue and said that whistleblowers should be encouraged to speak out on matters of public concern. OSC also requested the Department of Health and Human Services (HHS) to conduct an independent investigation about the allegations made and CDC's Associate Director of Laboratory Science and Safety, who conducted the investigation, found that the evidence did not support the allegations. OSC found the CDC investigation reasonable. CDC had three sources of data to compare the different tests' sensitivities. One was from the whistleblowers' laboratory, another from the creator of the Trioplex test that was alleged to be less sensitive, and the third was an independent laboratory that compared the Singleplex and Trioplex tests.	The CDC investigation into the whistleblower's claims did not attempt to gather additional information on comparing the tests from public health laboratories using the Singleplex test. According to CDC officials, they could not do a direct comparison of the two tests because the equipment required for both tests did not exist at either location. The agency acknowledged that the original Trioplex test was authorized only a smaller input volume while the Singleplex is not subject to such limitation because it had never been submitted to the Food and Drug Administration (FDA) for review and was used only as a laboratory-developed test. CDC submitted a substantial amendment to the Trioplex test for FDA's authorization to increase the input volume of the test in August 2016, and in January 2017 the authorization was amended again to allow laboratories to use a singleplex reaction on the Trioplex assay. According to CDC, the larger input volume has been demonstrated to increase the sensitivity of the Trioplex assay. According to a CDC website, a "head-to-head comparison of the Trioplex test and the Zika-only assay" has not been conducted. In HHS' technical comments they stated that a "head- to-head comparison of the Trioplex and the Singleplex laboratory developed test" has been performed and showed equivalent performance. A journal article later showed that the original Trioplex test was less sensitive than the Singleplex test. Increasing the input volume of the test increased the limit of detection of the Trioplex test approximately 20 to 50 times.

Source: GAO analysis of HHS and Office of Special Counsel documents; CDC "Updated Laboratory Guidance: Frequently Asked Questions" https://www.cdc.gov/zika/laboratories/lab-guidance-faq.html (assessed May 18, 2017); M. Stone and others, "Relative Analytical Sensitivity of Donor Nucleic Acid Amplification Technology Screening and Diagnostic Real-Time Polymerase Chain Reaction Assays for Detection of Zika Virus RNA," Transfusion, (2017) | GAO-17-445.

CDC did not make publically available data comparing the performance characteristics of different CDC diagnostic tests that it distributed during the outbreak. CDC's website has information about the performance of its two authorized diagnostic

[89] GAO, *Standards for Internal Control in the Federal Government,* GAO-14-704G (Washington, D.C.: September 2014).

tests and the PRNT technique, but not the laboratory- developed test it distributed, called the Singleplex laboratory developed test (Singleplex). According to a HHS report, CDC did not provide information about one of its diagnostic tests because it could potentially create confusion and could have caused public health laboratories to discontinue use of the Trioplex test, and it had not done a comprehensive comparison of the Trioplex and Singleplex assay. Because CDC did not publically provide performance information about its laboratory developed test—which was distributed to some public health laboratories—questions arose regarding the sensitivity of the two CDC tests (Singleplex and Trioplex, see text box).

Representatives of three scientific professional societies told us that information about the development and verification of CDC's diagnostic test should be made available to the scientific and medical communities. Access to such data would provide transparency and allow for optimal patient care, according to these representatives. According to these societies' representatives, the lack of access to data on test performance prevented users from making informed decisions about which test to adopt or recommend during the outbreak. Without including information on the performance characteristics of tests it is distributing, CDC cannot ensure that healthcare providers and the public have the information they need to make informed decisions about which test is best for their use.

MOSQUITO CONTROL METHODS HAVE STRENGTHS AND LIMITATIONS, AND FEDERAL AGENCIES FACE SEVERAL CHALLENGES ASSISTING THESE EFFORTS

Mosquito Control Methods in the United States Are Often Combined under Integrated Vector Management

Types of mosquito control methods available in the United States include: (1) physical control, or nonchemical mosquito control, (2) larval mosquito control, (3) adult mosquito control, and (4) personal protection. Mosquito control entities and literature identified available methods that may control mosquitoes in general. However, not all methods presented in this chapter specifically apply to *Aedes aegypti* mosquitoes, in part because not all such entities we spoke with had *Aedes aegypti* in their area. For example, HHS identified ditching as irrelevant for *Aedes aegypti* mosquitoes.[90] These methods can

[90] Discussion targeted more to *Aedes aegypti* mosquitoes is in (1) National Science and Technology Council, *A Strategy for Integrating Best Practices with New Science to Prevent Disease Transmission by* Aedes *Mosquito Vectors*, (Washington, D.C.: December, 2016); (2) Centers for Disease Control and Prevention, *Surveillance and Control of* Aedes aegypti *and* Aedes albopictus *in the United States*, accessed October, 17, 2016, https://www.cdc.gov/chikungunya/pdfs/surveillance-and-control-of-aedes-aegypti-and-aed es-albopictus-

be combined with surveillance of the mosquito population, using integrated vector management (IVM) to optimize the application of multiple methods, depending on knowledge of mosquito biology and distribution.[91]

Different mosquito control methods target different stages of the mosquito lifecycle. The mosquito's lifecycle has two stages—an aquatic stage in which eggs develop into larvae and pupae and a terrestrial stage in which the mosquito leaves the water, can fly, and can transmit pathogens and lay eggs. Figure 7 depicts major lifecycle steps encompassing these stages.

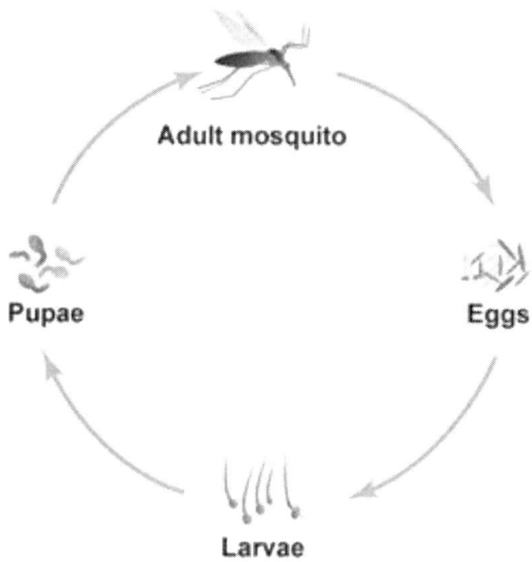

Source: GAO, adapted from CDC. | GAO-17-445.

Figure 7. The Lifecycle of a Mosquito.

Available Methods for Physical Control of Mosquitoes and Their Strengths and Limitations

Physical control, or the use of physical or mechanical means to remove water sources serving as larval development sites or prevent mosquito entry into buildings, includes (1) controlling water sources needed for mosquito breeding and (2) using barriers, such as window screens, to keep mosquitoes away from people.[92] A National Science and Technology Council (NSTC) report stated that physical control includes removing

---

us.pdf; or (3) Department of Defense, Armed Forces Pest Management Board, *Technical Guide No. 47:* Aedes *Mosquito Vector Control*. (Silver Spring, MD: March 2, 2016).

[91] IVM is sometimes referred to as integrated pest management or integrated mosquito management (IMM). According to CDC, IMM combines methods to prevent and control mosquitoes that spread viruses, like Zika, dengue, and chikungunya. IMM is based on an understanding of mosquito biology, the mosquito lifecycle, and the way mosquitoes spread viruses. IMM uses methods that have been scientifically proven to reduce mosquito populations and, when followed correctly, are safe.

[92] These categorizations and the methods they include can vary. For example, physical control and water source control are sometimes separated. One textbook categorizes the latter as "environmental management." See Norbert Becker and others. *Mosquitoes and Their Control,* Second Edition (Berlin: Springer, 2010). HHS officials also told us that bed nets and screening may be considered personal protection methods.

standing sources of water, such as from containers, old tires, or blocked drains, and using well-fitted and intact screens on all house doors and windows.[93]

Mosquito control entity officials we interviewed told us that they use a variety of physical control methods. For example, one told us that his mosquito control program still benefits from ditching projects completed in the 1960s and is continuing to use excavators to ditch areas to enhance water run-off.[94] Another official told us that his program includes a "drain and cover" community outreach approach, asking residents to drain standing water, use window screens, and wear long-sleeved clothing. A third official we interviewed included a program for swimming pool management by helping identify and fill in abandoned swimming pools.

Each of these physical control methods has strengths and limitations. Specifically, officials from mosquito control entities told us that water- source control such as by large-scale ditching is very effective and avoids the use of chemicals for certain types of mosquitoes. However, a mosquito control entity official also said that this method is probably challenged in the current regulatory environment. According to a NSTC report, large-scale outdoor water source control may have limited effectiveness against *Aedes aegypti* mosquitoes because breeding requires only small volumes of water (for example, one tablespoon, under certain conditions). Another mosquito control entity stated that inspections of property by mosquito control personnel may be effective but are time-consuming.[95] According to a NSTC report and mosquito control entity officials we interviewed, such property inspections can be challenged by privacy and property rights.

In addition, while physical control of larval development sites can reduce or eliminate mosquito larvae, the local environment may not be suited to such measures if extensive water bodies are present. It may be impractical or impossible to remove or move volumes of water. For example, a mosquito control entity official told us that since nearby swampland cannot be removed, physical control through water management is not an option for them.

Available Methods for Controlling Mosquito Larvae and Their Strengths and Limitations

Controlling immature mosquitoes includes using chemical or biological control methods. Chemical larvicides include methoprene and pyriproxyfen, and biologically based larvicides include *Bacillus thuringiensis israelensis* (Bti).[96] CDC guidance includes

---

[93] National Science and Technology Council. *A Strategy for Integrating Best Practices with New Science to Prevent Disease Transmission by* Aedes *Mosquito Vectors*, (Washington, D.C.: December 2016).

[94] This official said that the goal of ditching projects is to eliminate or reduce the number, size and frequency of mosquito breeding sites.

[95] These inspections are intended to identify mosquito breeding sites such as sources of water.

[96] Literature indicated limited effectiveness of some types of larval control for reducing dengue transmission or morbidity. R. Boyce and others, "Bacillus thuringiensis israelensis (Bti) for the control of dengue vectors: systematic literature review," *Tropical Medicine & International Health*, vol. 18, no. 5 (2013); and Leyanna

another method of larvae control—applying certain oils on water surfaces to suffocate mosquito larvae and pupae.[97] Mosquito control entity officials we spoke with all told us they use larviciding, such as with Bti, or with mosquito fish that eat mosquito larvae.

The "mosquito fish" eats mosquito larvae

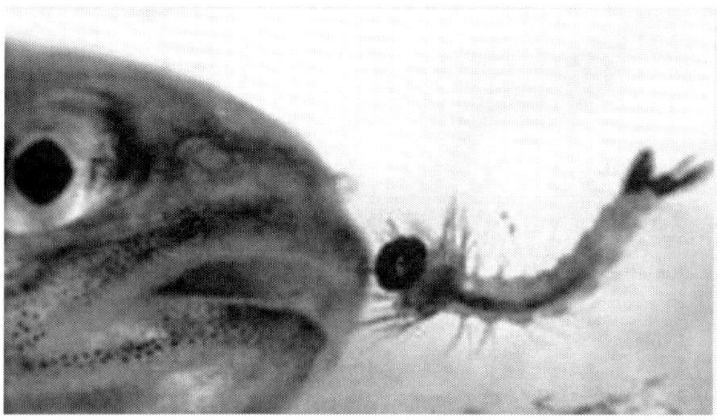

A "mosquito fish" prepares to ingest a mosquito larva. This tiny fish, which can eat its own weight in mosquito larvae each day, has been introduced into waterways throughout the world to aid in controlling mosquitoes, especially where malaria and yellow fever are a threat.

Source: CDC, Office of the Associate Director for Communications, Division of Public Affairs, Public Health Image Library, ID #4958. | GAO-17-445.

Using larvicides has strengths and limitations. Specifically, using biologically based larvicides may be more accepted by the public than adult pesticides, but is limited by cost and effectiveness. Officials from mosquito control entities we spoke with told us that residents are more accepting of biologically-based larvicides because they consider them more natural. However, a mosquito control entity official added that larviciding tends to be more expensive than other techniques. A mosquito control official told us that mosquito-borne diseases have not been successfully controlled by using larvicide alone because, while it reduces the population by 70 percent to 80 percent, controlling a disease such as the Zika virus disease requires a population reduction greater than 80 percent to 90 percent.[98] Even very few mosquitoes can lead to an outbreak or epidemic.[99]

George and other,. "Community- effectiveness of Temephos for Dengue Vector Control; A Systematic Literature Review," *PLoS Neglected Tropical Disease*, vol. 9, no. 9 (2015).

[97] Centers for Disease Control and Prevention, Surveillance and Control of *Aedes aegypti* and *Aedes albopictus* in the United States, accessed October 17, 2016, https://www.cdc.gov/chikungunya/pdfs/surveillance-and-control-of-aedes-aegypti-and-aed es-albopictus-us.pdf.

[98] EPA officials told us they have issued a joint statement with CDC on mosquito control in the United States that states that mosquito control is based on the fact that the greatest control impact on mosquito populations occurs when they are concentrated, immobile and accessible. This emphasis focuses on habitat management and controlling immature stages before mosquitoes emerge as adults. See https://www.epa.gov/mosquitocontrol/joint-statement-mosquito-control-united-states, accessed April 18, 2017. According to EPA, larviciding is an important component, along with other techniques including source reduction, IVM and adulticiding, in mosquito vector population reduction.

[99] The mosquito control official said that the characterization of mosquito threat depends on factors such as the local temperature, mosquito number, and human exposure to mosquitoes.

A mosquito control entity official told us that larvicide also needs to be applied within a limited window of opportunity and that larvicide application is delayed in its effect. Similarly, control using mosquito fish appears to be "natural" to the public, but is time consuming and has limited applicability for *Aedes* mosquitoes that carry the Zika virus, because *Aedes* mosquito eggs can survive in small containers that dry out.

Available Methods for Controlling Adult Mosquitoes and their Strengths and Limitations

Adult mosquitoes can be controlled with certain pesticides, or adulticides, applied indoors or outdoors. An EPA official told us it has registered nine active ingredients for use as adulticides, including malathion, naled, and permethrin. CDC and NSTC documents indicate that some adulticides are intended for area-wide space spraying (fogging), while others are intended for residual spraying (in and around buildings), where the pesticide remains active on surfaces that mosquitoes land on.[100] Mosquito control entity officials we spoke with said they disperse a variety of adulticides using a variety of methods, including handheld units, helicopters, fixed wing aircraft, and trucks. CDC guidance includes additional methods such as nonpesticide traps—for example, CDC's Autocidal Gravid Ovitrap, which captures egg-laying mosquitoes on a sticky glue.[101]

Using adulticides also has strengths and limitations. Specifically, officials from mosquito control entities told us that adulticide spraying can be effective in controlling mosquito populations. One mosquito control professional noted that mosquito-borne diseases such as West Nile virus disease have historically been controlled by adulticides. However, we identified several limitations with adulticide spraying. One limitation mosquito control entity officials and CDC staff identified is public resistance to pesticides.[102] Another limitation is that adulticiding effectively requires control over droplet size; mosquito control entity officials we spoke with told us they required special equipment to control the dispersal rate and properties of the adulticides. Other limitations include limited effectiveness under certain weather conditions and the potentially deleterious effect of broad-spectrum adulticides on other insects such as bees.

---

[100] According to WHO documentation, space spraying is technically a fog (sometimes referred to as an aerosol); it entails dispersing a liquid insecticide into the air in the form of hundreds of millions of tiny droplets.

[101] Centers for Disease Control and Prevention. *Surveillance and Control of* Aedes aegypti *and* Aedes albopictus *in the United States*, accessed October 17, 2016, https://www.cdc.gov/chikungunya/pdfs/surveillance-and-control-of-aedes-aegypti-and-aed es-albopictus-us.pdf. CDC guidance breaks down control methods differently and refers to these traps as physical control, but HHS officials told us that these traps should be considered adult mosquito control methods.

[102] An expert from our meeting told us that the effectiveness of aerial spraying against *Aedes aegypti* lacks robust, evidence-based support which may affect future response capabilities.

The correct application of mosquito repellant spray

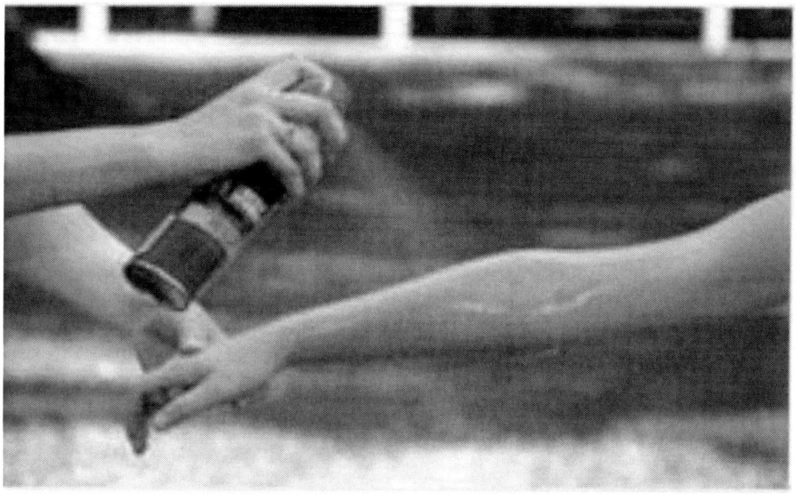

When someone spends long periods of time outdoors, insect repellent should be reapplied according to product label instructions. The best way to protect yourself and your family from chikungunya, as well as other mosquito-borne illnesses including the Zika virus, is to avoid being bitten by mosquitoes by using insect repellent, wearing long sleeves and pants, using air conditioning or window and door screens to keep mosquitoes outside, and reducing mosquito breeding grounds such as standing water.

Source: CDC, Office of the Associate Director for Communications, Division of Public Affairs, Public Health Image Library, ID #17796. | GAO-17-445.

Additionally, *Aedes aegypti* mosquitoes are primarily daytime biters, requiring spraying during certain times for optimal effectiveness.[103] However, one mosquito control entity official was reluctant to spray during commuting hours, including times when schoolchildren go to or return from schools. Further, increasing resistance of mosquitoes to existing active ingredients decreases the effectiveness of adulticiding and creates the need for new control methods. Finally, pesticide spraying over waters of the U.S. is subject to permit requirements under the Clean Water Act, which may present a challenge for mosquito control entities in applying pesticides for mosquito control (see appendix VI).

Alternative strategies may enhance the effectiveness of adulticide application. For example, one study demonstrated that data from "contact tracing"—which uses travel histories to help identify potential sites of infection—can be used to target locations for indoor spraying.[104] According to this study, this method may reduce mosquito-borne

---

[103] One expert from our meeting added that *Aedes* mosquitoes are found in and in close proximity to dwellings. Another expert from our meeting indicated that certain products, such as Duet and Suspect, may be effective against *Aedes albopictus*.

[104] Gonzalo Vazquez-Prokopec and others, "Combining Contact Tracing with Targeted Indoor Residual Spraying Significantly Reduces Dengue Transmission," *Science Advances,* vol. 3 (2017).

dengue transmission by about 90 percent. However, the method requires access to indoor environments and permission to spray inside homes.

Available Methods for Personal Protection against Mosquitoes and their Strengths and Limitations

Personal protection includes using repellents, wearing long-sleeved clothing, and using bed nets. Repellent ingredients can include dermally applied chemicals such as DEET.[105] Some repellents such as permethrin can be impregnated in clothing.

Personal protection methods also have strengths and limitations. Specifically, NSTC reports that using repellents permits individuals to remain protected as they conduct their daily routines. While personal protection methods are under the individual's control, they are effective only when properly and regularly applied. For example, one mosquito control expert at our meeting told us that despite having authority over a specific population, compliance related to the usage of bed nets or repellants is still difficult to enforce.

Other Issues Related to Available Mosquito Control Efforts

We identified three other related issues that affect available mosquito control efforts:

Community Awareness of Mosquito Control Efforts

NSTC reports that the effectiveness of public-health interventions, such as mosquito control, depends on community awareness and perception and the implementation of control practices. The risk of the Zika virus is generally under-perceived and misinformation is widespread about vector-control practices. Further, communication and outreach between the mosquito control entities and the community are necessary for effective mosquito control. Mosquito control entity officials we spoke with agreed, noting the importance of public education and outreach. For example, mosquito control entity officials sometimes use a variety of approaches for such efforts, such as going door to door, attending meetings and conferences, holding public events at schools, buying radio time, and communicating online. Mosquito control entity officials told us that two major challenges that mosquito control efforts face are educating the public and ensuring public compliance. One told us that the public generally misunderstands mosquito control methods. Additionally, while reducing sources of water can be effective and people tend to be receptive to such messages, they can forget to implement them.

---

[105] According to a CDC factsheet, DEET (or N,N-diethyl-meta-toluamide) is the active ingredient in many insect repellents. Experts from our meeting told us of additional repellent ingredients, including picaridin, IR3535 and para-methane 3-8, diol (PMD).

Example mosquito trap used to trap vectors to be tested for pathogens

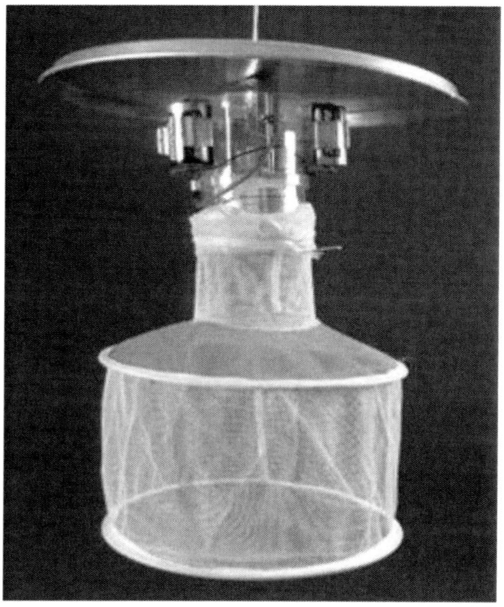

This "light trap" enabled CDC scientists to venture easily into dense, remote areas when conducting arbovirus epidemiological field work that included capturing mosquito vectors. The trap weighs only 1.75 pounds and is easily repaired. Different types of traps are used for different types of mosquitoes. For example, the "light trap" is not used for *Aedes aegypti* mosquitoes.

Source: CDC, Office of the Associate Director for Communications, Division of Public Affairs, Public Health Image Library, ID #6355. | GAO-17-445.

Mosquito Control Methods Can Be More Effective with an IVM Approach

IVM combines control methods with surveillance of the mosquito population.[106] A CDC website describes IVM as combining methods to control mosquitoes and prevent the spread of mosquito-borne viruses based on an understanding of mosquito biology, behavior, and spread of viruses.[107] IVM uses methods that are safe and scientifically proven to reduce mosquito populations when applied correctly, according to this website. An expert from our meeting included education as a critical component of IVM; an NSTC report describes education as a prerequisite for successful IVM. Officials from all the mosquito control entities we spoke with told us they use some form of IVM, and

[106] Integrated Vector Management can be defined as "the rational combination of all available control methods in the most effective, economical and safe manner to maintain mosquito vector populations at acceptable levels." Surveillance is considered a prerequisite for successful IVM programs. Norbert Becker and others. Mosquitoes and Their Control, Second edition. (Berlin: Springer, 2010).

[107] Centers for Disease Control and Prevention, "Integrated Mosquito Management," accessed January 31, 2017, https://www.cdc.gov/zika/vector/integrated_mosquito_management.html. HHS officials told us that IVM includes mosquito species surveillance as well as insecticide resistance monitoring in the surveilled species. They added that vector control methods are specific to each type of mosquito.

include surveillance of the mosquito population. One mosquito control official also noted that IVM is sometimes tailored to specific mosquito species.[108]

Additional methods being developed may eventually be incorporated into IVM strategies.

Mosquito control methods under development show promise but their effectiveness remains to be established
Mosquito control methods under development include the use of genetically-engineered mosquitoes and mosquitoes infected with the *Wolbachia* bacterium, among others. Some of these approaches can decrease the number of offspring that survive to adulthood. Other approaches under development can decrease the transmission of disease-causing virus. An NSTC report stated that some reported strengths of these approaches include potentially lower impact on other species and minimizing collateral risks to humans by more specific targeting of mosquito species. Some potential limitations include public opposition to some of the methods as well as a lack of studies demonstrating their effect on mosquito-borne disease transmission.

Source: GAO analysis of literature and agency information | GAO-17-445.

Surveillance Helps Inform Mosquito Control Efforts

All mosquito control entity officials we spoke with told us that they use surveillance of the mosquito population to assess the presence and abundance of mosquitoes and to direct the use of mosquito control methods. Traps can be used to perform surveillance. Different traps are suited to different species—for example, mosquito control entity officials told us that they use BioGents-Sentinel traps to specifically target Zika virus vectors such as *Aedes aegypti* and *Aedes albopictus*. Mosquito control entity officials also said that sentinel animals, such as regularly monitored chickens, are used for surveillance of mosquitoes that carry West Nile virus. One mosquito control entity uses landing counts, which enumerate the number of mosquitoes landing on a human volunteer over some period such as 1 minute. Finally, mosquito control entities can rely on reported mosquito complaints from the community as part of their surveillance.

The Federal Government Faced Challenges Supporting Mosquito Control Efforts

The federal government has a limited role in implementing mosquito control because mosquito control efforts are implemented at the state and local levels. However, the federal government faced a number of challenges in supporting these mosquito control efforts. According to CDC documentation, the agency developed technical guidance and provides funding and technical assistance to support state and local mosquito control activities.[109] We identified four challenges to the federal government's efforts to support mosquito control activities: (1) the timing of the availability of funds and sustaining

---

[108] According to EPA officials, different mosquito species have different behaviors (e.g., daytime feeding versus morning and evening feeding) and understanding them is key to effective control, and important to successful IVM.

[109] Centers for Disease Control and Prevention. *Draft Programmatic Environmental Assessment. Mosquito Control Activities Funded by CDC to Combat Zika Virus Transmission in the United States*, (Jan. 9, 2017).

expertise, (2) communication of data about mosquito distribution, (3) linking the effects of mosquito control to disease outcomes, and (4) limited information about mosquito control entities.

The Timing of the Availability of Funds and Sustaining Expertise

Federal agencies faced challenges related to the cyclic nature of mosquito-borne diseases, including recruiting and maintaining expertise. For example, part of IVM is matching specific methods or tools to specific situations and requires an understanding of mosquito biology.[110] However, experts at our meeting identified two issues in implementing IVM. First, one expert at our meeting said that vector biology is " kind of a dying field" in which "trained people cannot get jobs," and another expert at our meeting indicated that vector biology program support has not been sustained.[111] CDC officials agreed, stating that it is challenging to study cyclic diseases such as West Nile virus. When the disease fades, the jobs and resources also go away, so that the next time the disease appears, staff must be retrained or new staff trained.

Second, CDC officials told us that mosquito control needs vary with seasonal cycles, resulting in periods of several months that require more resources followed by some periods when little or no resources are needed. For example, CDC officials told us that even though surveillance traps are not perishable, mosquito control entities ran out of certain traps during the 2016 mosquito season and had to wait 6-months to acquire new traps.[112] According to CDC officials, funds for purchasing traps were not available until summer.

Further, grant funds awarded for mosquito control may not make it to some local mosquito control districts. CDC staff stated that CDC awarded funds to combat the Zika virus, including $56 million between August and December 2016 for mosquito control and surveillance. However, an expert at our meeting told us that CDC does not directly fund specific mosquito control entities but instead provides funds to grant recipients, typically states.[113] Since the states submit the grant applications and direct the use of certain grant funds after the award, and CDC does not directly monitor mosquito control entities, CDC may face challenges addressing entity needs.[114]

---

[110] For example, an Armed Forces Pest Management Board official told us that mosquito species number 3,000, with 300 of them transmitting disease.

[111] According to a CDC website, CDC is funding Centers for Excellence in Vector-Borne Disease. The funding period for the Centers of Excellence is 5 years. CDC told us its Strategic Plan for establishing a new "systems approach" to vector control relies on these centers, among other things. See https://www.cdc.gov/media/releases/2016/p1222-zika-funding.html, accessed April 6, 2017.

[112] CDC officials told us that mosquito traps have only one domestic manufacturer.

[113] Certain cities, such as New York City, and U.S. territories can apply for funding directly from CDC, independently of the states.

[114] For example, one entity official we interviewed told us of restrictions, including not being able to use funds for public education or having rigid deadlines for expenditures, that decreased the flexibility of their control program.

CDC Faced Challenges Communicating the Presence of Mosquitoes

CDC faced challenges in communicating the presence of mosquitoes in a manner that was clear and useful to different groups such as mosquito control entities and the general public. CDC distributed maps of the estimated potential range of the primary Zika virus vector mosquitoes on its webpage and in guidance, but imprecision in the maps can lead to confusion, according to some mosquito control officials. According to CDC officials, the maps allowed states to determine the level of effort needed for more precise mosquito surveillance as well as to show the public where they may encounter certain mosquito species.

One mosquito control official told us that confusion about CDC's maps resulted from people failing to look at the qualifications stated in the map captions and mistakenly concluding that an entire state was infested with Zika virus vector mosquitoes. This official said that CDC's maps of the range of *Aedes* mosquitoes may be unhelpful since they are intended to show the mosquitoes' potential range while some residents who saw the maps were worried that they were in an area with Zika virus.[115] This official also told us the maps created a challenge of reconciling information that their own mosquito control program staff had gathered with that presented on a highly publicized CDC map. For example, one mosquito control entity official we spoke with told us that it has not had *Aedes aegypti* in its county since 2012. However, the state where the mosquito control entity is located is entirely within the potential range identified by the CDC map. An expert from our meeting told us that the CDC map showed regions painted with a broad brush, and such information could spread fear.

To illustrate some differences between CDC's estimated potential range of *Aedes aegypti* mosquitoes and locations with reported occurrence of the mosquito, we compared the CDC map to a map of historical mosquito data compiled from multiple sources and published in a recent article written by CDC scientists. The map from the article shows a different, much sparser, pattern of recorded presence than CDC's estimated potential range (Figure 8).[116]

Experts identified limitations with both maps. For example, one expert from our meeting told us that the CDC map may extend the potential mosquito range too far north in some locations. Another expert stated that the CDC map does not account for all the factors that affect mosquito distribution. In addition, one expert told us that the data for the map on the right in Figure 8 may be incomplete, and a mosquito control official told

---

[115] One CDC map had an explanation in the footnote and caption that readers ignored, giving the mosquito control official a public relations challenge.

[116] Micah B. Hahn and others, "Reported Distribution of *Aedes* (*Stegomyia*) *aegypti* and *Aedes* (*Stegomyia*) *albopictus* in the United States, 1995-2016 (Diptera: Culicidae)," *Journal of Medical Entomology,* vol. 53, no. 5 (2016): 1169-75. The mosquito data were compiled from multiple sources, including existing collection records and a survey that the authors designed to capture additional surveillance records from vector control districts, university researchers, and local health departments.

us that the map did not convey whether an area reporting no mosquitoes had performed mosquito surveillance.[117]

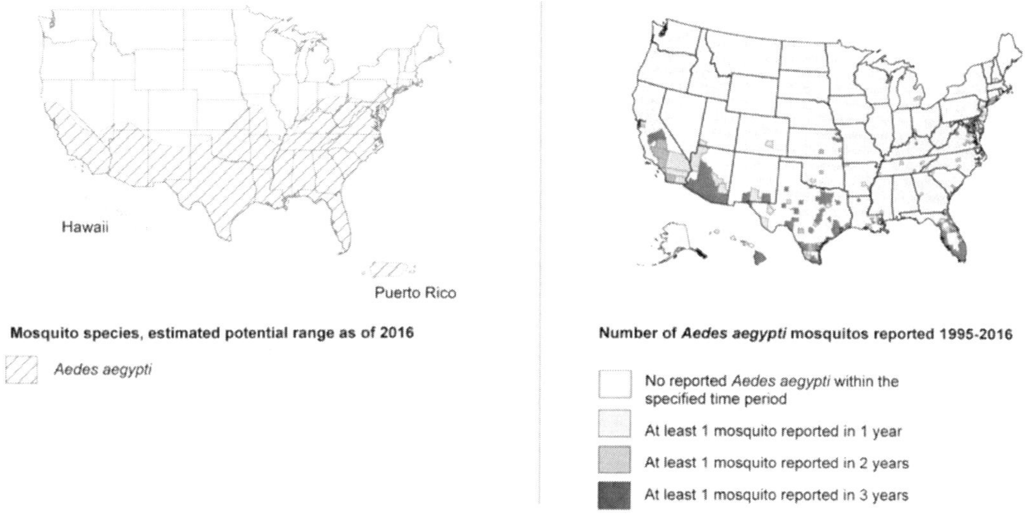

Source: GAO. Map 1 adapted from CDC, map 2 adapted from Micah B. Hahn. | GAO-17-445.

Figure 8. *Aedes aegypti* in the United States - A Comparison of Estimated Potential Range and Reported Presence.

CDC officials told us that their map was generated with data ranging as far back as 1995, and was sourced from a combination of published records and an understanding of species ecology and U.S. geography.

However, the detailed information was not posted on the CDC website or in documentation associated with the map.[118] As a result, the map may not be useful for all of its intended purposes. According to *Standards for Internal Control in the Federal Government*, management should use quality information to achieve the agency's objectives and should select appropriate methods to communicate externally.[119] Additionally, the standards state that agency management should externally communicate necessary quality information to achieve those objectives. This includes selecting appropriate methods to communicate externally, considering factors such as the intended recipients and the nature of the information being communicated. With regards to the information presented on CDC maps, experts suggested including more details, such as (1) collection records, (2) measures of the stability of the mosquito populations (showing how long populations of such mosquitoes would be expected to persist in a given

[117] According to Micah B. Hahn and others, "Reported Distribution of *Aedes (Stegomyia) aegypti* and *Aedes (Stegomyia) albopictus* in the United States, 1995-2016 (Diptera: Culicidae)," *Journal of Medical Entomology*, vol. 53, no. 5 (2016): 1169-75, incomplete information is a known limitation. They stated that "lack of collection records for *Aedes aegypti* . . . should not be interpreted as absence of that mosquito."

[118] The CDC website at https://www.cdc.gov/zika/vector/range.html, (accessed January 27, 2017), for example, states only that the maps have been updated "from a variety of published and unpublished sources."

[119] GAO, *Standards for Internal Control in the Federal Government*, GAO-14-704G (Washington, D.C.: September 2014).

location), and (3) areas of risk for transmission of mosquito-borne diseases. Additionally, understanding the date range and sources of the data can help place map information in context. Without such context, CDC's maps could generate confusion about mosquito presence, resulting in concern among residents and public relations challenges, among other things.

Challenges in Linking Mosquito Control Efforts to Disease Outcomes

CDC faced challenges in determining whether mosquito control efforts are associated with the reduction of mosquito-borne disease. For example, mosquito control entity officials told us the entity's mosquito control efforts are not directly linked to disease reduction. An official from another mosquito control entity told us that it links mosquito control only to the mosquito population. Another said that it links mosquito control to the presence of West Nile virus in sentinel chickens.[120] Additionally, West Nile virus, CDC officials told us, is a bird disease, so CDC can surveil for West Nile virus and detect this virus 2 weeks before it can affect people.[121] However, Zika virus lacks this environmental component and enters a country with human travelers. Zika virus is thus picked up by human surveillance before mosquito surveillance and lacks a similar 2- week delay.[122]

Other challenges to analyzing the relationships between mosquito control methods and disease reduction include the dependence of reported disease cases on weather, human susceptibility and immunity. According to CDC officials, data were insufficient to create an analogous link for the Zika virus, in part because the specific data needed to demonstrate the effect were not available, due to privacy considerations for individuals' health records. Therefore, it will be difficult to tease out the effect of mosquito control methods on disease reduction.

CDC Had Limited Information on Mosquito Control Entities

CDC's capacity to develop a national strategy for mosquito control is limited and depends on its knowledge of mosquito control entities and their capabilities. CDC relied on external sources such as the National Pesticide Information Center, the American Mosquito Control Association, or the National Association of County and City Health

---

[120] According to a mosquito control district webpage, sentinel chicken serology is performed by placing chickens in an area over an extended period and testing their blood for the presence of antibodies to different viruses. See http://www.wumcd.org/surveillance/chicken.html, accessed April 6, 2017.

[121] Studies have demonstrated reductions in West Nile Virus disease due to aerial pesticide spraying. Duke Ruktanonchai and others. "Effect of Aerial Insecticide Spraying on West Nile Virus Disease- North-Central Texas, 2012." *The American Journal of Tropical Medicine and Hygiene*, vol. 91, no.2 (2014); and Ryan Carney and others.
Efficacy of Aerial Spraying of Mosquito Adulticide in Reducing Incidence of West Nile Virus, California, 2005. *Emerging Infectious Diseases*, vol. 14, no. 5 (2008.).

[122] CDC officials told us they use ArboNET, an online reporting tool for mosquito-borne diseases, to track virus infection in mosquito numbers. They have now launched MosquitoNET, which will include additional information such as mosquito presence, mosquito abundance, and insecticide resistance.

Officials to compile a list of mosquito control entities. CDC staff told us that this list is likely to capture the larger, well-funded entities but may miss some smaller ones.

Further, mosquito control capabilities in the United States are variable. According to an assessment by the National Association of County and City Health Officials, 68 percent of the responding mosquito control entities in 10 priority jurisdictions were rated as "needs improvement."[123] A mosquito control official we interviewed agreed that variability in mosquito control entity capacities is significant. This means that it is challenging for CDC to determine the status of mosquito control efforts in different regions of the United States and to identify regions that may need additional technical guidance or assistance.[124]

CONCLUSION

Emerging infectious diseases such as influenza, Ebola and Zika viruses represent an ongoing threat to the health of people in the United States and worldwide. The recent Zika virus outbreak presented some challenges, some of which are unique to Zika virus disease, in relation to epidemiology, diagnostic tests, and federal agencies' role in vector control strategies.

With regard to the epidemiology of the Zika virus, CDC and its public health partners established standardized Zika case definitions. However, the estimated high rate of infected persons who had mild or no symptoms and, as a result, did not seek medical treatment made it challenging to obtain an accurate measure of the magnitude and impact of Zika virus in the United States.

With regard to the availability of accurate and reliable diagnostic tests for the Zika virus, FDA authorized several diagnostic tests under EUA, but some performance characteristics were not consistently reported across different diagnostic tests, making it more challenging to compare tests. Information on performance characteristics presented in each diagnostic test product label was not consolidated across available tests, and the identity of the comparator assay was not listed on some labels, making it challenging for users to make informed decisions about which test to adopt or recommend to patients.

---

[123] NACCHO Mosquito Surveillance and Control Assessment in Zika Virus Priority Jurisdictions, 2016. NACCHO surveyed 10 jurisdictions that were deemed "high priority for assessing necessary support for Zika response" by CDC and its collaborators. These jurisdictions are Alabama, Arizona, California, Florida, Georgia, Hawaii, Los Angeles County, Louisiana, Mississippi, and Texas. A rating of "needs improvement" signifies a negative answer to at least one of five core questions regarding mosquito control program actions and capabilities. About half the surveyed mosquito control entities responded, with 21 percent of the respondents being rated "fully capable." The survey was conducted during the latter half of 2016.

[124] CDC's MosquitoNET can help address this challenge but mostly relies on self-reporting by Epidemiology and Laboratory Capacity for Infectious Diseases Cooperative Agreement (ELC) awardees and may continue to contain gaps in knowledge. ELC funds all 50 state health departments, six of the nation's largest local health departments (Chicago, the District of Columbia, Houston, Los Angeles County, New York City and Philadelphia), and eight territories or U.S. affiliates, including U.S. Virgin Islands, Puerto Rico and Guam. There are 64 grantees.

CDC developed the first two authorized diagnostic tests for the Zika virus and offered these tests to public health laboratories, but not to some manufacturers. Some manufacturers did not have access to the authorized CDC tests and encountered difficulty acquiring authorized tests from other manufacturers. Without a clear and transparent process for distributing CDC diagnostic tests, the agency may not be able to develop the capacity of the commercial sector to be able to meet the needs during an outbreak.

In addition, users were not able to compare clinical performance across authorized diagnostic tests in the absence of a diagnostic test reference standard that all manufacturers use. CDC has not provided detailed information on its website for all the diagnostic tests it distributed during the Zika virus outbreak. Until CDC lists information about all the diagnostic tests it distributes, it may be more challenging for users to determine which test to use.

With regard to vector control methods, federal agencies can provide important information to assist mosquito control efforts implemented at the state and local levels. However, the information that CDC included in its maps did not include sufficient details on its estimates of potential distribution of mosquitoes that carry the Zika virus, which made it challenging for mosquito control experts and the public to correctly interpret and use such data.

Recommendations for Executive Action

We recommend that the Secretary of Health and Human Services direct the Commissioner of the Food and Drug Administration to take the following two actions:

- Consolidate information from individual diagnostic test labels and make this information available in a form that enables users to more readily compare information across tests.
- Require manufacturers to list the identity of comparator assays on their diagnostic test labels.

We also recommend that the Secretary of Health and Human Services direct the Director of Centers for Disease Control and Prevention to take the following three actions:

- Establish a transparent process to provide CDC diagnostic tests, upon request, to manufacturers that are in the final stages of diagnostic test authorization.

- Include information on CDC-developed tests distributed to or shared with public health laboratories on CDC's website, including laboratory developed tests.
- Provide details such as collection records, dates, and data limitations on posted and disseminated mosquito distribution maps to better inform mosquito control experts and the general public.

AGENCY COMMENTS AND OUR EVALUATION

We provided a draft of this chapter for review and comment to HHS and EPA. HHS's written response is reprinted in appendix III. EPA did not provide a written response. HHS agreed with four of our recommendations, partially agreed with one of our recommendations and provided information on actions it is taking to address these recommendations. HHS and EPA also provided technical comments, which we incorporated as appropriate.

- HHS concurred with our recommendation for FDA to consolidate information from individual product labels and said that this information would be available on FDA's website.
- In response to our recommendation that FDA require manufacturers to list the identity of the comparator assay, HHS stated that it would recommend that manufacturers describe the test used for comparison in order to reduce the risk of confusion by diagnostic test users.
- In response to our recommendation to establish a transparent process to provide CDC diagnostic tests to manufacturers, HHS stated that CDC will work with its existing Technology Transfer Office to implement a transparent process for providing manufacturers with approved CDC diagnostic assays.
- In response to our recommendation that CDC provide details such as collection records, dates, and data limitations on posted and disseminated mosquito distribution maps to better inform mosquito control experts and the general public, HHS described several actions taken by CDC to help improve the quality of the data that is used to develop estimated potential ranges of the mosquitoes that spread Zika virus disease, including conducting a rapid review of available data on the mosquitoes that can transmit the Zika virus and conducting surveys to record the location of mosquitoes capable of spreading different diseases.

- In response to our recommendation to include information on CDC-developed tests distributed to public health laboratories, HHS partially concurred and provided clarifying information. HHS agreed that it should share information on CDC-developed tests that have received EUA. However, regarding this recommendation, HHS did not agree that it should share information on CDC's laboratory-developed tests that have not received EUA because CDC is unable to provide detailed information on characteristics of these unstandardized tests. We maintain that sharing information about these laboratory developed tests that are used for comparison testing is important because of the concerns that were raised regarding the sensitivity of one of CDC's EUA tests. We recognize that laboratory- developed tests that have not received EUA are not standardized, but we believe that CDC can provide certain information on the performance characteristics and quality of these tests based on its knowledge about these tests. Sharing this information could help other diagnostic test users make informed decisions about which test to adopt or recommend. HHS also noted that CDC does not distribute laboratory developed tests that have not received EUA but in some circumstances shares them with public health laboratories. In response to this comment, we have modified our recommendation to reflect this information.

As agreed with your offices, we will send copies of this chapter to appropriate congressional committees, the Secretary of Health and Human Services, and the Administrator of the Environmental Protection Agency, and other interested parties.

Timothy M. Persons, PhD.
Chief Scientist

APPENDIX I: PARTICIPANTS IN GAO'S EXPERT MEETING

This appendix lists the experts, and their affiliations, who participated in the Zika Virus Expert Meeting held with the assistance of the National Academies of Sciences, Engineering, and Medicine, on November 9–10, 2016, at 500 5th Street, N.W., Washington, D.C.[125]

- Amy L. Altman, PhD, Vice President, Biodefense and Protein Diagnostics, Luminex Corporation

[125] At the outset of the meeting on November 9, 2016, GAO advised participants that they would not be identified, that no quotes would be attributed to any person, and that they were not expected to speak for their institutions.

- Jamie A. Blow, PhD, Director, Armed Forces Pest Management Board, Defense Pest Management, Department of Defense
- Michael Callahan, MD, MSPH, Director of Translational Therapeutics, Vaccine, and Immunotherapy Center, Massachusetts General Hospital, Harvard Medical School
- Joseph M. Conlon, MSc, BCE, Technical Adviser, American Mosquito Control Association
- Durland Fish, PhD, Honorary DSc, Emeritus Professor, Yale School of Public Health
- Eva Harris, PhD, Professor, Division of Infectious Diseases and Vaccinology, School of Public Health and Director, Center for Global Public Health, University of California at Berkeley
- Anna M. Likos, MD, MPH., State Epidemiologist and Interim Deputy, Secretary for Health, Florida Department of Health
- Jorge L. Munoz-Jordan, PhD., Chief, Molecular Diagnostics and Research Laboratory, Division of Vector Borne Infectious Diseases, Dengue Branch, Centers for Disease Control and Prevention
- Benjamin Pinsky, MD, PhD, Medical Director, Clinical Virology Laboratory, Stanford University School of Medicine
- Brenda Rivera-García, DVM, MPH, Territorial Epidemiologist, Puerto Rico Department of Public Health
- Alfonso J. Rodriguez-Morales, MD, PhD, Chair, Colombian Collaborative Network of Zika (RECOLZIKA)
- Daniel A. Strickman, PhD, Senior Program Officer of Vector Control, Global Health Program, Bill and Melinda Gates Foundation
- Jill Taylor, PhD, Director, Wadsworth Center, New York State Department of Health
- Gonzalo Vazquez-Prokopec, PhD, Assistant Professor, Department of Environmental Sciences, Emory University
- Scott C. Weaver, PhD, Professor and Chair, Department of Microbiology and Immunology, University of Texas Medical Branch
- Kelly Wroblewski, MPH, MT, Director, Infectious Disease Programs, Association of Public Health Laboratories

Appendix II: Objectives, Scope, and Methodology

The objectives of this review were to (1) provide information on what is known and not known about the epidemiology of the Zika virus and determine the challenges, if any, in conducting surveillance and epidemiological studies, (2) determine the characteristics of different Zika virus authorized diagnostic tests and any challenges manufacturers and users faced, and the extent to which Food and Drug Administration (FDA) and Centers for Disease Control and Prevention (CDC) followed their own communication guidance during the U.S. outbreak, and (3) identify available mosquito control methods, describe their strengths and weaknesses, and identify any challenges federal agencies and others face in assisting mosquito control efforts.[126]

To conduct this work, we reviewed relevant laws, regulations, and guidance. We reviewed relevant documentation such as, FDA's guidance to the manufacturers, product labels, and agencies reports on the epidemiology of the Zika virus, and interviewed officials from key federal agencies that are involved in the domestic Zika virus response. With the assistance of the National Academy of Sciences, we convened a meeting with 16 experts to discuss issues related to the Zika virus outbreak. These experts represented academia, the federal government, and industry and had combined expertise in epidemiology, diagnostics, and mosquito control.

The Forum on Microbial Threats within the National Academies of Sciences, Engineering, and Medicine solicited nominations for the expert panel from its extensive contacts in academia, government, foundations, and other organizations interested in vector borne diseases, particularly Zika virus disease. These contacts include current and past members of National Academies of Science's Forum on Microbial Threats, selected members of the National Academy of Medicine, and other National Academies of Science stakeholders. The result was approximately 109 nominees. From this initial list, experts were selected for their knowledge and expertise in the science and epidemiology of Zika virus, Zika virus diagnostics, and mosquito control, as well as their experience in the academic, industry, nonprofit, and government sectors.

We chose two U.S. cities to visit to interview about their experiences and challenges in terms of Zika virus epidemiology, diagnostic users, and mosquito control—namely, New York City, which had the largest reported number of travel-associated cases, and Miami, Florida, for the largest reported number of locally transmitted cases.[127] For both site visits, we interviewed and collected information from city and state public health and mosquito officials. We also conducted site visits to three agencies within the Department of Health and Human Services (HHS): CDC, FDA, and National Institutes of Health (NIH).

To provide information on what is known about Zika virus epidemiology and the challenges in conducting surveillance and epidemiologic studies, we reviewed surveillance case data from CDC, the Pan American Health Organization (PAHO), and the World Health Organization (WHO). We reviewed peer-reviewed journal articles and

---

[126] For the purpose of this chapter, users of diagnostic tests include laboratory personnel, health care providers, and others in the medical and scientific communities.

[127] We did not visit Puerto Rico (or other U.S. territories) but we were able to meet with Puerto Rican scientists for our National Academies of Science expert group meeting.

reports about the Zika virus and associated health outcomes. We interviewed federal and selected state and city public health officials about Zika virus surveillance and epidemiology.

We also interviewed representatives from public health organizations, including the Association of State and Territorial Health Officials (ASTHO), Council of State and Territorial Epidemiologists (CSTE), and National Association of County and City Health Officials (NACCHO). We asked the representatives about the roles of their organizations in Zika virus surveillance and epidemiologic studies and any challenges they encountered.

To determine the characteristics of different Zika virus diagnostic tests, we focused on those diagnostic tests that were authorized for use under FDA's Emergency Use Authorizations (EUA). This excluded laboratory developed tests. We reviewed and compared the product labels available on FDA's website for 16 diagnostic tests with EUAs as of April 12, 2017. We reviewed product labels and determined the reported limit of detection for each molecular diagnostic test. We reviewed the product labels for information about the FDA reference samples. We also reviewed the letter of authorization and factsheets for healthcare providers and patients available on FDA's website for each authorized diagnostic test.

To determine the strengths and limitations of different diagnostic tests and the challenges associated with Zika virus diagnostic testing, research, development, and regulatory approval, we interviewed several manufacturers that had an EUA diagnostic test for the Zika virus. We attempted to interview the manufacturers of the 14 different Zika virus diagnostic tests that had a EUA, including CDC, which manufactured two of the diagnostic tests. We interviewed CDC officials about their tests in site visits to Atlanta, Georgia, and Fort Collins, Colorado. We also contacted the 14 commercial manufacturers of the EUA diagnostic tests through email and were able to interview 10 of them that responded to our inquiry.[128] We used a structured set of interview questions to obtain data from the eight manufacturers that included questions on performance characteristics, operational characteristics, types of samples, strengths and weakness of the diagnostic test as well as limitations, and challenges associated with Zika diagnostic test development, research, testing, and regulatory processes.

We also spoke with various users of the authorized diagnostic tests, including officials from selected state public health laboratories and CDC and Department of Defense (DOD) laboratories about the strengths and limitations of different tests. We selected diagnostic test users by emailing seven different entities that were listed in an HHS report as using a CDC test in their laboratories, and we were able to interview

---

[128] One company declined to be interviewed, and the remaining were unresponsive.

officials at five laboratories that responded to our inquiry.[129] We coordinated with DOD officials and submitted questions to their laboratories that use diagnostic tests for Zika.

We asked users of diagnostic tests about the type or types of tests they used, how they decided on which test(s) to use, the origin of specimens tested, the performance of comparison testing performed, and whether they had access to information regarding the potential risks and benefits of EUA tests and knowledge of available alternatives. We also asked for their interpretation of an adverse event for Zika diagnostic tests.

We compared information from our interviews with federal officials and our review of agency documents to internal controls from *Standards for Internal Control in the Federal Government*.[130] To determine current CDC and FDA practices and whether they follow of their own communication guidance, we compared information we collected from agency interviews and from our expert meeting and review of relevant documentation to internal agency guidance documents, such as the *Emergency Use Authorization of Medical Products and Related Authorities*.[131]

To identify available mosquito control methods and their strengths and weaknesses, we reviewed agency documents and peer-reviewed literature and conducted interviews with a nongeneralizable selection of mosquito control entities. We focused on entities with a high potential abundance of the mosquito species that transmit the Zika virus as reported in a journal article and areas where there was local Zika transmission, among other things. We emailed 13 mosquito control entities and were able to interview eight that responded to our inquiry. We asked these mosquito control entities about challenges with implementing their programs, technologies they use for mosquito control, how they select specific methods, sources of funding, and changes to their programs because of Zika. To assess the challenges that federal agencies face in assisting mosquito control efforts, we spoke with federal agency officials in CDC, EPA, and FDA; experts in federal government and academia; and members of our expert panel. The sample of mosquito control entities we selected for our review is nongeneralizable, meaning that information from our interviews cannot be used to make general statements about mosquito control entities across the United States.

We conducted this performance audit from June 2016 to May 2017 in accordance with generally accepted government auditing standards. Those standards require that we plan and perform the audit to obtain sufficient, appropriate evidence to provide a reasonable basis for our findings and conclusions based on our audit objectives.

---

[129] U.S. Department of Health and Human Services, *Report of Investigation*. OSC File Number DI-16-3709 (Washington, D.C.: 2016).

[130] Both the 1999 edition of GAO, *Standards for Internal Control in the Federal Government*, GAO/AIMD-00-21.3.1 (Washington, D.C.: November 1999), and the 2014 revision (GAO-14-704G).

[131] Food and Drug Administration, *Emergency Use Authorization of Medical Products and Related Authorities: Guidance for Industry and Other Stakeholders,* OMB Control 0910- 0595 (Washington, D.C.: U.S. Department of Health and Human Services, January 2017).

We believe that the evidence obtained provides a reasonable basis for our findings and conclusions based on our audit objectives.

APPENDIX III: COMMENTS FROM THE DEPARTMENT OF HEALTH AND HUMAN SERVICES

DEPARTMENT OF HEALTH & HUMAN SERVICES OFFICE OF THE SECRETARY

Assistant Secretary for Legislation
Washington, DC 20201

MAY 1 7 2017

Tim Persons
Director, Applied Research and Methods
U.S. Government Accountability Office
441 G Street NW
Washington, DC 20548

Dear Mr. Persons:

Attached are comments on the U.S. Government Accountability Office's (GAO) report entitled, "*Emerging Infectious Diseases: Actions Needed to Address the Challenges of Responding to Zika Virus Disease Outbreaks*" (GAO-17-445).

The Department appreciates the opportunity to review this report prior to publication.

Sincerely,

Barbara Pisaro Clark

Barbara Pisaro Clark
Acting Assistant Secretary for Legislation

GENERAL COMMENTS OF THE DEPARTMENT OF HEALTH AND HUMAN SERVICES (HHS) ON THE GOVERNMENT ACCOUNTABILITY OFFICE'S DRAFT REPORT ENTITLED: EMERGING INFECTIOUS DISEASES: ACTIONS NEEDED TO ADDRESS THE CHALLENGES OF RESPONDING TO ZIKA VIRUS DISEASE OUTBREAKS (GAO-17-445)

The U.S. Department of Health and Human Services (HHS) appreciates the opportunity from the Government Accountability Office (GAO) to review and comment on this draft report.

HHS notes that the report places significant weight on the ability of users to evaluate Zika tests based solely on performance, when in fact, there is little clinical significance. Although test performance is an important factor for a laboratory to consider when deciding which test to implement, other factors impact the relative utility of different tests for different settings, including whether the test fits the laboratory's needs or requires the laboratory to purchase new instrumentation. In addition, all authorized Zika molecular tests, regardless of the sensitivity, will miss some individuals who were exposed to the virus, given the short window of detection for Zika nucleic acid in symptomatic patients. For that reason, all molecular tests carry the requirement that negative test results be retested with a serological test following the Centers for Disease Control and Prevention (CDC)-issued algorithm. Differences in sensitivity for the authorized molecular tests are less significant than the report suggests, since following the CDC-issued algorithm should account for the relatively few people who were missed by the molecular test and instead were caught by follow up testing. Finally, the Food and Drug Administration (FDA) notes that the systematic use of the FDA Reference Material allows a more rigorous analysis of the comparative sensitivities of the assays from the various manufacturers.

Recommendation 1
GAO recommends that the Secretary of HHS direct the Commissioner of FDA to take the following two actions:

- Consolidate information from individual diagnostic test labels and make this information available in a form that enables users to more readily compare information across tests.
- Require manufacturers to list the identity of comparator assays on their diagnostic test labels.

HHS Response 1
HHS concurs with the GAO's recommendation. This information will be made available on FDA's website.

HHS also concurs with the GAO's recommendation regarding the inclusion of the identity of comparator assays on diagnostic test labeling, subject to the following clarification. To implement GAO's recommendation, FDA would recommend that sponsors of Zika diagnostic tests provide identification of the comparator assay by describing the assay(s), rather than provide the name of the assay in order to reduce the risk of confusion by end users. An example of a description of a comparator assay might be: "The comparator assay was an rRT-PCR assay authorized by FDA for detection of Zika RNA in serum with analytical sensitivity in the range XX-YY RNA Units/mL." FDA's recommendation is based on the Statistical Guidance on Reporting Results from Studies Evaluating Diagnostic Tests which states: "Comparing a new test to a non-reference standard does not yield true performance. If the new test is better than the non-reference standard, the agreement will be poor." Consequently a "new" device which has "better" sensitivity (lower LoD) than a "comparator" device may appear to have false positive results relative to the "comparator" assay depending on the level of Zika virus in the clinical specimens. End users may incorrectly infer that the "new" device is inferior to the "comparator" device. Alternatively, the agreement could be poor if the comparator is more accurate than the new test thereby compounding the challenges for the end users to decide which test has superior performance.

Recommendation 2
We also recommend that the Secretary of HHS direct the Director of CDC to take the following three actions:

- Establish a transparent process to provide CDC diagnostic tests, upon request, to manufacturers that are in the final stages of diagnostic test authorization.
- Include information on CDC-developed tests distributed to public health laboratories on CDC's website, including any laboratory developed tests.
- Provide details such as collection records, dates, and data limitations on posted and disseminated mosquito distribution maps to better inform mosquito control experts and the general public.

HHS Response 2

Establish a transparent process to provide CDC diagnostic tests, upon request, to manufacturers that are in the final stages of diagnostic test authorization.

HHS concurs with GAO's recommendation and efforts are underway to implement it. On January 15, 2016, CDC issued a Health Advisory encouraging healthcare providers to report suspected Zika virus disease cases to their state health departments to facilitate diagnosis and mitigate the risk of local transmission. At that time, there were no commercially available tests to diagnose Zika virus and tests were being performed using existing available nonspecific time-consuming PCR methods by state health departments and CDC. In March 2016, CDC secured FDA Emergency Use Authorization (EUA) for the Trioplex rRT-PCR assay, which was the first test that was able to detect and differentiate Zika virus, dengue virus, and chikungunya virus. The EUA permitted CDC to provide the Trioplex assay to qualified laboratories. CDC began manufacturing the Trioplex assay in March, and prioritized distribution of the assay to state/local health departments in geographic areas at greatest risk of Zika transmission.

CDC initially prioritized sharing of assays with state and local health departments for several reasons, including: (1) there was a limited supply of assays available; (2) CDC guidance to healthcare providers recommended that they screen for Zika and seek testing through a state/local health department; and (3) testing conducted by state/local health departments could be easily reported to CDC to help better understand the impact of Zika in the United States. Furthermore, many people infected with Zika do not show symptoms, and those that do have symptoms that are non-specific and similar to a cold or flu. Given the limited availability of the assay during the early part of 2016, CDC did not want to create circumstances where the supply of available assays was exhausted by testing low/no-risk people. This approach during the early part of 2016 ensured that there was a sufficient supply of available assays to screen and diagnose those most at risk. CDC did provide the Trioplex assay to commercial manufacturers for EUA comparison analysis once supplies were available. However, CDC does acknowledge it did not always utilize a transparent process to provide the Trioplex assay to manufacturers for comparison analysis.

Going forward, CDC will work with its existing Technology Transfer Office to implement a transparent process to provide manufacturers engaged in EUA-comparator analyses with approved CDC diagnostic assays. This process will ensure that intellectual property and materials transfer agreements are addressed appropriately, and will also allow CDC to clearly articulate any criteria under which the provision of diagnostic assays may be delayed such as limited availability or some other compelling public health interest.

Include information on CDC-developed tests distributed to public health laboratories on CDC's website, including any laboratory developed tests.

HHS partially concurs with GAO's recommendation related to sharing information on CDC-developed tests.

In early 2016, CDC received FDA Emergency Use Authorization (EUA) for two Zika diagnostic assays: Trioplex rRT-PCR assay and the Zika MAC-ELISA assay. In January 2017, FDA approved CDC's request to modify the Trioplex rRT-PCR assay to include a singleplex reaction option. These are the only CDC-developed Zika diagnostic assays that have received EUA. For these assays, CDC provided information consistent with the FDA-

Instructions for Use requirements for each EUA. This information was posted on CDC's website (https://www.cdc.gov/zika/hc-providers/types-of-tests.html) as well as on FDA's EUA website (https://www.fda.gov/MedicalDevices/%20Safety/EmergencySituations/ucm161496.htm).
For EUA assays, CDC provides information including but not limited to: specimen handling, materials/equipment requirements provided by CDC to approved external laboratories, quality control instructions, testing algorithms and test validity determination instructions, assay limitations, performance characteristics, clinical performance data and contact information.

For EUA assays, CDC provides the receiving laboratories the specified reagents and approved instructions for conducting the test. The receiving laboratories are required to demonstrate proficiency in order to continue receiving the reagents.

CDC concurs with GAO's recommendation to make this information available for all EUA assays developed by CDC. CDC does not concur with GAO's recommendation that CDC provide similar information for any CDC laboratory developed assays, including those that have not received EUA from the FDA.

CDC does not distribute laboratory-developed assays that have not received EUA. In some circumstances, CDC shares laboratory-developed assay protocols (generally through scientific publications) and laboratory controls with partner public health laboratories to advance technical cooperation.

CDC is unable to provide detailed information for non-EUA laboratory-developed assays on characteristics such as assay performance and quality control instructions because the assay is not standardized. Laboratory-developed assays are designed, manufactured and used within an individual laboratory. Each laboratory can therefore adapt the assays and utilize different products and protocols, which makes it impossible to develop a standardized set of performance and quality characteristics. As a result, each laboratory must determine these characteristics based on use in the individual laboratory.

Provide details such as collection records, dates, and data limitations on posted and disseminated mosquito distribution maps to better inform mosquito control experts and the general public.
HHS concurs with GAO's recommendation and efforts are underway to implement it. In the United States, surveillance for *Aedes aegypti* and *Aedes albopictus* mosquitoes was neither systematically nor routinely completed in recent decades. As a result, when the Zika virus outbreak began in the Americas, health departments and vector control districts in the United States did not have a good understanding of where *Ae. aegypti* and *Ae. albopictus* mosquitoes were found at a local or state level.

In early 2016, CDC undertook a rapid review of available data on *Aedes* distribution throughout the United States to provide an informed and timely estimate of the potential range of *Ae. aegypti* and *Ae. albopictus* given the growing concerns related to Zika and link to microcephaly in infants. In addition to publishing the maps that identified the estimated range of the mosquitoes, CDC conducted outreach to state and local partners and other stakeholders to explain the methodology as well as the intended uses of the maps. In these efforts, CDC's primary objectives were to provide clear, accurate and timely information about the potential range of *Aedes* distribution to the public.

In the spring and fall of 2016, CDC conducted surveys to record where these mosquitoes, capable of spreading chikungunya, dengue, and Zika viruses, had been collected from 1995 to 2016. In addition, additional intensified mosquito surveillance across the Southern United States in the summer of 2016 related to the Zika response indicates a substantial increase in the number of counties with records of the mosquitoes. This additional information will help improve the quality of data that is used to develop estimated potential range of these

mosquitoes. CDC will refine estimated distribution maps when new data warrant changes, and will continue to improve how it communicates data sources and methodology, dates and data limitations on the CDC website and in any outreach to state and local organizations and the general public.

Appendix IV: Zika Virus Case Definitions for National Notifiable Disease Reporting

The following are summarized descriptions of criteria and Zika case classifications that were effective in June 2016, which updated interim definitions published in February 2016.[132]

Criteria for a Zika Case

Criteria for laboratory evidence of recent Zika virus infection:

- culture of Zika virus from blood, body fluid, or tissue; OR
- detection of Zika virus antigen or viral ribonucleic acid (RNA); OR
- positive Zika virus immunoglobulin M (IgM) antibody test with positive Zika virus neutralizing antibody titers and negative neutralizing antibody titers against dengue or other flaviviruses[133] regularly found to the region where exposure occurred.

Criteria for laboratory evidence of recent flavivirus infection that is possibly Zika virus:

- positive Zika virus IgM antibody test with positive neutralizing antibody titers against Zika virus and dengue virus or other flaviviruses regularly found to the region where exposure occurred.
- positive Zika virus IgM antibody test AND negative dengue virus IgM antibody test with no neutralizing antibody testing performed.

Criteria for establishing an epidemiologic linkage:

- resides in or recent travel to an area with known Zika virus transmission; OR

---

[132] See https://wwwn.cdc.gov/nndss/conditions/zika/case-definition/2016/06/ (accessed March 27, 2017) for more details on these criteria and definitions, such as the specific types of specimens used for laboratory criteria.

[133] Flaviviruses are positive, single-stranded, enveloped RNA viruses found in arthropods (primarily ticks and mosquitoes).

- sexual contact with a confirmed or probable case within the infection transmission risk window of Zika virus infection or person with recent travel to an area with known Zika virus transmission; OR
- receipt of blood or blood products within 30 days of symptom onset; OR
- organ or tissue transplant recipient within 30 days of symptom onset; OR
- association in time and place with a confirmed or probable case; **OR**
- likely vector exposure in an area with suitable seasonal and ecological conditions for potential local vector-borne transmission.

Table 5. Non-congenital Zika virus case classifications and definitions for reporting to the national notifiable disease reporting system

Case classification[a]	Definition
Zika virus disease	Clinical criteria: A person with one or more of the following not explained by another cause: Clinically compatible illness that includes acute onset of fever (measured or reported), OR certain type of rash, OR joint pain, OR conjunctivitis Complication of pregnancy fetal loss, OR fetus or neonate with congenital microcephaly or specified other abnormalities Guillain-Barré syndrome or other neurological symptoms
Confirmed case	Meets clinical criteria for non-congenital disease; AND Has specified laboratory evidence of recent Zika virus infection
Probable case	Meets specified clinical criteria; AND Has an epidemiologic linkage; AND Has specified laboratory evidence of recent Zika virus or flavivirus infection
Zika virus infection	
Confirmed case	A person who does not meet specified clinical criteria; AND Has specified laboratory evidence of recent Zika virus infection
Probable case	A person who does not meet specified clinical criteria; BUT Has an epidemiologic linkage; AND Has specified laboratory evidence of recent Zika virus infection

Source: CSTE and CDC established Zika Virus Disease and Zika Virus Infection 2016 Case Definitions, Approved June 2016. CSTE approved position statement 16-ID-01 in June 2016, which modified the previous February 2016 interim case definitions. I GAO-17-445.

[a]There are also specific definitions for these case classifications for newborn infants, referred to as "congenital" cases. See https://wwwn.cdc.gov/nndss/conditions/zika/case-definition/2016/06/ (accessed March 27, 2017) for these definitions and for more details for the definitions in the table.

Appendix V: Performance Characteristics Information Presented in EUA Molecular Diagnostic Tests Labels for Zika Virus

Table 6. Confirmed limits of detection (LOD) results using the food and drug administration (FDA) reference materials as reported on product labels

Diagnostic Test and Manufacturer	Sample type	S1	S2
Zika Virus Real-time RT-PCR: Viracor-IBT Laboratories, Inc.	Plasma	1000	500
	Urine	1000	500
VERSANT® Zika RNA 1.0 Assay (kPCR) Kit: Siemens Healthcare Diagnostics Inc.	Serum	1000	5000
	Urine	3000	5000
xMAP® MultiFlex™ Zika RNA Assay: Luminex® Luminex Corporation	Serum	3000	5000
	Urine	3330	5000
Sentosa® SA ZIKV RT-PCR Test (4x24): Vela Operations Singapore Pte Ltd	Serum	30000	15000
	Urine	10000	5000
Zika Virus Detection by RT-PCR: ARUP Laboratories	Plasma	3000	1650
	Urine	3300	4500
RealTime ZIKA: Abbott	Serum	1000	500
	Urine	300	500
Molecular Diagnostics Zika ELITe MGB® Kit U.S.: ELITechGroup Inc.	Plasma	3300	5560
Zika Virus RNA Qualitative Real-Time RT-PCR: Focus Diagnostics, Inc.	Serum	1000	500
	Urine	1000	1000
Aptima® Zika Virus Assay: Hologic, Inc.	Plasma	100	150
	Processed urine	300	150
Trioplex Real-time RT-PCR Assay: Centers for Disease Control and Prevention	Serum	3300	1670
	Urine	1000	1670
RealStar® Zika Virus RT-PCR Kit U.S.: altona Diagnostics GmbH	Serum	3162	5000
	Urine	3162	1581, 5000[a]
Gene-RADAR® Zika Virus Test: Nanobiosym Diagnostics, Inc.	Serum	3333	5000

Source: GAO analysis based on product labels. | GAO-17-445.

Note: S1 is concentrated stock 1 (FSS13025: Cambodia, 2010 provided by UTMB. GenBank#JN860885).

S2 is concentrated stock 2 (PRAVABC59: Puerto Rico, 2015 provided by CDC. GenBank#KU501215.

The table lists currently authorized molecular test EUA for Zika virus as of April 12, 2017. On March 13, 2017, FDA "revoked the EUA for emergency use" of one Zika virus test because the company requested the test be withdrawn from authorization due to technical performance and business considerations.

[a]1581 and 5000 were reported as point values which differed because two different extraction methods were used.

Table 7. Value ranges for limit of detection of Zika virus in plasma, serum, and urine in selected emergency use authorized diagnostic tests

Diagnostic test	Plasma	Serum	Urine
Aptima Zika Virus Assay: Hologic, Inc.	5.9 copies/mL - 13.4 copies/mL[a]	n/a	n/a
RealStar® Zika Virus RT-PCR Kit U.S.: altona Diagnostics GmbH	251.62 geq/mL	251.62 geq/mL	79.57 geq/mL
Trioplex Real-time RT-PCR Assay[d]: Centers for Disease Control	n/a	1.51×10^4 (GCE/mL) - 3.11×10^4 (GCE/mL)[b]	1.79×10^4 (GCE/mL) - 4.20×10^4 (GCE/mL)[b]
VERSANT® Zika RNA 1.0 Assay (kPCR) Kit: Siemens Healthcare Diagnostics Inc.	721 copies/mL or 0.05 TCID50/mL	721 copies/mL or 0.05 TCID50/mL	721 copies/mL or 0.05 TCID50/mL
Zika Virus RNA Qualitative Real-Time RT-PCR: Focus Diagnostics, Inc.	n/a	250 RNA copies/mL	n/a
Zika Virus Real-time RT-PCR: Viracor-IBT Laboratories, Inc.	97 copies/mL	n/a	98 copies/mL
xMAP® MultiFLEX™ Zika RNA Assay: Luminex Corporation	687 copies/mL	687 copies/mL	687 copies/mL
Zika Virus Detection by RT-PCR: ARUP Laboratories	160 copies/mL	160 copies/mL	160 copies/mL
Sentosa® SA ZIKV RT-PCR Test (4x24): Vela Operations Singapore Pte Ltd	3×10^3 copies/mL - 6×10^3 copies/mL[c]	3×10^3 copies/mL - 6×10^3 copies/mL[c]	3×10^3 copies/mL - 6×10^3 copies/mL[c]
RealTime ZIKV: Abbott	40 copies/mL	30 copies/mL	40 copies/mL
Molecular Diagnostics Zika ELITe MGB® Kit U.S.: ELITechGroup Inc.	270 copies/mL	n/a	n/a
Gene-RADAR® Zika Virus Test: Nanobiosym Diagnostics, Inc.	n/a	200 PFU/mL	n/a

Source: GAO analysis based on product labels. | GAO-17-445.

Note: n/a means that the test is not authorized for the specimen type listed (serum, plasma, or urine) and therefore the LOD is not listed in the product label. The table lists currently authorized molecular test EUA for Zika virus as of April 12, 2017. On March 13, 2017, FDA "revoked the EUA for emergency use" of one Zika virus test because the company requested the test be withdrawn from authorization due to technical performance and business considerations.

[a]Two different LOD were listed for plasma based on Brazilian donor plasma 2015 and *in vitro* transcript.

[b]Range based on four different LOD listed for different extraction methods.

[c]LOD was determined for two different Zika strains (MR-766 and PRVABC59).

[d]CDC Trioplex assay is also approved for cerebrospinal fluid and amniotic fluid, but the LOD is not listed in product label.

Table 8. Six of 12 authorized Zika molecular diagnostic test labels that did not list the comparator assay for clinical performance

Reference assay and Manufacturer	Comparator assay listed[a]	Comparator assay type[b]	Comparator assay[d]
Zika Virus RNA Qualitative Real-Time RT- PCR: Focus Diagnostics, Inc.	Yes	EUA	Trioplex Real-time RT-PCR Assay: Centers for Disease Control
	Yes	LDT	Lanciotti Test[c]
Aptima® Zika Virus Assay: Hologic, Inc.	Yes	EUA	Trioplex Real-time RT-PCR Assay: Centers for Disease Control
Zika Virus Real-time RT-PCR: Viracor-IBT Laboratories, Inc.	No	EUA	n/a
VERSANT® Zika RNA 1.0 Assay (kPCR) Kit: Siemens Healthcare Diagnostics Inc.	Yes	LDT	Lanciotti Test[c]
xMAP® MultiFlex™ Zika RNA Assay: Luminex Corporation	No	EUA	n/a
Sentosa® SA ZIKV RT-PCR Test (4x24): Vela Operations Singapore Pte Ltd	Yes	EUA	RealStar® Zika Virus RT-PCR Kit U.S.: altona Diagnostics
Zika Virus Detection by RT-PCR: ARUP Laboratories	No	EUA	n/a
Abbott RealTime ZIKA	No	EUA	n/a
Molecular Diagnostics Zika ELITe MGB® Kit U.S.: ELITechGroup Inc.	Yes	EUA	LightMix® Zika rRT-PCR Test: Roche[e]
	No	LDT	n/a
Trioplex Real-time RT-PCR Assay: Centers for Disease Control	No	In-House Assay	n/a
RealStar® Zika Virus RT-PCR Kit U.S.: altona Diagnostics GmbH	Yes	LDT	Lanciotti Test[c]
Gene-RADAR® Zika Virus Test: Nanobiosym Diagnostics, Inc.	No	EUA	n/a

Source: GAO analysis based on product labels. | GAO-17-445.

Note: The table lists currently authorized molecular test EUA for Zika virus as of April 12, 2017. One Zika virus EUA has been revoked because the company requested the test be withdrawn from authorization due to technical performance and business considerations.

[a]6 of 12 labels did not list the comparator assay for clinical specimens. Note that the Molecular Diagnostics Zika ELITe MGB® Kit U.S.: ELITechGroup Inc.has one of the comparator assays listed and one that is not so it is included in the labels that listed comparator assays.

[b]Comparator type is categorized as EUA=emergency use authorized; LDT=laboratory developed test; or an in-house assay.

[c]Performance of the Zika Virus RNA Qualitative Real-Time RT-PCR test was also referenced and reviewed from the publication in Robert S. Lanciotti and others, "Genetic and Serologic Properties of Zika Virus Associated with an Epidemic, Yap State, Micronesia, 2007," *Emerging Infectious Diseases,* vol. 14 (2008): 1232–1239.

[d]EUA Diagnostic Tests that do not have a comparator assay listed would not have a name listed and therefore are listed as "n/a."

[e]The LightMix® Zika rRT-PCR Test: Roche is no longer authorized as of March 13, 2017.

APPENDIX VI: ISSUES WITH MOSQUITO CONTROL PESTICIDE REGULATION

In discussion with mosquito control entities, we heard that certain federal regulations related to pesticide applications may create additional issues for mosquito control. Pesticide use for mosquito control, among other uses, is regulated by the Federal Insecticide, Fungicide, and Rodenticide Act (FIFRA),[134] under which vendors register pesticides for sale or distribution and pesticide users are required to follow the labeling for the pesticide application.[135] In addition to using products that have been registered under FIFRA, mosquito control entities must obtain a permit to spray pesticides on or near waters of the United States under the Clean Water Act.[136] Some mosquito control entity officials we spoke with told us the National Pollution Discharge Elimination System (NPDES) permit process has led to an increase in ongoing administrative burdens, such as reporting requirements, with one stating that their burden has increased from 1 hour of daily paperwork to 6 hours.[137]

Mosquito control officials we interviewed told us that some mosquito control entities have discontinued their programs, at least partly because of additional reporting requirements under NPDES permitting. However, an American Mosquito Control Association official told us that while they had a number of second-hand reports, they could not specify actual instances of entities ceasing operations because of NPDES costs. One mosquito control official told us that NPDES permitting burdens will largely affect smaller mosquito control entities that may not be as well funded, many of which shut down and have not been replaced with another entity.[138] This official added that the entities shut partially because of the economic downturn and that NPDES paperwork

---

[134] 7 U.S.C. § 136 *et. seq.*

[135] The Environmental Protection Agency (EPA) regulates the use of pesticides. EPA officials told us that one of their major challenges is communicating their role to the U.S. public. EPA officials told us the EPA role is to evaluate pesticides and their uses. EPA officials told us that they review and analyze data submitted by pesticide manufacturers for safety approval. EPA does not (1) oversee or perform mosquito control, (2) design or create pesticides, or (3) provide guidance on use of specific pesticides because of factors such as pesticide resistance.

[136] The Clean Water Act prohibits the discharge of pollutants into waters of the United States from point sources unless EPA or a state issues a National Pollutant Discharge Elimination System (NPDES) permit for the discharge. 33 U.S.C. § 1342. EPA issued a final rule in 2006 excluding FIFRA-registered pesticides from the NPDES permitting requirements. 71 Fed. Reg. 68,483 (Nov. 27, 2006). In 2009, the 6th Circuit Court of Appeals vacated EPA's final rule and all persons discharging chemical pesticides that leave a residue or biological pesticides into waters of the U.S. must now obtain a NPDES permit. *Nat'l Cotton Council of Am. V. United States EPA*, 553 F.3d 927 (Jan. 7, 2009).

[137] In 2011, EPA issued a final NPDES Pesticide General Permit (PGP) to alleviate some of the administrative burden associated with individual NPDES permitting on pesticide operators. Reissued in 2016, the PGP provides a mechanism for certain dischargers to comply with the Clean Water Act requirements for pesticides for the geographic area where EPA is the NPDES permitting authority. Most states have also developed PGPs for pesticide discharges into waters in their states.

[138] According to EPA, there is no de minimus exemption in the CWA. All mosquito control districts or similar pest control districts need an NPDES permit to discharge biological pesticides and chemical pesticides that leave a residue to waters of the U.S. However, EPA and most states, in their NPDES permits, provide for automatic coverage under their permits if pesticide applicators do not exceed certain annual treatment area thresholds.

burden was a possible, but not exclusive, cause. A mosquito control professional told us that his program discontinued applying pesticides partly as a result of NPDES permitting, but since the program still supplies pesticides, they know that the use of pesticides has increased.[139] This professional questioned the benefit of NPDES permits if pesticide applicators react by taking actions that result in the use of more pesticides. The American Mosquito Control Association stated that NPDES permits duplicate FIFRA processes, create new avenues for lawsuits, and have no substantive or foreseeable environmental benefit. [140]

A mosquito control official expressed support for NPDES permitting, because following NPDES permitting guidelines allowed his program to minimize adulticide discharges as a first response and to develop a more desirable IVM plan. From 2012 to 2016, this entity was able to reduce adulticiding acres by more than 30 percent, despite an increase in citizen requests for service. However, another official stated that encouraging larvicide use or IVM can be done more effectively than through NPDES permitting, such as through federal funding of programs that implement best practices.

Environmental group representatives we spoke with agreed that documented evidence is scarce on the effects of NPDES permits on pesticide levels in water. However, environmental group representatives told us of benefits to the permit process, including (1) encouraging nonchemical means of control, (2) establishing a limit on the amount of pesticides in specific bodies of water, and (3) enabling the monitoring of pesticide use. Representatives from one group told us that the Clean Water Act fills a regulatory gap that FIFRA does not address. Representatives from another group stated that the permitting application is simple.

Further, an environmental group representative told us NPDES notification and reporting requirements allow the public to be aware of what is being sprayed and how much. One representative told us her office received calls from residents wondering what was being sprayed and saying they are not aware of requirements regarding who notifies the public about spraying.

EPA officials told us that they have not documented evidence that (1) pesticide use has decreased or (2) water quality has changed, in response to NPDES permits for FIFRA-compliant pesticide application. However, an EPA notice states that the cost of compliance with NPDES permits is minimal.[141]

---

[139] According to EPA, it is difficult to make any definitive conclusions regarding the increase or reduction of pesticide use as a result of NPDES permits. This is because the prevalence of mosquitoes and the need for pesticide use varies due to several factors such as the amount of rainfall, temperature and other weather variables annually. An NPDES permit neither prohibits nor encourages the use of pesticides. An NPDES permit is only required when pesticides are selected as the control method and their application would result in a discharge to waters of the U.S.

[140] EPA officials said they were aware of one ongoing lawsuit related to use of pesticides under a NPDES permit.

[141] Cost analysis EPA presented as part of the 2016 Reissuance for the NPDES Pesticide General Permit was restricted to the areas of EPA permitting authority, including Idaho, Massachusetts, New Hampshire, New Mexico, the District of Columbia, and other federal and Native American territories. Therefore, the results of

Further, EPA documentation states that EPA disagrees that FIFRA and NPDES requirements are duplicative. According to this documentation, NPDES permits minimize discharges of pesticides to waters of the United States beyond FIFRA requirements, among other things.

this analysis do not apply to the remaining states, except for federal and Native American territories within them.

In: Infectious Diseases
Editor: Philippe Georges
ISBN: 978-1-53616-401-5

Chapter 3

ZIKA SUPPLEMENTAL FUNDING: STATUS OF HHS AGENCIES' OBLIGATIONS, DISBURSEMENTS, AND THE ACTIVITIES FUNDED*

United States Government Accountability Office

ABBREVIATIONS

BARDA	Biomedical Advanced Research and Development Authority
BRFSS	Behavioral Risk Factor Surveillance System
CDC	Centers for Disease Control and Prevention
CMS	Centers for Medicare & Medicaid Services
ELC	Epidemiology and Laboratory Capacity for Infectious Diseases
HHS	Department of Health and Human Services
HRSA	Health Resources and Services Administration
NIH	National Institutes of Health
PHPR	Public Health Preparedness and Response
PHSSEF	Public Health and Social Services Emergency Fund
PRAMS	Pregnancy Risk Assessment Monitoring System

WHY GAO DID THIS STUDY

Zika—a virus primarily transmitted through mosquito bites—can cause symptoms that include fever, rash, and joint and muscle pain. In pregnant women, the Zika virus can

* This is an edited, reformatted and augmented version of the United States Government Accountability Office Report to Congressional Committees, Publication No. GAO-18-389, dated May 2018.

be passed to the fetus and cause severe brain defects. In response to an outbreak in the United States and its territories, Congress appropriated $932 million in September 2016 through the Zika Response and Preparedness Act to HHS and its agencies to prevent, prepare for, and respond to the Zika virus and its related health conditions, and conduct related research.

The act also included a provision that GAO study the activities supported with the appropriated funds. This chapter describes (1) the status of funds obligated and disbursed from the Zika supplemental funding appropriated to HHS and its agencies; and (2) how selected awardees used their Zika supplemental funding, and their experiences with applying for and managing the funding. To do this work, GAO reviewed agency documents on Zika supplemental funding and activities, and interviewed officials from the HHS agencies and selected awardees. To select awardees, GAO identified states based on the amount of initial Zika supplemental funding they received from CDC, the Centers for Medicare & Medicaid Services, and the Health Resources and Services Administration; and selected states with the highest and lowest funding. In total, GAO selected 12 awardees: 10 states, as well as one county and one city from 2 of the 10 states.

GAO provided a draft of this chapter to HHS. In response, HHS provided technical comments, which were incorporated as appropriate.

WHAT GAO FOUND

As of September 30, 2017, Department of Health and Human Services' (HHS) agencies had obligated nearly all of the $932 million of Zika supplemental funding Congress appropriated in 2016 through the use of multiple funding mechanisms, including cooperative agreements, grants, and contracts. Four HHS agencies had small unobligated balances as of the September 30, 2017, obligation deadline; these balances cannot be used to incur new obligations, but may be used to adjust award amounts in future years. Disbursement of the obligated funds was ongoing, with about 21 percent of the Zika supplemental funding (approximately $195.5 million) disbursed as of December 31, 2017. The agencies have until September 30, 2022, to disburse the remainder.

The 12 awardees GAO interviewed—officials from 10 states and two local entities—funded multiple activities with their Zika supplemental funding, and had varying experiences applying for and managing the funds.

- Awardees told GAO that they used their funding to support such activities as collection of information about individuals affected by the Zika virus (human surveillance), mosquito control activities, laboratory capacity building, public outreach, and health care services. For example, Florida used Zika supplemental funding in its state-run laboratories to purchase materials for testing Zika virus-related specimens.

- A majority of the awardees GAO spoke with reported positive experiences applying for and managing the Zika supplemental funding, including good communication with agency officials and awardees' familiarity with the mechanisms used to make the awards. However, some awardees noted challenges, such as time frames to use the funding that varied among multiple awards and identifying the activities that could be funded. These challenges added administrative burdens to applying for and managing the Zika supplemental funding while officials were responding to the outbreak, according to the awardees. In October 2017, the Centers for Disease Control and Prevention (CDC) issued a new notice of funding opportunity that agency officials said is intended to help minimize the administrative burden on states and certain localities during emergencies—such as preparing applications—by pre-approving public health departments in these jurisdictions to be eligible to rapidly receive future awards.

Zika supplemental obligations as of September 30, 2017

		In dollars (rounded)	
HHS agency	Total supplemental funding	Amount obligated	Unobligated balance
Biomedical Advanced Research and Development Authority	245,000,000	245,000,000	0
Centers for Disease Control and Prevention	394,000,000	393,706,358	293,642
Centers for Medicare & Medicaid Services	75,000,000	74,982,493	17,508
Health Resources and Services Administration	66,000,000	65,978,442	21,558
National Institutes of Health	152,000,000	151,998,591	1,409
Total	932,000,000	931,665,883	334,117

Source: GAO analysis of Department of Health and Human Services (HHS) data. | GAO-18-389.

May 14, 2018

The Honorable Roy Blunt
Chairman

The Honorable Patty Murray
Ranking Member
Subcommittee on Labor, Health and Human Services,
Education, and Related Agencies
Committee on Appropriations
United States Senate

The Honorable Tom Cole
Chairman

The Honorable Rosa DeLauro
Ranking Member
Subcommittee on Labor, Health and Human Services,
Education, and Related Agencies
Committee on Appropriations
House of Representatives

The Zika virus outbreak in 2015 affected individuals infected with the virus in ways that had not been seen with other infectious disease outbreaks. Zika—a virus primarily transmitted through mosquito bites—can cause symptoms that include fever, rash, conjunctivitis (red eyes), and joint and muscle pain, though many infected individuals do not have symptoms or will only experience mild symptoms. However, in this outbreak, the Zika infection in pregnant women has been linked to adverse pregnancy and birth outcomes: the virus can be passed to the fetus and cause a birth defect of the brain called microcephaly and other severe brain defects, according to the Centers for Disease Control and Prevention (CDC).[1] CDC officials note that this is the first time in more than 50 years that aninfectious pathogen has been identified as the cause of birth defects. The virus is also linked to other problems, such as miscarriage, stillbirth, and other birth defects, as well as Guillain-Barré syndrome, an uncommon sickness of the nervous system.[2] In the western hemisphere, the first cases of locally transmitted Zika virus disease were confirmed in Brazil in May 2015; in the continental United States, the first locally transmitted cases were confirmed in Florida during June to August 2016.[3] The World Health Organization declared the Zika virus a Public Health Emergency of International Concern from February to November 2016, and maintains that it is a significant, enduring public health challenge.

As of January 24, 2018, about 5,600 cases involving Zika virus disease have been reported in the United States and about 37,000 cases have been reported in the U.S. territories, primarily in Puerto Rico. In response to the outbreak, Congress appropriated

[1] Microcephaly is a rare nervous system disorder that causes a baby's head to be smaller than expected and not fully developed, which can lead to impaired thought processes, delayed motor function, and other adverse outcomes. A study published in December 2017 found that 19 children ages 19 to 24 months born with microcephaly and with laboratory evidence of Zika virus infection experienced problems including an inability to sit independently, difficulties with sleeping and feeding, seizures, and hearing and vision problems. Ashley Satterfield-Nash et al., "Health and Development at Age 19-24 Months of 19 Children Who Were Born with Microcephaly and Laboratory Evidence of Congenital Zika Virus Infection During the 2015 Zika Virus Outbreak—Brazil, 2017," Morbidity and Mortality Weekly Report, vol. 66, no. 49 (Dec. 15, 2017): 1347-1351.

[2] Guillain-Barré syndrome is a rare disorder in which the body's immune system attacks the nervous system outside the brain and spinal cord, causing muscle weakness and in some cases paralysis, although most people recover.

[3] While the continental United States' first locally transmitted case was identified in Florida, locally transmitted Zika virus was reported in December 2015 in Puerto Rico.

$932 million in September 2016 through the Zika Response and Preparedness Act to the Department of Health and Human Services (HHS) and its agencies for activities such as responding to the Zika virus, developing vaccines, and reimbursement for health care costs related to the Zika virus.[4] Specifically, the act appropriated $394 million to CDC, $152 million to the National Institutes of Health (NIH), and $387 million to HHS's Public Health and Social Services Emergency Fund (PHSSEF), of which $386 million was allocated to additional HHS agencies—the Biomedical Advanced Research and Development Authority (BARDA) within the Office of the Assistant Secretary for Preparedness and Response, the Centers for Medicare & Medicaid Services (CMS), and the Health Resources and Services Administration (HRSA).[5] The agencies had until September 30, 2017, to obligate the funding, for example, by awarding a contract or a grant to an entity (awardee). Agencies have until September 30, 2022, to disburse, or spend, the funding.

The Zika Response and Preparedness Act included a provision that we study activities supported with funds appropriated by the act. In this chapter, we describe

1. the status of obligations and disbursements of Zika supplemental funding by HHS agencies; and
2. how selected awardees used their Zika supplemental funding, and their experiences with applying for and managing the funding.

To describe the status of obligations and disbursements of Zika supplemental funding by HHS agencies, we analyzed BARDA, CDC, CMS, HRSA, and NIH obligation data as of September 30, 2017—the date funding had to be obligated—and disbursement data as of December 31, 2017—the first full quarter of data available at the time of our review. Each agency provided tabulated data that included information such as the award title, awardee name and location, award amount, award time frame, and the funding mechanism the agency used to award the funding. We interviewed officials from each agency to discuss the status of the agencies' obligations and disbursements of the Zika supplemental funding, the different mechanisms used to award the funding, and the various factors that influenced the obligation and disbursement of the funding to awardees. We also reviewed documentation of the funding opportunity announcements to obtain information such as the activities allowed under each type of award. To determine the reliability of the data provided, we compared the tabulated award amounts received from CDC and HRSA to the actual notices of award provided by both agencies, and

---

[4] Zika Response and Preparedness Act, Pub. L. No. 114-223, div. B, tit. I, 130 Stat. 857, 901 (2016). For the purposes of this chapter, we refer to funding appropriated in the Zika Response and Preparedness Act as Zika supplemental funding.

[5] The remaining $1 million appropriated to HHS's PHSSEF was to be divided equally between HHS's Office of Inspector General and GAO for oversight activities. Pub. L. No. 114-223, § 104, 130 Stat. at 904. Throughout this chapter we use "agency" to refer to agencies within HHS and the Office of the Secretary, except for HHS's Office of Inspector General.

compared NIH award data to the amounts reported in NIH's online database. We also obtained information from BARDA, CMS, and NIH officials regarding the underlying financial data systems used to compile the data and the controls in place for recording and maintaining the data. We reviewed the data from each agency for data discrepancies and obtained the information necessary to resolve the discrepancies from relevant agency officials. Furthermore, we interviewed officials from HHS's Office of the Assistant Secretary for Financial Resources on the accuracy of the data and the steps the office takes to verify agencies' obligation and disbursement data. On this basis, we determined that the data were sufficiently reliable for the purposes of our reporting objectives. Additionally, to describe the various factors that can affect the disbursement of funding after obligation, we interviewed officials representing selected awardees. To select awardees, we first identified states that were awarded Zika supplemental funding from HHS agencies (45 states) based on our review of the amount of initial Zika supplemental funding they received from CDC, CMS, and HRSA. From those 45 states, we judgmentally selected 10 states—5 states with the highest funding and 5 states with the lowest funding—which included the 2 states that experienced local Zika virus transmissions (Florida and Texas). Our selected states with the highest funding were Arizona, California, Florida, Louisiana, and Texas. Our selected states with the lowest funding were Alaska, Colorado, Iowa, Kansas, and Oklahoma.[6] To obtain perspectives of awardees at the local level, we judgmentally selected two local awardees within 2 of the selected states—Houston, Texas, and Los Angeles County, California. For each selected state or jurisdiction, we interviewed state, county, or city officials who could provide information about their Zika supplemental funding. The perspectives of the 12 awardees we interviewed cannot be generalized to other awardees.

To describe how selected awardees used their Zika supplemental funding and gain their perspectives on applying for and managing this funding, we reviewed documentation from the 12 selected awardees to identify the activities they funded. We also interviewed officials from the selected awardees (state officials and officials from one county and one city) about their experiences with using the Zika supplemental funding and to obtain examples of awardees' Zika activities. We conducted site visits to Florida and Texas, because at the time of our work, they alone had reported local Zika virus transmissions.[7] Additionally, we reviewed CDC and CMS documents to determine the amount of funding received and the purpose of the funding for each of the selected awardees. We also

[6] In determining states' respective funding levels under the Zika Response and Preparedness Act, we excluded funding awarded by NIH and BARDA to entities other than states. We also excluded a $44 million appropriation to CDC for the Public Health Emergency Preparedness cooperative agreement program. The Zika Response and Preparedness Act specified that this amount was to restore fiscal year 2016 funds that HHS had reprogrammed for Zika response activities prior to its enactment, which could be used for purposes other than Zika-related activities. See Pub. L. No. 114-223, 130 Stat. at 902.

[7] We planned to conduct a site visit to Puerto Rico, as it was the territory with the most Zika disease cases and also had reported active Zika transmissions. However, we were not able to speak to officials in Puerto Rico due to ongoing recovery efforts following hurricanes Irma and Maria.

interviewedCDC officials regarding any changes the agency has made to its plans for awarding funding in the future.

We conducted this performance audit from April 2017 to May 2018 in accordance with generally accepted government auditing standards. Those standards require that we plan and perform the audit to obtain sufficient, appropriate evidence to provide a reasonable basis for our findings and conclusions based on our audit objectives. We believe that the evidence obtained provides a reasonable basis for our findings and conclusions based on our audit objectives.

BACKGROUND

During a disease outbreak, including the Zika virus, HHS is the lead federal agency for public health and medical response, and it leverages national public health and medical resources to prepare for and respond to the outbreak.[8]

Zika Virus Transmission and Prevention

The Zika virus is primarily transmitted to humans by infected mosquitoes, but can also be transmitted from mother to child during pregnancy or around the time of birth, or from person-to-person through sexual contact or blood transfusion. According to CDC, once an individual has been infected with the Zika virus, they are likely to be protected from future infections. The *Aedes aegypti* mosquitoes are reportedly the primary mosquito spreading the Zika virus, while the *Aedes albopictus* mosquitoes, which share many of the same traits as *Aedes aegypti*, also have the ability to spread the virus.[9] Local transmission of the virus has occurred in American Samoa, Florida, Puerto Rico, Texas, and the U.S. Virgin Islands. Travel-associated cases of Zika virus infection have been reported in every state, with the largest numbers of cases reported in California, Florida, New York, and Texas.[10]

---

[8] Within HHS, the Office of the Assistant Secretary for Preparedness and Response leads and coordinates national preparedness and response to outbreaks in the United States. Within that office, BARDA coordinates and supports advanced research and development, manufacturing, and initial procurement of medical countermeasures, such as vaccines, drugs, therapies, and diagnostic tools. CDC monitors and responds to outbreaks by, for example, conducting studies to learn about the link between infection and health outcomes, monitoring and reporting cases of infection, and providing guidance to travelers and health care providers. According to officials, NIH funds and carries out basic and applied research to develop diagnostics, vaccines and therapeutics, as well as epidemiological studies to better understand disease progression and long-term health effects.

[9] Edward B. Hayes, "Zika Virus Outside Africa," Emerging Infectious Diseases, vol.15, no. 9 (2009): 1347–50; and National Science and Technology Council, A Strategy for Integrating Best Practices with New Science to Prevent Disease Transmission by Aedes Mosquito Vectors (Washington, D.C.: December 2016).

[10] CDC's case counts for travel-associated cases of Zika virus infection, by state, also include cases where the Zika virus was transmitted sexually, through a laboratory, and person-to-person through an unknown route.

There is no vaccine to prevent the Zika virus, so CDC guidance recommends preventing the spread of the virus by protecting against mosquito bites by wearing protective clothing, using insect repellant, and staying in places with air conditioning and window and door screens to keep mosquitoes outside, among other actions. Mosquito control in the United States is implemented and overseen at the state and local levels by entities such as mosquito control districts and health agencies. Federal agencies support such control entities with funding and subject matter experts, and may regulate some control methods such as pesticides.

Zika Funding Prior to September 2016

In April 2016, the Office of Management and Budget and the Secretary of Health and Human Services announced that they had identified \$589 million—\$510 million of it from existing Ebola virus disease resources within HHS, the Department of State, and the U.S. Agency for International Development—that could quickly be redirected and spent on immediate efforts to control and respond to the spread of the Zika virus. According to HHS, out of the \$589 million, \$374 million was redirected to domestic Zika virus control activities. HHS reports that almost all of this funding (\$354 million) was distributed to three HHS agencies, as follows:

- CDC received \$222 million for various activities including field staff, state response teams, Zika virus testing, tracking of pregnant women who were infected with the Zika virus, and grants for mosquito control and other Zika prevention activities;
- BARDA received \$85 million for private sector development of Zika vaccines, treatments, and technologies to protect the blood supply, and other countermeasures; and
- NIH received \$47 million for Zika medical countermeasure development, including clinical trials on the leading Zika vaccine candidate.

Additionally, according to HHS officials, in August 2016, the Secretary of Health and Human Services notified Congress of the department's intent to redirect an additional \$81 million in unobligated HHS funds for Zika vaccine development activities. Of this amount, \$34 million was drawn from accounts at NIH and \$47 million was drawn from funds transferred from other HHS agencies and reprogrammed from within PHSSEF.[11]

---

[11] Reprogramming is the shifting of funds within an appropriation or account to use them for purposes other than those contemplated at the time of appropriation; it is the shifting of funds from one object class to another or from one program activity to another. See GAO, *A Glossary of Terms Used in the Federal Budget Process*, GAO-05-734SP (Washington, D.C.: Sept. 1, 2005).

From these redirected funds, $34 million (i.e., the amount drawn from other NIH accounts) was to be used by NIH to continue clinical trials on its lead Zika vaccine candidate. The remaining $47 million was to be used by BARDA for continued private sector Zika vaccine development.

September 2016 Zika Supplemental Funding

In September 2016, Congress appropriated $932 million to HHS and its agencies in the Zika Response and Preparedness Act. Of that amount, $394 million was appropriated directly to CDC and $152 million was appropriated directly to NIH. The remainder was appropriated to HHS's PHSSEF, from which HHS allocated $245 million to BARDA within the Office of the Assistant Secretary for Preparedness and Response, $75 million to CMS, and $66 million to HRSA. (See fig. 1.)

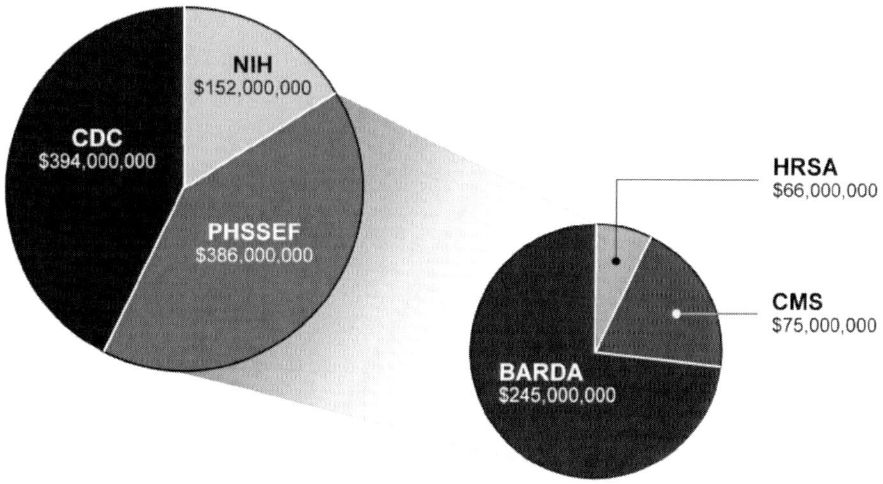

Legend:
BARDA = Biomedical Advanced Research and Development Authority
CDC = Centers for Disease Control and Prevention
CMS = Centers for Medicare & Medicaid Services
HRSA = Health Resources and Services Administration
NIH = National Institutes of Health
PHSSEF = Public Health and Social Services Emergency Fund

Source: Department of Health and Human Services document. | GAO-18-389.
Note: BARDA is within the Office of the Assistant Secretary for Preparedness and Response.

Figure 1. Total Zika Supplemental Funding by Agency.

The Zika supplemental funding remained available for obligation until September 30, 2017, for the following purposes:

- CDC: to prevent, prepare for, and respond to the Zika virus, health conditions related to the virus, and other vector-borne diseases, domestically and internationally.[12]
- NIH: for research on the virology, natural history, and pathogenesis of the Zika virus infection, and preclinical and clinical development of vaccines and other medical countermeasures for the Zika virus and other vector-borne diseases, domestically and internationally.
- respond to the Zika virus, health conditions related to the virus and other vector-borne diseases, domestically and internationally; and to develop necessary countermeasures and vaccines, including the development and purchase of vaccines, therapeutics, diagnostics, necessary medical supplies, and administrative activities.
- BARDA: HHS allocated funding to BARDA to support further development of Zika vaccine candidates, diagnostics, and pathogen reduction technologies initiated in fiscal year 2016 to advance these projects toward licensure or approval by the Food and Drug Administration.
- CMS: HHS allocated funding to CMS for expenses to support states, territories, tribes, or tribal organizations with active or local transmission cases of the Zika virus, as confirmed by CDC. The funding was allocated to reimburse the costs of health care for health conditions related to the Zika virus, other than costs that are covered by private health insurance, of which not less than $60 million were for territories with the highest rates of Zika virus transmission.
- HRSA: HHS allocated $20 million for projects of regional and national significance in Puerto Rico and other U.S. territories, $40 million to expand the delivery of primary health services in Puerto Rico and the other territories, and $6 million to be used to assign National Health Service Corps members to Puerto Rico and the other territories to provide primary health services in areas affected by the Zika virus or other vector-borne diseases through the National Health Service Corps Loan Repayment Program.[13]

Agencies have until September 30, 2022, to disburse the Zika supplemental funding appropriated by the Zika Response and Preparedness Act.

---

[12] Additionally, CDC was directed to use $44 million of the funding appropriated by the Zika Response and Preparedness Act to restore fiscal year 2016 funds that were reprogrammed from the Public Health Emergency Preparedness cooperative agreement program for Zika virus response prior to the act's enactment.

[13] The National Health Service Corps offers financial and other support to primary care providers and sites in underserved communities.

HHS Agencies Have Obligated Nearly All of the Zika Supplemental Funding; Disbursements Are Ongoing

Agencies Obligated Nearly All of Their Zika Supplemental Funding as of September 30, 2017, Primarily Through Cooperative Agreements, Grants, and Contracts

We found that as of September 30, 2017—the end of the Zika supplemental appropriation's period of availability—nearly all Zika supplemental funding had been obligated, primarily through cooperative agreements, grants, and contracts.[14] BARDA obligated 100 percent of its Zika supplemental funding, while CDC, CMS, HRSA, and NIH obligated over 99 percent of their funding.[15] (See table 1.)

Table 1. Zika supplemental funding obligations as of September 30, 2017

HHS agency	In dollars (rounded)		
	Total supplemental funding	Amount obligated	Unobligated balance
Biomedical Advanced Research and Development Authority (BARDA)	245,000,000	245,000,000	0
Centers for Disease Control and Prevention	394,000,000	393,706,358	293,642
Centers for Medicare & Medicaid Services	75,000,000	74,982,493	17,508
Health Resources and Services Administration	66,000,000	65,978,442	21,558
National Institutes of Health	152,000,000	151,998,591	1,409
Total	932,000,000	931,665,883	334,117

Source: GAO analysis of Department of Health and Human Services (HHS) data. | GAO-18-389.

Note: BARDA is within the Office of the Assistant Secretary for Preparedness and Response.

Three of the five agencies had obligated over half of their Zika supplemental funding by January 31, 2017, 4 months after enactment of the appropriation. For example, according to CDC officials, using cooperative agreements with application processes familiar to the awardees helped enable the agency to obligate its funding soon after receiving the appropriation.[16] Some agencies began obligating later in the one-year obligation time frame based on their approach to obligating the Zika supplemental

[14] A cooperative agreement is an alternative assistance instrument used instead of a grant whenever substantial federal involvement with the recipient during performance is anticipated. For grants, an agency's involvement is essentially administrative, which includes standard federal stewardship responsibilities, such as reviewing performance to ensure that the objectives, terms, and conditions of the grant are accomplished.

[15] These unobligated balances are not available after September 30, 2017, to incur new obligations. However, agencies can use unobligated balances to correct errors in recording obligations properly incurred during the period of availability or to cover legitimate cost adjustments in future years, such as those that may arise from contract modifications within the general scope of a prior year contract.

[16] Although CDC generally used existing mechanisms familiar to awardees, agency officials explained that the application process still needed to be completed—from creating and publishing notices of funding opportunities to issuing notices of award—prior to the obligation of funding.

funding. For example, CMS withheld a portion of its supplemental funds in the event additional awardees became eligible for funding within the obligation time frame—eligibility included having active or local transmission of the Zika virus.

Agency officials told us that they used cooperative agreements, grants, and contracts to award Zika supplemental funding to existing and new awardees. The agencies also used other mechanisms to obligate the Zika supplemental funding, such as interagency agreements, intramural research awards, and funding used within the agency for travel and other expenses.[17] According to officials, agencies used these mechanisms to award Zika supplemental funding in the following ways.

- BARDA executed new contracts and modified existing contracts through the agency's typical contracting process, officials said, for research in the areas of Zika clinical diagnostics and vaccine development. BARDA did not use any Zika supplemental funding to support internal administrative or personnel costs. (See app. I for the contracts BARDA awarded with its Zika supplemental funding.)
- CDC generally obligated Zika supplemental funding to current awardees through existing cooperative agreements, according to agency officials. (See app. II through VII for the cooperative agreements CDC used to award Zika supplemental funding to existing awardees.) CDC also awarded funding through contracts and interagency agreements, and obligated about $24 million for internal CDC expenses, such as salaries and benefits, travel, supplies, and equipment. (See app. VIII for the contracts and interagency agreements CDC awarded with its Zika supplemental funding.)
- CMS created a new program—the Zika Health Care Services Program—to award its Zika supplemental funding through cooperative agreements, according to agency officials. The purpose of the 3-year program is to support prevention activities and treatment services for women (including pregnant women), children, and men adversely or potentially affected by the Zika virus.[18] CMS awarded funding through the Zika Health Care Services Program to those states, territories, tribes, or tribal organizations with active or local transmission of the Zika virus, as confirmed by CDC. CMS awarded funding to the health departments in American Samoa, Florida, Puerto Rico, and the U.S. Virgin Islands in January 2017. In June 2017, CMS awarded funding to the health

---

[17] Intramural research entails government scientists working in their institutes' and centers' own laboratories and clinics. An interagency agreement occurs when one agency either places an order directly against another agency's contract or uses the contracting services of another agency to obtain supplies or services.

[18] According to CMS documentation, the Zika Health Care Services Program is intended to address four critical components of a comprehensive response to Zika: (1) increase access to contraceptive services for women and men; (2) increase access to and reduce barriers to diagnostic testing, screening, and counseling for pregnant women and newborns; (3) increase access to appropriate specialized health care services for pregnant women, children born to mothers with maternal Zika virus infection, and their families; and (4) improve provider capacity and capability. Awardee needs may vary and some awardees may not have unmet needs across each of the four areas.

department in Texas, the only new state or territory with local transmission of the Zika virus.[19] In both CMS award rounds, only states and territories received awards, because they were the only areas with active or local transmission of the Zika virus. CMS retained about $3.6 million of the Zika supplemental funding to use for administrative support services, as well as for travel for monitoring and oversight. (See app. IX for the awards CMS made with its Zika supplemental funding.)

- HRSA generally obligated Zika supplemental funding through grants to existing awardees, according to agency officials. HRSA did not retain any Zika supplemental funding for internal activities. (See app. X for the grants HRSA awarded.)
- NIH used grants and contracts to award its Zika supplemental funding to new and existing awardees. NIH also used about $95 million of the Zika supplemental funding for internal activities—studies conducted by NIH researchers. According to NIH officials, the somewhat unique aspects of the Zika virus as an arbovirus infectious disease led NIH to focus on vaccines as a priority, along with development of diagnostics, therapeutics, vector control, and surveillance.[20] (See app. XI for NIH's Zika supplemental awards.)

Officials from all five agencies cited coordination initiatives through regular interagency or organizational teleconferences and participation in working groups. According to CMS officials, during the Zika virus response, CDC, CMS, HRSA, and other federal partners held interagency Zika coordination calls to discuss ongoing developments related to the Zika virus. Additionally, because CMS and HRSA were both awarding funding for perinatal health care services, officials said they collaborated to ensure that activities available through the CMS grants complemented the activities available through HRSA's Special Projects of Regional and National Significance. In addition, HRSA officials reported conducting joint site visits with CDC and CMS, as well as streamlining reporting requirements to reduce grantee reporting burden. Furthermore, BARDA officials said that they awarded and administered a contract for CDC on the development of a vector control product. CDC provided the funding and topical subject matter expertise for the award, and BARDA provided management services for the contract, because of BARDA's experience with these types of contracts. BARDA and NIH officials also reported collaborating on vaccine development. BARDA officials explained that while the vaccine development process requires that different agencies

---

[19] According to officials, CMS issued supplemental awards to each of the five grantees in September 2017, using additional remaining funds.

[20] Arthropod-borne viruses (arboviruses) are transmitted to humans primarily through the bites of infected mosquitoes and ticks.

support multiple vaccine development candidates, the two agencies coordinated to avoid redundancy.

Agencies Had Disbursed About 21 Percent of the Zika Supplemental Funding as of December 31, 2017

We found that as of December 31, 2017, the HHS agencies had disbursed about 21 percent (approximately $195.5 million of $932 million) of the Zika supplemental funding. According to agency officials and selected awardees we spoke with, various factors can affect the disbursement of funding after obligation. These factors include time to draw down funding from the federal agencies, allowing for program implementation and a planning period, and awardees' internal administrative processes and unique characteristics, as described below.

Drawdown Procedures

CDC officials said that awardees draw down federal funding on their individual schedules based upon how they manage their federal funding. Some awardees draw down on a daily basis, as needed, while others draw down on a biweekly or monthly basis. Additionally, drawdowns for personnel costs coincide with payroll schedules, which could be biweekly or monthly. For example, in the case of monthly payroll, two awardees told us that the federal funding for a particular month's expenses would be drawn down the following month. Furthermore, selected awardees we spoke with said that they draw down federal funding after they have incurred an expense, such as when they receive an invoice. For example, Los Angeles County officials reported that in order to draw down the funds for the organization that is responsible for servicing their vector control activities, they have to first receive an invoice from the organization, which the county pays with its own funds. Only then can the county draw down the federal funding. This process usually results in at least a 3-month period between receiving the invoice and drawing down the federal funding, officials said.

Program Implementation and Planning Period

According to CMS officials, the agency awarded funding to health departments in American Samoa, Florida, Puerto Rico, Texas, and the U.S. Virgin Islands from the Zika Health Care Services Program, which was a new collaboration between CMS and these specific awardees. The officials said that the steps awardees needed to take to stand-up new programs—such as budget review and approval processes, selection of key personnel to administer the grant, grant activities related to contracting, and hiring and procurement—can delay start-up and implementation of the grant programs.

Additionally, CMS gave awardees in the Zika Health Care Services Program a 3-month planning period after they received their notices of award to amend their activities.[21] For example, Texas officials reported that they used the 3-month planning period to work on executing contracts with the local health departments in three counties bordering Mexico. Texas officials explained that collaborating with the local health departments entailed determining the greatest potential benefit of the use of the funds, because the award itself was not enough to cover all of the costs of direct health care services associated with the Zika virus.

Awardees' Processes and Characteristics

Local administrative processes for spending federal supplemental funds can result in varied disbursement time frames. For example, California received Zika supplemental funding for an award that required an amendment to an administrative contract, which state officials said takes about 7 to 8 months for internal state approval. Additionally, certain awardees' characteristics affect disbursements. For example, Houston officials said the city was eligible for and was directly awarded a CDC cooperative agreement, but because it does not conduct vector control activities itself, the city had to negotiate a contract with the surrounding county to conduct these activities, adding additional time before it could begin disbursements.

Officials also noted that awardees' personnel hiring issues can affect disbursement time frames. For example, CMS officials said that some territories experienced delays in carrying out activities due to provider shortages, particularly among specialists needed to care for children with developmental delays and birth defects caused by the Zika virus. CMS officials noted that island jurisdictions, such as the U.S. territories, can find hiring more difficult due to a shortage of health care professionals available within the territory, thus requiring individuals to be recruited from outside the territory, which adds time to the process and raises costs. In addition, Florida officials in Miami-Dade County reported that the necessary staff surge during the Zika response was challenging to fill, noting that it was particularly difficult to find phlebotomists and nurses, because they were in high demand.[22]

---

[21] CMS provided awardees with a 3-month planning period to fine tune the request for all specific activities funded under the award. CMS officials said that they provided this period because there was a limited time provided to submit an application due to the Zika virus being a public health emergency. According to CMS officials, the 3-month planning period enabled awardees to fully analyze and identify a comprehensive set of needs, to fine tune the request for all specific activities funded under the award; to begin the process for staffing, contracting, establishing reimbursement methodologies, and other procurement efforts; to ensure that CMS funding is coordinated with funding from other federal agencies; and to ensure non-duplication of funding from all sources.

[22] A phlebotomist is an individual trained to draw blood for tests, transfusions, research, or blood donations.

Standard vaccine development processes also influenced the rate of disbursement. Due to the long duration of the vaccine development process, BARDA officials said, disbursements to certain awardees have occurred at varying intervals. For example, some contract invoices are received on a monthly basis, or twice a month if the company is a small business. The invoices are then reviewed and if deemed acceptable, they are processed for payment.

The 2017 hurricane season may have affected certain awardees' use of their Zika supplemental funding, which prompted agencies to respond by approving various types of short-term relief for administrative, financial management, and audit requirements for awardees affected by the hurricanes. Three agencies—CDC, CMS, and HRSA—awarded Zika supplemental funding to areas affected by hurricanes Harvey, Irma, and Maria in 2017: Florida, Puerto Rico, Texas, and the U.S. Virgin Islands. CDC officials told us, for example, that because of the hurricanes they granted extensions at the request of the awardees for submitting financial and progress reports, and continuation of activities. Similarly, CMS offered hurricane-affected awardees of the Zika Health Care Services Program the option to extend the deadline for deliverables, if necessary. CMS officials told us that grant activities had been affected by the hurricanes, and all grantees had communicated the intent to fully resume activities as soon as they are able to do so. Due to the 3-year project period for grantees, CMS officials said that the affected entities can still accomplish programmatic responsibilities, even if there is a temporary halt in project activities. Furthermore, HRSA officials said that they provided Puerto Rico and the U.S. Virgin Islands with extensions on required program, financial, and audit reports.[23]

Selected Awardees Undertook Multiple Activities with Zika Supplemental Funding, and Had Varying Experiences Applying for and Managing Funds

Selected Awardees Used Zika Supplemental Funding for Activities Including Surveillance, Vector Control, Laboratory Capacity, and Health Care Services

Selected awardees we spoke with used Zika supplemental funding for a variety of activities. Collectively, the activities included four primary types: medical surveillance,

[23] On October 26, 2017, the Office of Management and Budget released a memorandum to federal agencies with guidance for administrative relief for grantees affected by hurricanes Harvey, Irma, and Maria. Under certain circumstances, agencies could provide flexibility with application deadlines, provide no-cost extensions on expiring awards, allow expenditure of award funds for salaries and other project activities, and waive prior approval requirement waivers, among other actions.

vector control, laboratory capacity building, and providing health care services, as described below.[24]

- Medical surveillance activities include identifying and reporting Zika virus disease cases to CDC, as well as reporting Zika virus infections in pregnant women and infants to the U.S. Zika Pregnancy Registry.[25]
- Vector control activities include detecting and monitoring *Aedes aegypti* and *Aedes albopictus* mosquito distribution and mosquito control, and monitoring of insecticide resistance and management.
- Laboratory capacity building activities include developing laboratory capacity to perform Zika virus testing.
- Health care service activities for those selected awardees that received funding from CMS (Florida and Texas) included increasing access to contraceptive services for men and women; increasing access to and reducing barriers to diagnostic testing, screening, and counseling for pregnant women and newborns; and increasing access to appropriate specialized health care services for pregnant women, children born to mothers with maternal Zika virus infection, and their families.

Table 2 provides examples of the types of activities funded by the selected awardees we interviewed. This table does not include a comprehensive list of all of the awardees' Zika activities—see appendixes II through VI, and appendix IX for more information on the Zika supplemental funding CDC and CMS awarded to states, territories, and local jurisdictions.

Of the awardees we spoke with, Florida and Texas were the only states that had experienced local mosquito-borne transmission of the Zika virus. Other selected awardees—which included Arizona, Los Angeles County, and Louisiana—were primarily responding to travel-related cases of Zika virus disease. The following are additional examples of activities funded using Zika supplemental funding. For more information on the types of activities authorized under each award, see appendixes II-VI and IX.

---

[24] The selected awardees we spoke with are Alaska; Arizona; California; Colorado; Florida; Iowa; Kansas; Louisiana; Oklahoma; and Texas; as well as Houston, Tex., and Los Angeles County, Calif.

[25] CDC collaborated with state, tribal, local, and territorial health departments to establish the U.S. Zika Pregnancy Registry as an enhanced national surveillance system to monitor pregnancy and fetal/infant outcomes among pregnancies with laboratory evidence of possible recent Zika virus infection. The U.S. Zika Pregnancy Registry includes data from all 50 states, Washington, D.C., and all U.S. territories except Puerto Rico; pregnancies in Puerto Rico are monitored separately by the Zika Active Pregnancy Surveillance System.

Table 2. Examples of activities of selected awardees that received direct Zika supplemental funding from CDC and CMS

Awardee	Funding received, in dollars, by award type	Examples of activities
Alaska	ELC: 36,867	Alaska's Zika activities include ensuring that procedures are in place to assist in the monitoring of potential Zika cases among pregnant women and their infants; and overseeing the development and dissemination of outreach materials.
Arizona	ELC: 5,161,956 Birth defects: 200,000 BRFSS: 26,000 PHPR: 388,273	Arizona's activities include using a Zika Pregnancy Registry coordinator to assist the local health jurisdictions with interviewing patients, contacting providers, and ensuring timely follow-up for individuals at critical points in time for data collection, as well as transmitting the data to CDC in a timely fashion. Additionally, Arizona officials said that funding will be used for prevention efforts, including producing materials, such as posters, to hand out at events.
California	ELC: 12,496,481 Birth defects: 360,000 PHPR: 2,658,839	California's Zika activities include providing consultation, training, and operational support to detect, monitor, and control Aedes aegypti and Aedes albopictusmosquitoes; providing on-site technical assistance inthe event of local transmission; and conducting field-based pesticide resistance testing. According to state officials, California is also conducting education and outreach activities.
Colorado	ELC: 230,065	Colorado's Zika activities include using staff to build and maintain relationships necessary for long-term follow-up of patients and consistent data transmission to the U.S. Zika Pregnancy Registry.
Florida	ELC: 38,298,440 Birth defects: 360,000 BRFSS: 124,976 PHPR: 4,999,979 PRAMS: 40,000 CMS: 2,991,000	Florida's Zika activities include supporting the prevention of active transmission of Zika through source reduction, communication, and control, including the application of ground adulticide treatments, ground larvicide treatments, and aerial adulticide treatments. Additionally, staff will support Zika epidemiology and outreach projects, including involvement with active surveillance, response to any local introductions, follow-up with potentially Zika infected infants, as well as assistance with development and distribution of Zika and mosquito bite prevention outreach to targeted audiences.

Awardee	Funding received, in dollars, by award type	Examples of activities
Houston, Texas	ELC: 2,475,899 Birth defects: 199,804	Houston's Zika activities include providing staff to improve surveillance to monitor the incidence of women and infants who meet the U.S. Zika Pregnancy Registry case definition, identify and report all data to the registry in a timely manner, increase provider support and education, and gather follow-up clinical data on infants to identify developmental delays. According to city officials, Houston also will use the funding for education and outreach, to investigate all reports of suspected Zika exposure and infection, to establish and provide Zika testing for the 16 counties served by the Houston Health Department Bureau of Laboratory Services, and to partner with Harris County, Texas, for vector control activities.
Iowa	ELC: 372,847	According to state officials, Iowa's Zika activities include surveillance and case follow-up.
Kansas	ELC: 85,658	According to state officials, Kansas' Zika activities include staff to work on submitting data to the U.S. Zika Pregnancy Registry, and to follow-up on pregnant women and infants.
Los Angeles County, California	ELC: 1,750,283 Birth defects: 360,000 PHPR: 504,855	Los Angeles County's Zika activities include assigning staff to conduct Zika testing and prepare testing reports, including distinguishing Zika from chikungunya and dengue infections. According to county officials,Los Angeles County also developed hospital protocols and conducted patient tracking and follow-up with pregnant women.
Louisiana	ELC: 3,559,243 Birth defects: 200,000 BRFSS: 100,000 PHPR: 1,437,361	Louisiana's Zika activities include staff to provide outreach to obstetricians and pediatricians in the state to disseminate information regarding the U.S. Zika Pregnancy Registry, proper diagnosis and clinical management of Zika, and how to participate in the registry; andfollow-up with health care providers and patients to collect clinical information at designated time intervals on pregnant women and infants meeting the registry inclusion criteria from the point of case identification through 12 months after delivery. According to state officials, Louisiana also added Zika exposure as a risk factor for hearing loss to the state's newborn hearing screening form, and addedcongenital Zika virus as a maternal risk factor on the state's birth certificate application.

Table 2. (Continued)

Awardee	Funding received, in dollars, by award type	Examples of activities
Oklahoma	ELC: 18,121 Birth defects: 108,262	According to state officials, Oklahoma added congenital Zika virus disease (including congenital Zika syndrome) as an automatic qualifier for the Sooner Start Early Intervention program.
Texas	ELC: 18,654,908 Birth defects: 360,000 BRFSS: 124,854 PHPR: 5,000,000 CMS: 2,491,000	According to state officials, Texas' Zika activities include awareness and education of the state's population about Zika risks and prevention; funding to local health departments for surveillance, case investigation, and vector control; providing education and outreach to health care providers to improve the quality of the data within the U.S.Zika Pregnancy Registry; and providing pesticide resistance training. Most of the laboratory funding is used by state-run or associated laboratories.

Legend:
CDC = Centers for Disease Control and Prevention.
CMS = Centers for Medicare & Medicaid Services.
ELC = Epidemiology and Laboratory Capacity for Infectious Diseases cooperative agreement.
Birth defects = Surveillance, Intervention, and Referral to Services Activities for Infants with Microcephaly or other Adverse Outcomes Linked with the Zika Virus cooperative agreement.
BRFSS = Behavioral Risk Factor Surveillance System cooperative agreement.
PHPR = Public Health Preparedness and Response Cooperative Agreement for All-Hazards Public Health Emergencies PRAMS = Pregnancy Risk Assessment Monitoring System cooperative agreement.
Source: CDC, CMS, and awardee documentation, and interviews with state, county, and city officials. | GAO-18-389.

Florida

Florida, which has a centralized health department with county-based offices, used Zika supplemental funding for laboratory capacity and vector control activities, among other activities. According to state officials, funding for state-run laboratories was used for purchasing materials, such as those used for testing urine for the Zika virus, and funding staff located in counties to assist with handling Zika samples and testing, data entry, and result reporting to surveillance networks. Additionally, Florida used Zika supplemental funding for local vector control activities. For example, Miami-Dade County officials said that they purchased mosquito traps and removed mosquito breeding grounds, including plants, tires, and other objects that can hold standing water. (See fig. 2 for examples of the mosquito control activities in Miami-Dade County.)

Through CMS's Zika Health Care Services Program, Florida received funding for, among other things, two part-time advanced registered nurse practitioners to provide consultation and technical assistance in family planning clinics, and assist in the prescribing and management of various birth control methods. Florida also funded a health educator for Zika prevention and response duties, which included assisting local health care organizations in the development of educational programming to ensure that health care services are provided in accordance with CDC guidelines. The health educator's duties also included ensuring that pregnant women with the Zika virus and infants with congenital Zika infection are referred to proper care and other available programs and resources.

Mosquito "Flowerpot" Trap

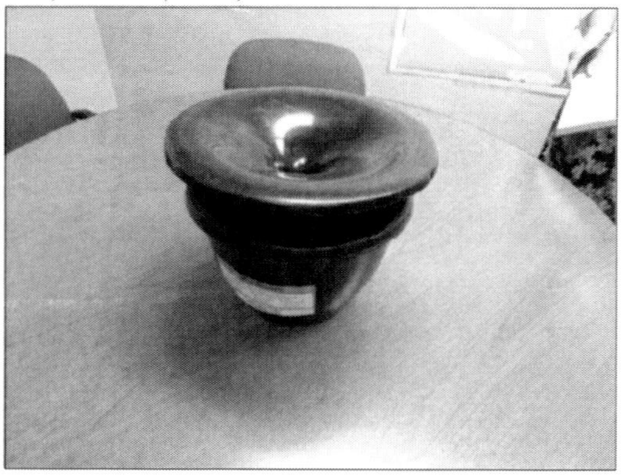

Employment of mosquito control traps: According to officials, Miami-Dade Mosquito Control Division employs a mosquito control trap that resembles a flower pot and uses larvicide on a floating gauze strip to kill mosquitoes and prevent their offspring from hatching or fully maturing. As of August 2017, there were about 300 of these traps in use by the agency in the areas of Miami-Dade County with identified Zika virus transmission.

Bromeliad plants

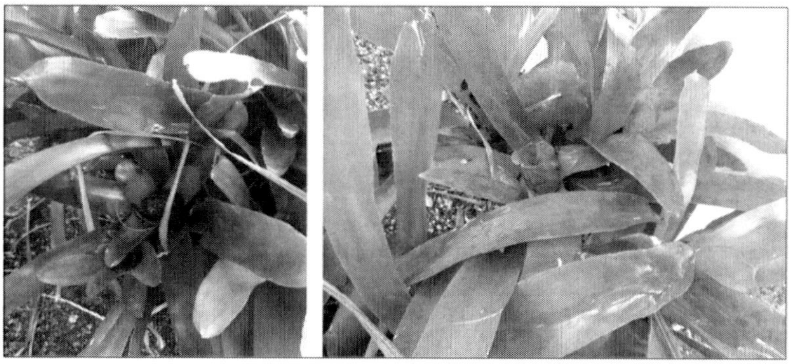

Removal of Bromeliad plants: According to officials, the Bromeliad—a member of the pineapple family that flourishes in tropical climates—is common throughout the Miami area in both public and residential areas. Bromeliads were a source of significant mosquito breeding in the Miami Beach botanical gardens, which had thousands of the plants; all of the plants were removed from the gardens in a two-day period.

Source: Interviews with officials in Miami-Dade County, Florida. | GAO-18-389.

Figure 2. Examples of Vector Control Activities in Miami-Dade County, Florida.

Texas

Texas officials said that the state used a CDC award to rapidly identify cases and conduct data analysis of Zika-related birth defects, to enhance surveillance of Zika virus-related birth defects by improving the Texas Birth Defects Registry database, and to facilitate remote access to electronic records. Texas also disseminated prevention materials and interviewed mothers of children with Zika-related birth defects about their experience in dealing with the health system in order to help identify developmental outcomes of the children.

Texas intends to use its CMS Zika Health Care Services Program funding—awarded on June 30, 2017—to increase clients' access to contraceptives; for care management, including counseling on Zika virus testing for pregnant women and their families; and for counseling to refer clients for services and support. State officials provided the following information on some of the activities intended for the program.

1. Increasing clients' access to contraceptives: Community health workers and case management staff will assist clinic providers with informing women and their partners about contraceptive availability and about the potential Zika virus risks during pregnancy. They will also work with the women to determine what messages work best with their partners regarding contraceptives.
2. Care management that includes pre- and post-test counseling on Zika virus testing for pregnant women and their families: Officials said that this activity is important because the CDC testing algorithm is complex, the results from various tests can be confusing, and there can be false positives from the tests. Generally, doctors do not have the time to go through the complexities of these issues with clients, such as how to understand the laboratory tests and results.
3. Counseling to refer clients for services and supports: This can include counseling about various types of resources to support clients pre-delivery, after delivery, and during the infant's first year of life.

Arizona

According to state officials, Zika supplemental funding was used to create an action plan with counties, and increase the state's ability to raise public awareness about the threat of the Zika virus, its transmission routes, and prevention measures. Officials stated that Arizona's border with Mexico makes communicating about Zika more complex, because individuals frequently cross the border for a variety of reasons including work, school, and to visit family, and do not necessarily consider themselves to be travelers. Additionally, the state used funding to increase the amount of personal protective equipment for the vector surveillance staff, and set up vector control contracts that could be accessed if the Zika virus spread locally, and in the event that vector control could not be handled at the local level. However, this contracting mechanism was not used, because there was no local transmission of the Zika virus in Arizona. According to state officials, Arizona plans to ask for an extension to use the funding in the next mosquito season. The state health department also sponsored training on mosquito identification.

Los Angeles County

County officials said that some funding was used to support personnel involved with Zika surveillance, testing, and case management. This included the detection of cases—individuals diagnosed with Zika infection—and also the dissemination of information to Los Angeles County's Maternal and Child Health group, which follows pregnant women through delivery and then transfers the cases to the county's Children's Medical Services group. For example, according to officials, once a case is identified, information is shared with the relevant vector control district about the location of the case, and the vector control district can then conduct inspection and abatement activities to reduce the risk of a local outbreak. Los Angeles County officials found that this process takes about one week from finding out about a case to completion of inspection and abatement. This included 1 day to get information to the vector control district and 1 to 5 days for completing inspection and abatement. The funding was also used to provide funds to the vector control districts to augment *Aedes* mosquito detection efforts and support outreach activities, according to county officials.

Louisiana

Louisiana officials said they used a CDC award, in part, to provide equipment and mileage reimbursement for nurses, who served as clinical liaisons between the birth defects surveillance program and hospitals and physicians statewide, to help enable rapid surveillance activities.

Awardees also funded other activities, such as outreach campaigns. See figure 3 for examples of outreach funded with Zika supplemental funding.

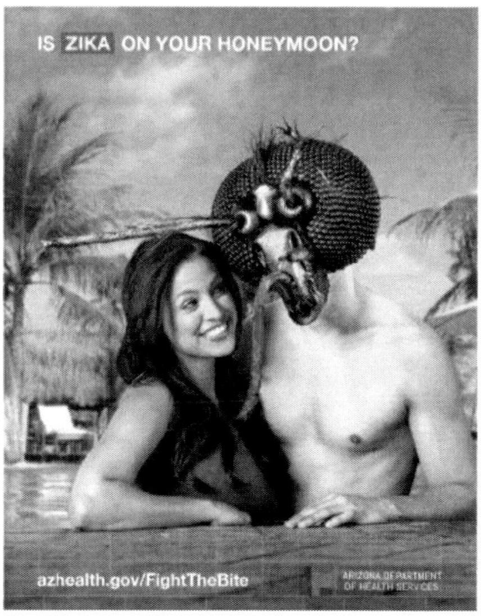

Communication campaign: Arizona Zika supplemental funding was used for prevention efforts, including producing materials to provide at events such as posters and handouts.

Text message campaign: Another health department, the Los Angeles County Department of Public Health, created a free text messaging and web-based public health awareness campaign to educate about and help prevent Zika virus and mosquito-borne infections. Once registered, subscribers received eight messages (two per week for four weeks). The messages covered general information, symptoms and testing, mosquito control, protecting children, travel, and pregnancy.

Source: Interviews with Arizona and Los Angeles County officials; Arizona Department of Health Services. (photo). | GAO-18-389.

Figure 3. Examples of Zika Outreach Activities.

Selected Awardees Had Mixed Experiences Applying for and Managing the Zika Supplemental Funding

While a majority of the 12 selected awardees we spoke with reported positive experiences with the process of applying for and managing the Zika supplemental funding, some awardees cited aspects of the process that were challenging. The awardees we spoke with received much of their supplemental funding from CDC and noted that the process went well: there was good communication with CDC officials; CDC's Epidemiology and Laboratory Capacity for Infectious Diseases cooperative agreement process to apply for Zika supplemental funds was more streamlined than the regular application process; and awardees said they were familiar with the mechanisms, which helped them navigate the process.[26]

Awardees we spoke to also cited some challenges to applying for and managing the Zika supplemental funding. These awardees noted that various time frames among multiple awards and restrictions on authorized activities under the awards added administrative burdens that officials had to deal with while responding to the outbreak. Florida officials said that the state received funding from different federal agencies, from different cooperative agreement awards, with different deadlines, and different rules on what the funding could be used for. For example, CDC distributed Zika supplemental funds to states and certain localities and territories through five cooperative agreements—some of which had multiple application rounds. Florida officials said that they had to track funding separately and identify the activities that could be funded under each award—administrative requirements that were burdensome during an emergency response. Figure 4 presents the period of time Florida had to use the Zika supplemental funding from multiple awards received from CDC.

In addition, awardees we spoke with cited challenges with adjusting their plans when federal funding was more or less than anticipated. For example, CDC officials said that they provided average award amount ranges as guidance for awardees as part of the application process for one of CDC's cooperative agreements.[27] Los Angeles County officials said that they applied for an amount that was near the limit, and county officials said that they had to adjust the activities they planned to fund when they received less than what they applied for. Iowa officials said that without knowing exactly how much funding would be available it was difficult to know what to apply for and made staffing changes difficult. Iowa officials had to adjust their initial plan when they later received additional unexpected funding.

---

[26] Awardees annually apply for and receive funding through CDC's Epidemiology and Laboratory Capacity for Infectious Diseases cooperative agreement. CDC provided additional awards through this cooperative agreement using its Zika supplemental funding.

[27] The approximate award range provided by CDC as guidance for three activities within the cooperative agreement was (1) $0 to $10,000,000; (2) $0 to $6,000,000; and (3) $0 to $550,000.

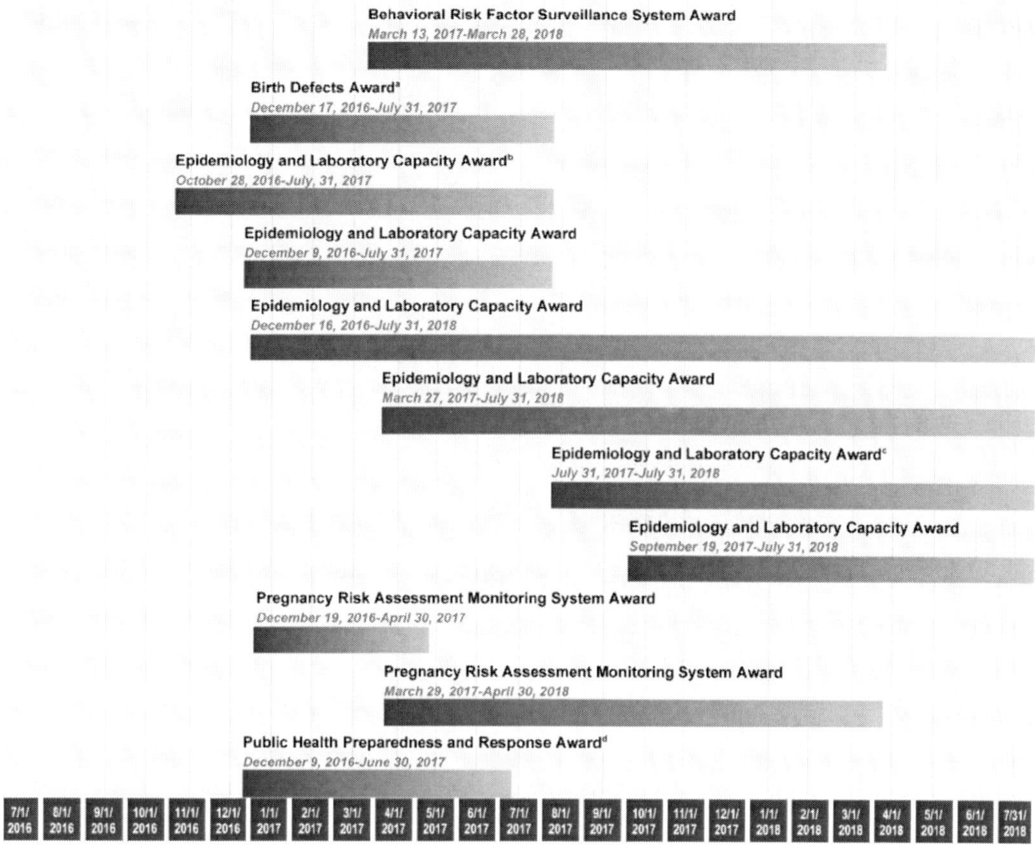

Source: Centers for Disease Control and prevention. | GAO-18-389.

[a] The title of the birth defects award is the Surveillance, Intervention, and Referral to Services Activities for Infants with Microcephaly or other Adverse Outcomes Linked with the Zika Virus award. According to officials from the Centers for Disease Control and Prevention (CDC), Florida received a no-cost extension for this award, which extends the period Florida has to use the funding to July 31, 2019.

[b] The title of this award is the Epidemiology and Laboratory Capacity for Infectious Diseases award.

[c] For this Epidemiology and Laboratory Capacity for Infectious Diseases award, CDC officials said that Florida could not begin using the funding until August 1, 2017.

[d] The title of this award is the Public Health Preparedness and Response Cooperative Agreement for All-Hazards Public Health Emergencies. According to CDC officials, Florida received a no-cost extension for this award, which extends the period Florida has to use the funding to June 30, 2018.

Figure 4. Timeline of Florida's Zika Supplemental Funding Awards.

In October 2017, CDC issued a new notice of funding opportunity that, according to agency officials, was intended to help minimize the administrative burden on these awardees (e.g., preparing applications and other paperwork) during significant public health emergencies by pre-approving public health departments in these jurisdictions to rapidly receive future awards.[28] This new notice of funding opportunity will be used to establish a list of awardees, with existing emergency preparedness and response capacity, that would be pre-approved for funding by CDC when a public health threat occurs, including infectious disease threats.[29] It requires that awardees have structures and plans in place to receive funding, as well as plans to respond to a public health threat. According to CDC officials, awards could potentially be provided within 2 weeks to pre-approved awardees after supplemental appropriations are enacted. According to CDC officials, as of February 2018, the agency had approved all 64 applicants for the notice of funding opportunity.[30] This means that CDC will consider these approved applicants for future funding if an emergency occurs and funding becomes available.

Agency and Third-Party Comments

We provided a draft of this chapter to HHS for review and comment. HHS provided technical comments, which we incorporated as appropriate.

We also provided relevant draft portions of this chapter to the Zika supplemental funding awardees we interviewed. Specifically, we provided the excerpts to officials in Alaska; Arizona; California; Colorado; Florida; Houston, Texas; Iowa; Kansas; Los Angeles County, California; Louisiana; Oklahoma; and Texas. All but one awardee responded. Awardees provided technical comments, which we incorporated as appropriate.

We are sending copies of this chapter to the appropriate congressional committees, the Secretary of Health and Human Services, and to other interested parties.

Marcia Crosse
Director,
Health Care

[28] According to CDC officials, they began thinking about creating the notice of funding opportunity during the 2009 H1N1 response.

[29] The notice of funding opportunity is open to all of CDC's Epidemiology and Laboratory Capacity for Infectious Diseases (ELC) and Public Health Emergency Preparedness awardees, as well as five tribes, which CDC defines as federally or state recognized American Indian or Alaska Native tribal governments serving a population of at least 50,000 members.

[30] According to CDC officials, as of December 2017, all of the ELC and Public Health Emergency Preparedness awardees had applied, but no tribes had applied. Agency officials told us that they were contacting the tribes to ensure they were aware of the opportunity. They also said that the application process for the notice of funding opportunity will be reopened at a later date and eligible tribes that are interested in applying will have the opportunity to do so at that time.

APPENDIX I: BIOMEDICAL ADVANCED RESEARCH AND DEVELOPMENT AUTHORITY'S ZIKA SUPPLEMENTAL AWARDS

The Biomedical Advanced Research and Development Authority (BARDA), within the Department of Health and Human Services' Office of the Assistant Secretary for Preparedness and Response, executed contracts to obligate its Zika supplemental funding for research in the areas of (1) vaccine development, (2) diagnostic development, and (3) pathogen reduction systems.

Table 3 presents information for each award as it was provided to us by BARDA.

Table 3. Biomedical advanced research and development authority's Zika supplemental funding contracts

Awardee	Activity description	Award (in dollars)
Battelle	Battelle will develop a passive transfer murinemodel to evaluate Zika vaccines.	1,468,809
Battelle	Battelle will conduct natural history studies for Zika infections in NHPs.	2,383,446
Cerus Corp[a]	This project will advance the INTERCEPT Blood System for pathogen reduction in donated red blood cells. It is already licensed and marketed for use platelets and plasma. The INTERCEPT Blood System is designed to reduce the risk of transfusion-transmitted infections by inactivating a broad range of pathogens such as viruses, bacteria, and parasites that may be present in donated blood. As a part of this project, a Phase 3 clinical study to evaluate safety and efficacy in acute care is being conducted in Puerto Rico.	57,421,416
InBios International Inc.	InBios is developing 2 different Zika IgM diagnostic tests under this contact, a semi-automated test for use in clinical laboratories, which is available under Emergency Use Authorization (EUA), and an easy-to-use lateral flow test for use in point of care settings. Development of both tests are funded through EUA to FDA 510(K) filing.	4,354,808
Moderna Therapeutics Inc[a]	Moderna is presently conducting a Phase 1 trial at three different clinical sites across the U.S. (first and second cohorts have been fully immunized) for an investigational mRNA Zika vaccine. Enrollment continues, and immunogenicity data (unblinded) from this study is expected later this year. Work is also ongoing at Moderna to scale up manufacturing in preparation for a large Phase 2/3 trial to initiate soon after the Phase 1 trial is completed in 2017.	109,112,211
Orasure Technologies Inc.	Orasureis developing a point of care Zika IgM diagnostic test for use in informing the care of pregnant women. The test is an easy-to-use lateral flow test. Development of data to support consideration by the FDA for an Emergency Use Authorization and continued development through FDA 510(K) clearance is included in the contract.	2,612,925
Sanofi Pasteur Inc[b]	Sanofi will complete Zika defined preclinical vaccine development activities. In addition, the Zika case definition study is being conducted in Central and South America. (As of 22 September 2017, 1,131 subjects have been enrolled).	7,500,000

Table 3. (Continued)

Awardee	Activity description	Award (in dollars)
Siemens Healthcare Diagnostics Inc.	Siemens is developing a laboratory Zika IgM blood test for use on 3 automated platforms in their Centaur product line. These are high throughput fully automated blood analysers. When available, this test will greatly increase the Zika testing capacity in the U.S. BARDA is fund work to support consideration of an Emergency Use Authorization by the FDA and continued development to FDA 510(K) approval.	8,945,785
Takeda Vaccines Inc.[a]	Takeda is developing aZika whole-virus inactivated vaccine which will be adjuvanted with aluminum hydroxide.	51,200,600

Source: Biomedical Advanced Research and Development Authority (BARDA). | GAO-18-389.

[a] This awardee received more than one award and funding amounts for awards for the same awardee and activity were added together in this table.

[b] Prior to September 30, 2017, Sanofi Pasteur decided to no longer develop a Zika vaccine. Non-Zika supplemental funding was de-obligated, according to BARDA officials, but the Zika supplemental funding was maintained by the agency to continue support of a Zika case definition study being conducted in Central and South America.

APPENDIX II: CENTERS FOR DISEASE CONTROL AND PREVENTION— EPIDEMIOLOGY AND LABORATORY CAPACITY FOR INFECTIOUS DISEASES AWARDEES

This appendix presents information on Zika supplemental funding awards made by the Centers for Disease Control and Prevention (CDC) through the Epidemiology and Laboratory Capacity for Infectious Diseases (ELC) cooperative agreement. CDC awarded Zika supplemental funding for the ELC cooperative agreement for the following activities:

- Zika vector surveillance and control,
- Zika epidemiology and laboratory surveillance, and
- U.S. Zika Pregnancy Registry.[31]

The Zika supplemental funding awarded through the ELC cooperative agreement was to further support and strengthen activities to protect the public's health, especially pregnant women, through epidemiologic surveillance and investigation, improving mosquito control and monitoring, and strengthening laboratory capacity. The funding will also support participation in the U.S. Zika Pregnancy Registry to monitor pregnant women with the Zika virus disease and their infants.

For each award, we present information as it was provided to us by CDC, as well as the activities funded. Table 4 provides information on ELC Zika supplemental funding

[31] Not all awardees received funding for each activity.

awarded to states and territories, and table 5 presents information on awards to local health departments.

Table 4. Epidemiology and laboratory capacity for infectious diseases cooperative agreement's Zika supplemental funding for states and territories, by awardee and activity funded

State/territory	Awardee	Activity funded	Award (in dollars)
Alabama	Alabama Department of Public Health	Zika vector surveillance and control	343,980
		Zika epidemiology and laboratory surveillance	584,738
		U.S. Zika Pregnancy Registry	549,996
		Total	1,478,714
Alaska	Alaska State Department of Health & Social Services	Zika epidemiology and laboratory surveillance	14,874
		U.S. Zika Pregnancy Registry	21,993
		Total	36,867
American Samoa	American Samoa Government	Zika vector surveillance and control	180,822
		Zika epidemiology and laboratory surveillance	454,563
		U.S. Zika Pregnancy Registry	136,200
		Total	771,585
Arizona	Arizona Department of Health Services	Zika vector surveillance and control	1,438,817
		Zika epidemiology and laboratory surveillance	3,615,719
		U.S. Zika Pregnancy Registry	107,420
		Total	5,161,956
Arkansas	Arkansas Department of Health	Zika vector surveillance and control	493,698
		Zika epidemiology and laboratory surveillance	129,539
		U.S. Zika Pregnancy Registry	516,579
		Total	1,139,816
California	Public Health Foundation Enterprises (California)	Zika vector surveillance and control	4,285,687
		Zika epidemiology and laboratory surveillance	7,058,745
		U.S. Zika Pregnancy Registry	1,152,049
		Total	12,496,481
Colorado	Colorado Department of Public Health and Environment	Zika epidemiology and laboratory surveillance	163,688
		U.S. Zika Pregnancy Registry	66,377
		Total	230,065
Connecticut	Connecticut State Department of Public Health	Zika epidemiology and laboratory surveillance	175,820
		U.S. Zika Pregnancy Registry	338,526
		Total	514,346

Table 4. (Continued)

State/territory	Awardee	Activity funded	Award (in dollars)
Delaware	Delaware Health & Social Services	Zika epidemiology and laboratory surveillance	12,791
		U.S. Zika Pregnancy Registry	435,759
		Total	448,550
Federated States of Micronesia	Federated States of Micronesia -FSM	Zika vector surveillance and control	68,717
		Zika epidemiology and laboratory surveillance	144,129
		U.S. Zika Pregnancy Registry	120,000
		Total	332,846
Florida	Florida Department of Health	Zika vector surveillance and control	25,590,915
		Zika epidemiology and laboratory surveillance	11,411,188
		U.S. Zika Pregnancy Registry	1,296,337
		Total	38,298,440
Georgia	Georgia Department of Public Health	Zika vector surveillance and control	302,612
		Zika epidemiology and laboratory surveillance	319,435
		U.S. Zika Pregnancy Registry	103,913
		Total	725,960
Guam	Guam Department of Public Health and Social Services	Zika vector surveillance and control	146,700
		Zika epidemiology and laboratory surveillance	299,191
		U.S. Zika Pregnancy Registry	266,201
		Total	712,092
Hawaii	Hawaii State Department of Health	Zika vector surveillance and control	273,306
		Zika epidemiology and laboratory surveillance	987,937
		Total	1,261,243
Illinois	Illinois Department of Public Health	Zika epidemiology and laboratory surveillance	598,160
		U.S. Zika Pregnancy Registry	566,770
		Total	1,164,930
Indiana	Indiana State Department of Health	Zika epidemiology and laboratory surveillance	43,407
		83,111	U.S. Zika Pregnancy Registry
		126,158	Total
Iowa	Iowa Department of Public Health	Zika epidemiology and laboratory surveillance	261,681
		111,166	U.S. Zika Pregnancy Registry
		372,847	Total

State/territory	Awardee	Activity funded	Award (in dollars)
Kansas	Kansas Department of Health and Environment	Zika epidemiology and laboratory surveillance	36,734
		U.S. Zika Pregnancy Registry	48,924
		Total	85,658
Kentucky	Kentucky Cabinet for Health & Family Services	Zika epidemiology and laboratory surveillance	249,384
		U.S. Zika Pregnancy Registry	164,822
		Total	414,206
Louisiana	Louisiana State Office of Public Health	Zika vector surveillance and control	1,450,246
		Zika epidemiology and laboratory surveillance	1,872,956
		U.S. Zika Pregnancy Registry	236,041
		Total	3,559,243
Maine	Maine Department of Health & Human Services	Zika epidemiology and laboratory surveillance	274,351
		U.S. Zika Pregnancy Registry	144,876
		Total	419,227
Marshall Islands	Republic of the Marshall Islands Ministry of Health	Zika vector surveillance and control	119,610
		Zika epidemiology and laboratory surveillance	91,293
		U.S. Zika Pregnancy Registry	83,418
		Total	294,321
Maryland	Maryland Department of Health and Mental Hygiene	Zika vector surveillance and control	137,817
		Zika epidemiology and laboratory surveillance	604,224
		U.S. Zika Pregnancy Registry	453,970
		Total	1,196,011
Massachusetts	Massachusetts Department of Public Health	Zika epidemiology and laboratory surveillance	434,761
		U.S. Zika Pregnancy Registry	546,183
		Total	980,944
Michigan	Michigan Department of Health & Human Services	Zika epidemiology and laboratory surveillance	277,714
		U.S. Zika Pregnancy Registry	218,757
		496,471	Total
Minnesota	Minnesota Department of Health	Zika epidemiology and laboratory surveillance	344,105
		U.S. Zika Pregnancy Registry	95,231
		Total	439,336
Mississippi	Mississippi State Department of Health	Zika vector surveillance and control	1,311,838
		Zika epidemiology and laboratory surveillance	447,215
		U.S. Zika Pregnancy Registry	249,701
		Total	2,008,754
Missouri	Missouri Department of Health & Senior Services	Zika epidemiology and laboratory surveillance	169,373
		U.S. Zika Pregnancy Registry	124,903
		Total	294,276

Table 4. (Continued)

State/territory	Awardee	Activity funded	Award (in dollars)
Montana	Montana State Department of Public Health & Human Services	Zika epidemiology and laboratory surveillance	17,137
Nebraska	Nebraska Department of Health and Human Services	Zika epidemiology and laboratory surveillance	21,073
		U.S. Zika Pregnancy Registry	456,365
		Total	477,438
Nevada	Nevada Division of Public and Behavioral Health	Zika epidemiology and laboratory surveillance	227,645
		U.S. Zika Pregnancy Registry	95,409
		Total	323,054
New Hampshire	New Hampshire Department of Health and Human Services	Zika epidemiology and laboratory surveillance	123,684
		U.S. Zika Pregnancy Registry	114,811
		Total	238,495
New Jersey	New Jersey Department of Health	Zika vector surveillance and control	67,500
		Zika epidemiology and laboratory surveillance	733,627
		U.S. Zika Pregnancy Registry	1,080,245
		Total	1,881,372
New Mexico	New Mexico Department of Health	Zika vector surveillance and control	490,684
		Zika epidemiology and laboratory surveillance	843,826
		U.S. Zika Pregnancy Registry	513,799
		Total	1,848,309
New York	Health Research, Inc. (New York State)	Zika epidemiology and laboratory surveillance	1,469,169
		U.S. Zika Pregnancy Registry	642,324
		Total	2,111,493
North Carolina	North Carolina Department of Health and Human Services	Zika epidemiology and laboratory surveillance	137,539
		U.S. Zika Pregnancy Registry	74,359
		Total	211,898
North Dakota	North Dakota State Department of Health	Zika epidemiology and laboratory surveillance	46,648
Northern Mariana Islands	Commonwealth Healthcare Corporation	Zika vector surveillance and control	16,882
		Zika epidemiology and laboratory surveillance	93,355
		U.S. Zika Pregnancy Registry	97,780
		Total	208,017
Ohio	Ohio State Department of Health	Zika epidemiology and laboratory surveillance	411,193
		U.S. Zika Pregnancy Registry	97,757
		Total	508,950

State/territory	Awardee	Activity funded	Award (in dollars)
Oklahoma	Oklahoma State Department of Health	Zika epidemiology and laboratory surveillance	18,121
Oregon	Oregon Health Authority, Public Health Division	Zika epidemiology and laboratory surveillance	134,598
		U.S. Zika Pregnancy Registry	159,138
		Total	293,736
Palau	Republic of Palau	Zika vector surveillance and control	90,000
		Zika epidemiology and laboratory surveillance	21,401
		U.S. Zika Pregnancy Registry	35,000
		Total	146,401
Pennsylvania	Pennsylvania State Department of Health	Zika epidemiology and laboratory surveillance	700,766
		U.S. Zika Pregnancy Registry	280,035
		Total	980,801
Puerto Rico	Puerto Rico Department of Health	Zika epidemiology and laboratory surveillance	2,038,276
		U.S. Zika Pregnancy Registry	741,967
		Total	2,780,243
Rhode Island	Rhode Island Department of Health	Zika epidemiology and laboratory surveillance	212,557
		U.S. Zika Pregnancy Registry	140,879
		Total	353,436
South Carolina	South Carolina Department of Health and Environmental Control	Zika epidemiology and laboratory surveillance	136,644
		U.S. Zika Pregnancy Registry	283,230
		Total	419,874
South Dakota	South Dakota Department of Health	U.S. Zika Pregnancy Registry	168,893
Tennessee	Tennessee State Department of Health	Zika epidemiology and laboratory surveillance	497,947
		U.S. Zika Pregnancy Registry	550,000
		Total	1,047,947
Texas	Texas Department of State Health Services	Zika vector surveillance and control	3,662,766
		Zika epidemiology and laboratory surveillance	13,978,845
		U.S. Zika Pregnancy Registry	1,013,297
		Total	18,654,908
Utah	Utah Department of Health	Zika epidemiology and laboratory surveillance	206,704
		U.S. Zika Pregnancy Registry	45,242
		Total	251,946
Vermont	Vermont Agency of Human Services	Zika epidemiology and laboratory surveillance	15,661
Virginia	Virginia Department of Health	Zika epidemiology and laboratory surveillance	708,799
		U.S. Zika Pregnancy Registry	189,447
		Total	898,246

Table 4. (Continued)

State/territory	Awardee	Activity funded	Award (in dollars)
U.S. Virgin Islands	Virgin Islands Department of Health	Zika vector surveillance and control	984,690
		Zika epidemiology and laboratory surveillance	865,970
		U.S. Zika Pregnancy Registry	1,169,735
		Total	3,020,395
Washington	Washington State Department of Health	Zika epidemiology and laboratory surveillance	476,691
		U.S. Zika Pregnancy Registry	118,618
		Total	595,309
West Virginia	West Virginia Department of Health and Human Services	Zika epidemiology and laboratory surveillance	168,241
		U.S. Zika Pregnancy Registry	108,262
		Total	276,503
Wisconsin	Wisconsin Department of Health Services	Zika epidemiology and laboratory surveillance	443,218
		U.S. Zika Pregnancy Registry	113,636
		Total	556,854

Source: Centers for Disease Control and Prevention. | GAO-18-389.

In addition to states and territories, six large city and county local health departments—Chicago, the District of Columbia, Houston, Los Angeles County, New York City, and Philadelphia—received ELC Zika supplemental awards.

Table 5. Epidemiology and laboratory capacity for infectious diseases cooperative agreement's Zika supplemental funding for local health departments, by awardee and activity funded

City/county	Awardee	Activity funded	Award (in dollars)
Chicago	City of Chicago Department of Public Health	Zika epidemiology and laboratory surveillance	157,889
		U.S. Zika Pregnancy Registry	182,496
		Total	340,385
District of Columbia	District of Columbia Department of Health	Zika epidemiology and laboratory surveillance	839,959
		U.S. Zika Pregnancy Registry	219,113
		Total	1,059,072
Houston	Houston Department of Health and Human Services	Zika vector surveillance and control	1,250,000
		Zika epidemiology and laboratory surveillance	723,104
		U.S. Zika Pregnancy Registry	502,795
		Total	2,475,899
Los Angeles County	County of Los Angeles Department of Public Health	Zika vector surveillance and control	614,952
		Zika epidemiology and laboratory surveillance	585,331
		U.S. Zika Pregnancy Registry	550,000
		Total	1,750,283

City/county	Awardee	Activity funded	Award (in dollars)
New York City	New York City Department of Health & Mental Hygiene	Zika epidemiology and laboratory surveillance	854,650
		U.S. Zika Pregnancy Registry	521,554
		Total	1,376,204
Philadelphia	Philadelphia Department of Public Health	Zika epidemiology and laboratory surveillance	237,516
		U.S. Zika Pregnancy Registry	215,103
		Total	452,619

Source: Centers for Disease Control and Prevention. | GAO-18-389.

APPENDIX III: CENTERS FOR DISEASE CONTROL AND PREVENTION—BIRTH DEFECTS AWARDEES

This appendix presents information on Zika supplemental funding awards made by the Centers for Disease Control and Prevention (CDC) through the Surveillance, Intervention, and Referral to Services Activities for Infants with Microcephaly or other Adverse Outcomes Linked with the Zika Virus (birth defects) cooperative agreement.[32]

Table 6. Birth defects cooperative agreement Zika supplemental funding by awardee state/territory

State/territory	Awardee	Award (in dollars)
Alabama	Alabama Department of Public Health	199,952
American Samoa	American Samoa Government	200,000
Arizona	Arizona Department of Health Services	200,000
Arkansas	Arkansas Children's Hospital Research	200,000
California	California Department of Public Health	360,000
California	County of Los Angeles Department of Public Health	360,000
Federated States of Micronesia	Federated States of Micronesia -FSM	137,437
Florida	Florida Department of Health	360,000
Georgia	Georgia Department of Public Health	280,000
Guam	Guam Department of Public Health and Social Services	163,340
Hawaii	Hawaii State Department of Health	200,000
Illinois	City of Chicago Department of Public Health	100,000
Illinois	Illinois Department of Public Health	180,000
Indiana	Indiana State Department of Health	200,000
Iowa	University of Iowa	100,000
Kentucky	Kentucky Cabinet for Health & Family Services	200,000
Louisiana	Louisiana State Office of Public Health	200,000
Marshall Islands	Republic of the Marshall Islands Ministry of Health	200,000
Massachusetts	Massachusetts Department of Public Health	100,000
Minnesota	Minnesota Department of Health	100,000
Mississippi	Mississippi State Department of Health	200,000

[32] The birth defects award for cities and counties is the Surveillance, Intervention, and Referral to Services Activities for Infants with Microcephaly or other Adverse Outcomes Linked with the Zika Virus - High Risk Local Areas Cooperative Agreement.

Table 6. (Continued)

State/territory	Awardee	Award (in dollars)
Missouri	Missouri Department of Health & Senior Services	200,000
Nebraska	Nebraska Department of Health and Human Services	77,427
Nevada	Southern Nevada Health District	200,000
New Jersey	New Jersey Department of Health	280,000
New York	Health Research, Inc. (New York State)	359,999
New York	New York City Department of Health & Mental Hygiene	352,287
North Carolina	North Carolina Department of Health and Human Services	280,000
Northern Mariana Islands	Commonwealth Healthcare Corporation	200,000
Ohio	Ohio State Department of Health	280,000
Oklahoma	Oklahoma State Department of Health	108,262
Pennsylvania	Pennsylvania State Department of Health	280,000
Pennsylvania	Philadelphia Department of Public Health	174,093
Puerto Rico	Puerto Rico Department of Health	200,000
Rhode Island	Rhode Island Department of Health	100,000
South Carolina	South Carolina Department of Health and Environmental Control	200,000
Tennessee	Tennessee State Department of Health	200,000
Texas	Houston Health Department	199,804
Texas	Texas Department of State Health Services	360,000
U.S. Virgin Islands	Virgin Islands Department of Health	199,885
Utah	Utah Department of Health	100,000
West Virginia	West Virginia Department of Health and Human Services	192,150
Wisconsin	Wisconsin Department of Health Services	100,000

Source: Centers for Disease Control and Prevention. | GAO-18-389.

The Zika supplemental funding awarded through the birth defects cooperative agreement was to provide additional resources to better establish, enhance, and maintain rapid population-based surveillance of microcephaly and other adverse outcomes (especially central nervous system defects) possibly linked to Zika virus infection during pregnancy using an active case-finding methodology; participation in centralized pooled clinical and surveillance data projects; ensuring affected infants and families are referred to services; and assessing health and developmental outcomes of these children.

Appendix IV: Centers for Disease Control and Prevention—Behavioral Risk Factor Surveillance System Awardees

This appendix presents information on Zika supplemental funding awards made by the Centers for Disease Control and Prevention (CDC) through the Behavioral Risk Factor Surveillance System (BRFSS) cooperative agreement.

The Zika supplemental funding awarded through the BRFSS cooperative agreement was to conduct a rapid population-based assessment of women and couples using or in need of contraceptives in order to provide comprehensive contraceptive services related to Zika virus exposure.

Table 7 presents information for each award as it was provided to us by CDC.

Table 7. Behavioral risk factor surveillance system cooperative agreement state/territory

State/territory	Awardee	Award (in dollars)
Alabama	Alabama Department of Public Health	104,641
Arizona	Arizona Department of Health Services	26,000
District of Columbia	District of Columbia Department of Health	116,618
Florida	Florida Department of Health	124,976
Georgia	Georgia Department of Public Health	100,000
Guam	Guam Department of Public Health and Social Services	73,111
Louisiana	Louisiana State Office of Public Health	100,000
Maryland	Maryland Department of Health and Mental Hygiene	65,139
Mississippi	Mississippi State Department of Health	100,000
New Mexico	New Mexico Department of Health	125,000
New York	Health Research, Inc. (New York State)	125,000
Puerto Rico	Puerto Rico Department of Health	124,294
Texas	Texas Department of State Health Services	124,854
U.S. Virgin Islands	Virgin Islands Department of Health	50,756

Source: Centers for Disease Control and Prevention. | GAO-18-389.

APPENDIX V: CENTERS FOR DISEASE CONTROL AND PREVENTION—PREGNANCY RISK ASSESSMENT MONITORING SYSTEM AWARDEES

This appendix presents information on Zika supplemental funding awards made by the Centers for Disease Control and Prevention (CDC) through the Pregnancy Risk Assessment Monitoring System (PRAMS) cooperative agreement.

The Zika supplemental funding awarded through the PRAMS cooperative agreement was to assess maternal behaviors and experiences related to Zika virus exposure among recently pregnant women who deliver a live-born infant in the United States.

Table 8 presents information for each award as it was provided to us by CDC.

Table 8. Pregnancy risk assessment monitoring system cooperative agreement's Zika supplemental funding by awardee

State/territory	Awardee[a]	Award (In dollars)
Alabama	Alabama Department of Public Health	29,993
Connecticut	Connecticut State Department of Public Health	40,000
District of Columbia	District of Columbia Department of Health	29,916
Florida	Florida Department of Health	40,000
Georgia	Georgia Department of Public Health	40,000
Illinois	Illinois Department of Public Health	40,000
Indiana	Indiana State Department of Health	30,000
Massachusetts	Massachusetts Department of Public Health	40,000
Missouri	Missouri Department of Health & Senior Services	30,000
New Jersey	New Jersey State Department of Health & Senior Services	40,000
New York	Health Research, Inc. (New York State)	30,000
Pennsylvania	Pennsylvania State Department of Health	29,830
Puerto Rico	Puerto Rico Department of Health	830,000
South Carolina	South Carolina Department of Health and Environmental Control	39,975
Tennessee	Tennessee State Department of Health	40,000
Virginia	Virginia Department of Health	39,953
Wisconsin	Wisconsin Department of Health Services	24,171

Source: Centers for Disease Control and Prevention. | GAO-18-389.

[a] These awardees received more than one award and funding amounts for awards for the same awardee were added together in this table.

APPENDIX VI: CENTERS FOR DISEASE CONTROL AND PREVENTION—PUBLIC HEALTH PREPAREDNESS AND RESPONSE AWARDEES

This appendix presents information on Zika supplemental funding awards made by the Centers for Disease Control and Prevention (CDC) through the Public Health Preparedness and Response (PHPR) Cooperative Agreement for All-Hazards Public Health Emergencies.

According to CDC officials, the Zika supplemental funding awarded through the PHPR cooperative agreement was to enable identified state, territorial, and local jurisdictions to address Zika virus disease planning and operational response gaps.

Table 9 presents information for each award as it was provided to us by CDC.

Table 9. Public health preparedness and response cooperative agreement for all-hazards public health emergencies cooperative agreement's Zika supplemental funding by awardee

State/territory	Awardee	Award (in dollars)
Alabama	Alabama Department of Public Health	522,093
American Samoa	American Samoa Government	453,009
Arizona	Arizona Department of Health Services	388,273
Arkansas	Arkansas Department of Health	212,707
California	California Department of Public Health	2,658,839
California	County of Los Angeles Department of Public Health	504,855
Federated States of Micronesia	Federated States of Micronesia -FSM	289,088
Florida	Florida Department of Health	4,999,979
Georgia	Georgia Department of Public Health	203,738
Guam	Guam Department of Public Health and Social Services	134,614
Hawaii	Hawaii State Department of Health	58,603
Kentucky	Kentucky Cabinet for Health & Family Services	428,132
Louisiana	Louisiana State Office of Public Health	1,437,361
Marshall Islands	Republic of the Marshall Islands Ministry of Health	86,300
Maryland	Maryland Department of Health and Mental Hygiene	288,558
New Jersey	New Jersey Department of Health	933,995
New York	Health Research, Inc. (New York State)	1,086,913
New York	Public Health Solutions (NYC)	1,294,244
Northern Mariana Islands	Commonwealth Healthcare Corporation	86,976
Puerto Rico	Puerto Rico Department of Health	3,931,723
Texas	Texas Department of State Health Services	5,000,000

Source: Centers for Disease Control and Prevention. | GAO-18-389.

APPENDIX VII: CENTERS FOR DISEASE CONTROL AND PREVENTION—OTHER COOPERATIVE AGREEMENTS' AWARDEES

This appendix presents information on Zika supplemental funding awards made by the Centers for Disease Control and Prevention (CDC) through additional cooperative agreements.

Tables 10-17 present information for each award as it was provided to us by CDC.

Administrative Support for the Zika Supplemental for Sentinel Enhanced Dengue Surveillance System Project

The Zika supplemental funding awarded through the Sentinel Enhanced Dengue Surveillance System Project cooperative agreement was to support sites working to provide new information on dengue and other acute febrile illnesses in Puerto Rico, which is located in the subtropics and where dengue epidemiology is similar to dengue endemic areas worldwide. The Zika supplemental funding was for two studies: (1) pregnant women with Zika infection, and (2) postnatal Zika infection by following 0-5 year old children.

Table 10. Sentinel enhanced dengue surveillance system project cooperative agreement's Zika supplemental funding by awardee

State/territory	Awardee	Award(in dollars)
Puerto Rico	Ponce School of Medicine	500,000

Source: Centers for Disease Control and Prevention. | GAO-18-389.

Vector-Borne Disease Regional Centers of Excellence

The Zika supplemental funding awarded through the Vector-Borne Disease Regional Centers of Excellence cooperative agreement is to establish regional centers of excellence aimed at building the capacity to address the problem of emerging and exotic vector-borne diseases in the United States, including Zika virus infection.

Table 11. Vector-borne disease regional centers of excellence cooperative agreement's Zika supplemental funding by awardee

State/territory	Awardee	Award(in dollars)
California	University of California –Davis	8,000,000
Florida	University of Florida	9,999,628
New York	CornellUniversity	9,999,936
Texas	University of Texas Medical Branch, Galveston	9,995,253
Wisconsin	University of Wisconsin	9,999,491

Source: Centers for Disease Control and Prevention. | GAO-18-389.

Enhancing Capacity for Vector Surveillance and Control to Prevent Zika, Dengue and Chikungunya Infection in Puerto Rico

The Zika supplemental funding awarded through the Enhancing Capacity for Vector Surveillance and Control to Prevent Zika, Dengue and Chikungunya Infection in Puerto Rico cooperative agreement is to fund activities to increase the surveillance and control of vectors, specifically *Aedes aegypti* mosquitoes (the vector of dengue, chikungunya, and Zika). The purpose of the program is to establish a vector control unit to oversee and implement comprehensive vector control activities in Puerto Rico.

Table 12. Enhancing capacity for vector surveillance and control to prevent zika, dengue and chikungunya infection in Puerto Rico cooperative agreement's Zika supplemental funding by awardee

State/territory	Awardee	Award (in dollars)
Puerto Rico	Puerto Rico Science, Technology & Research Trust	14,000,000

Source: Centers for Disease Control and Prevention. | GAO-18-389.

Immunization Grants-CDC Partnership: Strengthening Public Health Laboratories

The Zika supplemental funding awarded through the Immunization Grants-CDC Partnership: Strengthening Public Health Laboratories cooperative agreement is to promote quality and safe public health laboratory practice, improve public health laboratory infrastructure, strengthen the public health laboratory system, and develop a well-trained public health laboratory workforce.

Table 13. Immunization Grants-CDC Partnership: strengthening public health laboratories cooperative agreement's Zika supplemental funding by awardee

Awardee	Award (in dollars)
Association of Public Health Laboratories (APHL)	250,000

Source: Centers for Disease Control and Prevention. | GAO-18-389.

Building Capacity of the Public Health System to Improve Population Health through National, Nonprofit Organizations

Table 14. Building capacity of the public health system to improve population

Awardee	Award (in dollars)
American Academy of Pediatrics	740,000
Association of State & Territorial Health Officials (ASTHO)	1,150,000
Council of State& Territory Epidemiologists (CSTE)	500,000
March of Dimes Birth Defects Foundation	914,757
National Association of City & County Health Officials (NACCHO)[a]	900,000
National Indian Health Board (NIHB)	500,000

Source: Centers for Disease Control and Prevention. | GAO-18-389,

[a] This awardee received more than one award and funding amounts for these awards were added together in this table.

According to CDC officials, the Zika supplemental funding awarded through the Building Capacity of the Public Health System to Improve Population Health through National, Nonprofit Organizations cooperative agreement is to ensure national capacity for responding to the Zika outbreak and meeting the needs of those affected, such as by reaching out to specialized constituents to ensure they were informed on epidemiology and practice guidelines.

Strengthening the Public Health System in the U.S.- Affiliated Pacific Islands

The Zika supplemental funding awarded through the Strengthening the Public Health System in the U.S.-Affiliated Pacific Islands cooperative agreement is to provide capacity building assistance through a regional, nonprofit organization to strengthen the U.S.-Affiliated Pacific Islands' public health leadership, workforce, and public health systems and infrastructure in response to Zika virus within the U.S. Pacific territories.

Table 15. Strengthening the Public Health System in the U.S.-affiliated pacific islands cooperative agreement's Zika supplemental funding by award

Awardee	Award (in dollars)
Pacific Island Health Officers Association (PIHOA)[a]	400,000

Source: Centers for Disease Control and Prevention. | GAO-18-389.

[a] This awardee received more than one award and funding amounts for these awards were added together in this table.

Pan American Health Organization: Building Capacity and Networks to Address Emerging Infectious Diseases in the Americas

The Zika supplemental funding awarded through the Pan American Health Organization: Building Capacity and Networks to Address Emerging Infectious Diseases in the Americas cooperative agreement is for various activities including technical assistance, such as to develop standard operating procedures for diagnostic and integrated surveillance activities, as well as to support the development, implementation, and evaluation of diagnostic and surveillance guidelines.

Table 16. Pan American Health Organization: building capacity and networks to address emerging infectious diseases in the America's cooperative agreement's Zika supplemental funding by awardee

Awardee	Award (in dollars)
Pan American Health Organization	500,000

Source: Centers for Disease Control and Prevention. | GAO-18-389.

Global Health Security Partner Engagement: Expanding Efforts and Strategies to Protect and Improve Public Health Globally

According to CDC officials, the Zika supplemental funding awarded through the Global Health Security Partner Engagement: Expanding Efforts and Strategies to Protect and Improve Public Health Globally cooperative agreement is for enhanced surveillance for pregnant women in Colombia, including laboratory testing and case investigations.

Table 17. Global health security partner engagement: expanding efforts and strategies to protect and improve public health globally cooperative agreement's Zika supplemental funding by awardee

Awardee	Award(in dollars)
Vysnova Partners, Inc.	999,790

Source: Centers for Disease Control and Prevention. | GAO-18-389.

Appendix VIII: Centers for Disease Control and Prevention—Contracts and Interagency Agreements

This appendix presents information on Zika supplemental funding awards made by the Centers for Disease Control and Prevention (CDC) through additional contracts and interagency agreements.

Tables 18 and 19 present information for each award as it was provided to us by CDC, as well as the activity funded.

Table 18. Centers for disease control and prevention Zika supplemental funding contracts by awardee and activity funded

Awardee	Activity funded	Award (in dollars)
AB Sciex	Laboratory Capacity, Acceleration, Equipment	21,403.00
ABT Associates[a]	Public Health Outreach and Control	10,658,187.99
ABT Associates[b]	Public Health Emergency Preparedness	(1,082,005.00)
Agilent Technologies	Laboratory Capacity, Acceleration, Equipment	32,440.49
Air Science USA	Laboratory Capacity, Acceleration, Equipment	7,355.99
Alivepromo, Inc	Public Health Emergency Preparedness	728,736.08
All Business Machines, Inc	Laboratory Capacity, Acceleration, Equipment	66,823.20
Altus Technical Solutions	Laboratory Capacity, Acceleration, Equipment	108,000.00
Amdex Corporation	Public Health Emergency Preparedness	261,424.80
American Toner & Ink	Public Health Emergency Preparedness	3,827.25
AP&G Co, Inc	Vector Surveillance and Control	32,505.80
Applied Medical Technologies, Inc.	Laboratory Capacity, Acceleration, Equipment	7,889.16
Aprisa Technology	Vector Surveillance and Control	8,671.23
Arist Medical Sciences University	Laboratory Capacity, Acceleration, Equipment	52,800.00

Table 18. (Continued)

Awardee	Activity funded	Award (in dollars)
Aspen Commercial Group	Vector Surveillance and Control; Surveillance, Epidemiology, and Public Health Investigations	818,731.41
Aspen Commercial Group	Laboratory Capacity, Acceleration, Equipment	71,139.96
Atlanta Biologicals	Laboratory Capacity, Acceleration, Equipment	6,173.82
Awardee	Activity funded	Award (in dollars)
AUS Marketing Research Systems, Inc.	Surveillance, Epidemiology, and Public Health Investigations	100,000.00
Battelle Memorial Institute	Laboratory Capacity, Acceleration, Equipment	187,952.00
Becton, Dickson & Co.[a]	Laboratory Capacity, Acceleration, Equipment	404,651.87
BioAnalytical Instrumentsa	Laboratory Capacity, Acceleration, Equipment	450,766.67
BioAnalytical Instruments	Surveillance, Epidemiology, and Public Health Investigations	25,200.00
Biocare Medical	Laboratory Capacity, Acceleration, Equipment	55,366.00
Biocold Environmental, Inc	Laboratory Capacity, Acceleration, Equipment	15,025.00
Bio-Nuclear	Laboratory Capacity, Acceleration, Equipment	149,951.19
Bio-Rad Laboratories	Laboratory Capacity, Acceleration, Equipment	24,950.00
Bio-Rad Laboratories	Vector Surveillance and Control	3,741.00
Biotek Instruments[a]	Laboratory Capacity, Acceleration, Equipment	75,486.93
Booz Allen Hamiltona	Laboratory Capacity, Acceleration, Equipment	452,966.45
Booz Allen Hamilton	Public Health Emergency Preparedness	1,145,449.43
Booz Allen Hamilton	Vector Surveillance and Control	3,500.00
Bruker Daltonics	Laboratory Capacity, Acceleration, Equipment	20,281.00
Caduceus Healthcare[a]	Laboratory Capacity, Acceleration, Equipment	1,949,351.04
Caduceus Healthcare	Vector Surveillance and Control; Laboratory Capacity, Acceleration, Equipment; Public Health Outreach and Control	374,336.60
Caduceus Healthcare, Inc	Public Health Outreach and Control	249,956.60
Caduceus Healthcare, Inc	Laboratory Capacity, Acceleration, Equipment	483,573.33
Canona	Public Health Emergency Preparedness	69,526.24
Carl Zeiss Microscopy, LLC	Laboratory Capacity, Acceleration, Equipment	194,126.64
Carter Consulting	Surveillance, Epidemiology, and Public Health Investigations	120,497.00
CDI Laboratories, Inc.	Vector Surveillance and Control	16,800.00
Certified Technical Experts[a]	Laboratory Capacity, Acceleration, Equipment	229,142.00
Chenega Government Consulting, LLC[a]	Laboratory Capacity, Acceleration, Equipment	132,902.62
Chickasaw Health Consulting	Public Health Emergency Preparedness	31,820.00
Chickasaw Management Services, LLC	Public Health Outreach and Control	193,477.20
CNI Advantage, LLC[a]	Public Health Emergency Preparedness	2,068,011.79
CNI Advantage, LLC	Public Health Emergency Preparedness; Surveillance, Epidemiology, and Public Health Investigations	89,403.31
CNI Advantage, LLC[a]	Surveillance, Epidemiology, and Public Health Investigations	7,893,052.52
Communications Professionals, Inc.	Vector Surveillance and Control	15,620.00
Crimson Imaging Supplies, LLC	Public Health Emergency Preparedness	11,073.34
CTG Associates	Public Health Emergency Preparedness	75,699.00

Awardee	Activity funded	Award (in dollars)
Davis, James	Public Health Emergency Preparedness	6,689.85
Deloitte Consulting	Surveillance, Epidemiology, and Public HealthInvestigations	1,381,711.80
Diagger Scientific, Inc.[a]	Laboratory Capacity, Acceleration, Equipment	21,687.00
Digital Video Group, Inc	Public Health Emergency Preparedness	96,389.90
DOC Development, Inc[a]	Laboratory Capacity, Acceleration, Equipment	12,395.72
Eagle Medical Services	Public Health Emergency Preparedness; Surveillance, Epidemiology, and Public Health Investigations	931,963.19
Eagle Medical Services	Surveillance, Epidemiology, and Public Health Investigations	1,999,961.12
Elsevier Limited	Laboratory Capacity, Acceleration, Equipment	5,000.00
EMD Millipore Corporation	Laboratory Capacity, Acceleration, Equipment	22,972.80
Entomological Society of America	Vector Surveillance and Control	151,000.00
Environmental Systems Research Institute	Public Health Emergency Preparedness	49,391.00
Evolution Management, Inc	Public Health Outreach and Control	300,526.00
FedEx	Public Health Emergency Preparedness	37,429.17
Fisher Scientific Company[a]	Laboratory Capacity, Acceleration, Equipment	306,124.39
Fisher Scientific Company	Surveillance, Epidemiology, and Public Health Investigations	16,669.48
Fisher Scientific Company	Vector Surveillance and Control	10,125.85
Fitzgerald Industries International, Inc	Laboratory Capacity, Acceleration, Equipment	23,850.00
G2S Corporation	Public Health Emergency Preparedness	39,200.00
G2S Corporation	Public Health Emergency Preparedness; Surveillance, Epidemiology, and Public Health Investigations	3,918,687.12
G2S Corporation[a]	Surveillance, Epidemiology, and Public Health Investigations	3,391,153.86
G2S Corporation	Vector Surveillance and Control	1,509,787.25
GAP Solutions, Inc.[a]	Public Health Emergency Preparedness	626,343.67
GAP Solutions, Inc.	PublicHealth Outreach and Control	60,408.00
Gem Laser Express, Inc.	Public Health Emergency Preparedness	16,136.82
Geographic Mapping Technologies Corp.	Vector Surveillance and Control	14,850.00
Georgia State University Research Foundation, Inc	Laboratory Capacity, Acceleration, Equipment	1,530,000.00
Government Scientific Source[a]	Laboratory Capacity, Acceleration, Equipment	212,643.83
Helmer Scientific	Laboratory Capacity, Acceleration, Equipment	11,679.85
Hyclone Laboratories, Inc	Laboratory Capacity, Acceleration, Equipment	2,716.36
ICF Incorporated[a]	Public Health Outreach and Control	2,304,697.14
IHRC	Laboratory Capacity, Acceleration, Equipment	1,356,070.32
Illumina, Inc[a]	Laboratory Capacity, Acceleration, Equipment	101,132.07
Illumina, Inc	Public Health Emergency Preparedness; Vector Surveillance and Control; Public Health Outreach and Control	189,732.00
Impres Technology Solutions	Surveillance, Epidemiology, and Public Health Investigations	59,675.94
InBios International[a]	Laboratory Capacity, Acceleration, Equipment	323,184.00
InBios International	Surveillance, Epidemiology, and Public Health Investigations	6,963.00

Table 18. (Continued)

Awardee	Activity funded	Award (in dollars)
InBios International	Surveillance, Epidemiology, and Public Health Investigations; Vector Surveillance and Control	18,731.00
JC Gonzalez, Inc.[a]	Vector Surveillance and Control	40,970.70
Johns Hopkins University	Vector Surveillance and Control	500,000.00
Karn[a]	Laboratory Capacity, Acceleration, Equipment	35,668.42
Karn[a]	Public Health Emergency Preparedness	115,000.00
Karna[b]	Surveillance, Epidemiology, and Public Health Investigations	(16,568.10)
Karn[a]	Surveillance, Epidemiology, and Public Health Investigations; Public Health Outreach and Control	2,138,919.00
Leica Microsystems	Laboratory Capacity, Acceleration, Equipment	34,442.52
Leidos, Inc	Surveillance, Epidemiology, and Public Health Investigations	621,000.00
Life Technologies Corporation[a]	Laboratory Capacity, Acceleration, Equipment	79,918.85
Awardee	Activity funded	Award (in dollars)
Life Technologies Corporation	Vector Surveillance and Control	45,776.40
Lonza Walkersville, Inc.	Laboratory Capacity, Acceleration, Equipment	6,483.30
Luminex Corporation	Laboratory Capacity, Acceleration, Equipment	28,086.80
Madison Cloud IT Solutions, LLC	Public Health Emergency Preparedness	14,471.06
Mapbox Inc	Public Health Emergency Preparedness	25,000.00
McKing Consulting Corporation	Surveillance, Epidemiology, and Public Health Investigations	894,403.64
Microptics Service, Inc	Laboratory Capacity, Acceleration, Equipment	6,384.35
Molecular Devices[a]	Laboratory Capacity, Acceleration, Equipment	154,923.70
Mosquito Mate Inc	Vector Surveillance and Control	999,994.02
Multisystems, Inc	Laboratory Capacity, Acceleration, Equipment	10,031.80
Nexcelom Bioscience	Laboratory Capacity, Acceleration, Equipment	139,400.00
Nightingale Corp	Laboratory Capacity, Acceleration, Equipment	3,637.40
Nikon Inc[a]	Laboratory Capacity, Acceleration, Equipment	150,978.71
Northrop Grumman[a]	Public Health Outreach and Control	835,000.00
Northrop Grumman	Surveillance, Epidemiology, and Public Health Investigations	175,000.00
Northrop Grumman[a]	Vector Surveillance and Control	729,436.00
NuAire, Inc.	Laboratory Capacity, Acceleration, Equipment	8,698.40
OAG Aviation Worldwide LLC	Public Health Outreach and Control	147,000.00
Onset Computer Corporation	Vector Surveillance and Control	4,500.00
Pacific Biosciences of California	Public Health Emergency Preparedness; Laboratory Capacity, Acceleration, Equipment; Vector Surveillance and Control; Surveillance, Epidemiology, and Public Health Investigations	168,889.71
Pacific Link International, Corp[a]	Public Health Emergency Preparedness	34,374.00
Panasonic Healthcare Corporation of North America	Laboratory Capacity, Acceleration, Equipment	9,334.00
Premier & Companies	Laboratory Capacity, Acceleration, Equipment	4,653.94
P3S Corporation	Laboratory Capacity, Acceleration, Equipment	115,000.00
Qiagen, Inc[a]	Laboratory Capacity, Acceleration, Equipment	175,958.27
Red River Computer Co., Inc	Laboratory Capacity, Acceleration, Equipment	2,473.19

Awardee	Activity funded	Award (in dollars)
Rentokil North America, Inc	Surveillance, Epidemiology, and Public Health Investigations; Public Health Emergency Preparedness; Public Health Outreach and Control; Vector Surveillance and Control	1,382,575.00
Rentokil North America, Inc[a]	Vector Surveillance and Control	4,700,097.00
Roche Diagnostics Corporation[a]	Laboratory Capacity, Acceleration, Equipment	602,679.70
Roche Diagnostics Corporation[a]	Surveillance, Epidemiology, and Public Health Investigations	98,987.30
RTI International	Surveillance, Epidemiology, and Public Health Investigations	67,948.00
Rumph & Associates[a]	Laboratory Capacity, Acceleration, Equipment; Surveillance, Epidemiology, and Public Health Investigations	2,377,501.00
SBC Technology Partners, Inc	Public Health Emergency Preparedness	3,748.75
SDL Government, Inc.[a]	Public Health Outreach and Control	25,155.25
Sheknows LLC	Public Health Outreach and Control	15,000.00
Siemens Healthcare Diagnostics[a]	Laboratory Capacity, Acceleration, Equipment	357,540.66
Awardee	Activity funded	Award (in dollars)
Sigma-Aldrich	Laboratory Capacity, Acceleration, Equipment	5,317.62
Smith Travel Research, Inc	Public Health Outreach and Control	4,950.00
Southland Instruments, Inc.	Laboratory Capacity, Acceleration, Equipment	10,909.00
Springstar[a]	Vector Surveillance and Control	551,294.30
SRA International	Public Health Emergency Preparedness; Public Health Outreach and Control; Vector Surveillance and Control; Laboratory Capacity, Acceleration, Equipment; Surveillance, Epidemiology, and Public Health Investigations	500,000.00
SRA International	Public Health Outreach and Control	1,344,852.00
Steris Corporation	Laboratory Capacity, Acceleration, Equipment	51,836.58
Steris Corporation[a]	Vector Surveillance and Control	52,586.58
Strategic Communications, LLC	Laboratory Capacity, Acceleration, Equipment	2,067.96
Synergy America[a]	Public Health Emergency Preparedness	203,000.00
Synergy Group	Public Health Emergency Preparedness	48,020.29
Tanaq Government Services	Public Health Outreach and Control	284,990.00
Texas A&M Agrilife Research	Vector Surveillance and Control	1,200,923.00
The Cresston Company, LLC	Public Health Outreach and Control	40,194.00
Thermo Electron North America	Public Health Outreach and Control	990,122.21
Thomson Reuters (Scientific) LLC	Public Health Outreach and Control	23,588.00
Three Wire Systems, LLC	Public Health Emergency Preparedness	1,970.00
Three Wire Systems, LLC	Vector Surveillance and Control	19,339.77
Total Solutions	Surveillance, Epidemiology, and Public Health Investigations	550,184.67
Total Solutions	Surveillance, Epidemiology, and Public Health Investigations; Laboratory Capacity, Acceleration, Equipment	1,001,674.00
Triad Technology Partners, LLC	Public Health Outreach and Control	3,564.00
TWD Tradewinds, Inc	Laboratory Capacity, Acceleration, Equipment	145,569.00
Unicom	Surveillance, Epidemiology, and Public Health Investigations	140,158.00

Table 18. (Continued)

Awardee	Activity funded	Award (in dollars)
University of Arizona	Vector Surveillance and Control	1,250,000.00
University of New Mexico	Vector Surveillance and Control	1,301,000.00
University of North Carolina at Chapel Hill	Laboratory Capacity, Acceleration, Equipment	3,279,000.00
Veterans4you Corporation	Public Health Emergency Preparedness	3,620.00
VWR International	Laboratory Capacity, Acceleration, Equipment	84,490.13
VWR International	Vector Surveillance and Control	19,203.93
Vysnova	Surveillance, Epidemiology, and Public Health Investigations	7,281,151.00
Westat, Inc	Public Health Outreach and Control	94,026.00
Wright Line, LLC	Laboratory Capacity, Acceleration, Equipment	11,072.98
3M Company	Laboratory Capacity, Acceleration, Equipment	4,918.40

Source: Centers for Disease Control and Prevention (CDC). | GAO-18-389.

Note: Awards that included a change in the funding amount are reflected in the table, unless the change resulted in a zero balance. For example, CDC provided funding to one company, but later rescinded the same amount. Therefore, this award does not appear in the table as the resulting award is $0. CDC officials said that these types of actions are standard, particularly in an emergency situation when the needs of the response are rapidly evolving. Changes to awards can occur because there is a change in need for services, a vendor not having the needed items in stock, a reduction in the price of the contract, changes after the contract was awarded, and administrative corrections of a funding source.

[a] This awardee received more than one award and funding amounts for awards for the same awardee and activity were added together in this table.

[b] This awardee had funding that was rescinded. The rescinded funding was not combined with the awardee's other awards because it was for a different activity.

Table 19. Centers for disease control and prevention Zika supplemental funding interagency agreements by awardee and activity funded

Awardee	Activity funded	Award (in dollars)
BARDA	Vector Control	9,000,000.00
NIHa	Laboratory Capacity, Acceleration, Equipment	450,000.00
U.S. Department of Commerce	Public Health Outreach and Control	8,574.72
U.S. Department of Energy[a]	Laboratory Capacity, Acceleration, Equipment	779,856.91
U.S. Department of Energy[a]	Public Health Emergency Preparedness	134,278.80
U.S. Department of Energy[a]	Surveillance, Epidemiology, and Public Health Investigations	821,452.78
Verizon Business Services	Public Health Emergency Preparedness	112,000.00

Source: Centers for Disease Control and Prevention (CDC). | GAO-18-389.

Note: Awards that included a change in the funding amount are reflected in the table, unless the change resulted in a zero balance. For example, CDC provided $550,000 to the Health Resources and Services Administration, but later rescinded the same amount. Therefore, this award does not appear in the table as the resulting award is $0. CDC officials said that these types of actions are standard, particularly in an emergency situation when the needs of the response are rapidly evolving. Changes to awards can occur because there is a change in need for services, a vendor not having the needed items in stock, a reduction in the price of the contract, changes after the contract was awarded, and administrative corrections of a funding source.

[a] This awardee received more than one award and funding amounts for awards for the same awardee and activity were added together in this table.

APPENDIX IX: CENTERS FOR MEDICARE & MEDICAID SERVICES—ZIKA HEALTH CARE SERVICES PROGRAM AWARDS

This appendix presents information on Zika supplemental funding awards made by the Centers for Medicare & Medicaid Services (CMS) through the Zika Health Care Services Program. The Zika Health Care Services Program is aimed at supporting prevention activities and treatment services for women (including pregnant women), children, and men adversely or potentially affected by the Zika virus. According to CMS documentation, the Zika Health Care Service Program is intended to address four critical components of a comprehensive response to Zika:

1. Increase access to contraceptive services for women and men.
2. Increase access to and reduce barriers to diagnostic testing, screening, and counseling for pregnant women and newborns.
3. Increase access to appropriate specialized health care services for pregnant women, children born to mothers with maternal Zika virus infection, and their families.
4. Improve provider capacity and capability.

Table 20. Centers for medicare & medicaid services' Zika health care services program awardees

State/territory	Awardee	Award Amount
American Samoa	American Samoa Government Department of Health	1,791,000
Florida	Florida Department of Health	2,991,000
Puerto Rico	Puerto Rico Department of Health	61,291,000
Texas	Texas Department of State Health Services	2,491,000
U.S. Virgin Islands	U.S. Virgin Islands Department of Health	2,791,000

Source: Centers for Medicare & Medicaid Services. | GAO-18-389.

CMS awarded funding through the Zika Health Care Services Program, in two award rounds, to states, territories, tribes, or tribal organizations with active or local transmission of the Zika virus, as confirmed by the Centers for Disease Control and Prevention. In January 2017, CMS awarded funding to American Samoa, Florida, Puerto Rico, and the U.S. Virgin Islands.

In June 2017, CMS awarded funding to Texas, the only new area with local transmission of the Zika virus. Table 20 presents the awards CMS made through its Zika Health Care Services Program.

APPENDIX X: HEALTH RESOURCES AND SERVICES ADMINISTRATION'S ZIKA SUPPLEMENTAL AWARDS

This appendix presents information on Zika supplemental funding awards made by the Health Resources and Services Administration (HRSA) to health centers and for Special Projects of Regional and National Significance.[33]

- Health centers: HRSA provided awards to health centers through supplemental grant awards to support existing health centers in Puerto Rico and other territories in their efforts to expand the delivery of health care services, including the prevention of Zika and prevention and treatment of Zika-related illness. HRSA also provided supplemental grant awards to existing Health Center Program cooperative agreement awardees for efforts to provide training and technical assistance for Zika-related health center expansion activities.
- Special Projects of Regional and National Significance: HRSA provided awards for Special Projects of Regional and National Significance to support public health departments and other entities in Puerto Rico and other territories in efforts to ensure access to recommended services for pregnant women, infants, and children infected by the Zika virus in the prenatal, perinatal, and neonatal period. Activities include early identification through developmental screening, regular assessments and monitoring, telemedicine, care coordination, enabling services, family engagement and family-tofamily support; purchasing of diagnostic equipment and health information technology; and the training of health care providers, care coordinators, and other health care and public health professionals to ensure delivery of comprehensive, interdisciplinary health and social services for this population.

[33] HRSA also provided student loan repayment to qualified health professionals through the National Health Services Corps. We do not present this information by awardee in this appendix, as that data contains personal information.

Tables 21 and 22 present information for each award as it was provided to us by HRSA.

Table 21. Health resources and services administration Zika supplemental funding for health centers by awardee

State/territory	Awardee	Award (in dollars)
American Samoa	American Samoa Government Dept of Health	2,336,253
Hawaii	Pacific Islands Primary Care Association	250,000
Puerto Rico	Asociacian de Salud Primaria de Puerto Rico, Inc	750,000
Puerto Rico	Municipality of San Juan (HOMIS)	1,058,362
Puerto Rico	Consejo de Salud de Puerto Rico, Inc.	2,556,580
Puerto Rico	Centro de Servicios Primarios de Salud Inc	1,555,327
Puerto Rico	Concilio de Salud Integral de Loiza, Inc	1,577,352
Puerto Rico	Centro de Salud Familiar (PALMIERI)	1,563,775
Puerto Rico	Corporacion de Servicos Medicos Primarios y Prevencion de Hatillo	1,895,792
Puerto Rico	Centro de Salud de Lares, Inc.	1,668,179
Puerto Rico	Castaner General Hospital	1,428,258
Puerto Rico	Costa Salud Community Health Centers Inc	1,517,755
Puerto Rico	Corporacion de Servicios de Salud y Medicina Avanzada - COSSMA	1,938,143
Puerto Rico	Morovis Community Health Center, Inc.	1,482,153
Puerto Rico	Barceloneta Primary Health Services, Inc.	1,540,884
Puerto Rico	Camuy Health Services, Inc.	1,542,118
Puerto Rico	Salud Integral enla Montana, Inc.	2,089,258
Puerto Rico	Migrant Health Center, Western Region, Inc.	1,821,303
Puerto Rico	NeoMed Center Inc	2,285,262
Puerto Rico	HPM Foundation, Inc.	1,590,023
Puerto Rico	PryMed Medical Care, Inc.	1,532,746
Puerto Rico	Patillas Community Governing Board	1,868,331
Puerto Rico	Corporacion SANOS	1,266,725
U.S. Virgin Islands	Frederiksted Health Care Inc.	1,459,507
U.S. Virgin Islands	St. Thomas East End Medical Center Corporation	1,425,914

Source: Health Resources and Services Administration. | GAO-18-389.

Note: The Zika Response and Preparedness Act required that $40 million be used to expand the delivery of primary health services in Puerto Rico and other territories. According to officials from the Health Resources and Services Administration, the Pacific Islands Primary Care Association in Hawaii was funded to support health centers within the Pacific Basin based on their Zika-related needs.

Table 22. Health resources and services administration Zika supplemental funding for special projects of regional and national significance by awardee

State/territory	Awardee	Award (in dollars)
American Samo[a]	Dept of Health[a]	923,142
California	Children's Hospital of Los Angeles	333,333
Florida	University ofMiami	333,333
Illinois	American Academy of Pediatrics	250,000
Indiana	Indiana University	333,333
New Mexico	Family Voices, Inc	250,000
Puerto Rico	Parents Training Parents	150,000
Puerto Rico	Puerto Rico Department of Healtha	16,202,850
U.S. Virgin Islands	Virgin Islands Advocacy, Inc	150,000
U.S. Virgin Islands	Virgin Islands Department of Health Groupa	1,074,008

Source: Health Resources and Services Administration. | GAO-18-389.

Note: The Zika Response and Preparedness Act required that $20 million be awarded for projects of regional and national significance in Puerto Rico and other territories. The projects located in California, Florida, Illinois, Indiana, and New Mexico focus on the territories.

[a] This awardee received more than one award and funding amounts for these awards were added together in this table.

APPENDIX XI: NATIONAL INSTITUTES OF HEALTH ZIKA SUPPLEMENTAL AWARDS

The National Institutes of Health (NIH) awarded Zika supplemental funding to support research to better understand Zika and its complications, and inform the development of new interventions.

The three primary activities of funding include (1) vaccine development; (2) Zika in Infants and Pregnancy study; and (3) diagnostics, therapeutics, vector control, and other interventions.[34] NIH used contracts, grants, intramural research awards, and other awards to provide funding for research on the Zika virus and its complications.

Tables 23-26 present information for each award as it was provided to us by NIH.

[34] The Zika in Infants and Pregnancy study aims to improve understanding of the health effects of Zika virus infection in pregnant women and infants by following 10,000 pregnant women for the duration of their pregnancies and their infants at several intervals for at least one year after birth.

Table 23. National institutes of health's Zika supplemental funding contracts

Awardee	Activity description	Award (in dollars)
Advanced Bioscience Laboratories	Support the production and development of a recombinant subunit vaccine consisting of a portion of the Zika virus envelope protein developed by Hawaii Biotech.	455,190.00
Advanced Bioscience Laboratories	PCSs to develop a vaccine production master cell bank for MVA-CHIK/Zika vaccine (Sementis).	445,190.00
American Type Culture Collection	Reagent purchases to support ZIP studies in various countries.	1,370,000.00
Battelle	Support the development of virus neutralizing assay for the assessment of Zika Vaccines.	880,000.00
Baylor College of Medicine	Conduct an epidemiological trial in Guatemala to study the prevalence of microcephaly in a newborn population, viral transmission of Zika and to follow patients diagnosed with ZIKV infection for the development of neurologic manifestations of disease.	5,702,861.00
Deloitte Consulting LLP	Enhance the U.S. Government's partners' (NIH, BARDA, CDC, WRAIR (DoD) and FDA) capabilities in developing vaccine candidates and advancing the most promising to licensure. The ultimate objective is to accelerate the process and reduce costs, not only for Zika but for other vaccines for emerging or reemerging vector borne infectious diseases.	64,589.70
Emory University -Vaccine Trial and Evaluation Units (VTEU)	To Support study of U.S. travelers infected with Zika virus while abroad.	980,000.00
Emory University	Support T-cell assays of samples from 16-0033/34 trials to assess vaccine response.	258,122.01
Saint Louis University - Vaccine Trial and Evaluation Units (VTEU)	Support Phase1 ZPIV Clinical Trials.	2,479,304.00
Southern Research Institute	Support the testing of vaccine candidates against Zika virus infection in the Indian Rhesus macaque model.	1,319,631.00
Southern Research Institute	Southern Research Institute to manufacture and test monoclonal antibody and synthetic compounds as therapeutics against Zika infection.	400,000.00
St. Jude Children's Research Hospital	To continue support the Zika in Infants and Pregnancy (ZIP) study in Colombia.	962,066.00
The Emmes Corporation	Data management and support for clinical studies with NIAID developed Inactivated Zika Vaccine.	3,000,000.00
University of Alabama at Birmingham	Support the Zika in Infants and Pregnancy (ZIP) study in Peru.	997,527.00

Source: National Institutes of Health. | GAO-18-389.

Table 24. National institutes of health's Zika supplemental funding grants

Awardee	Activity description	Award (in dollars)
Beth Israel Deaconess Medical Center	To support the development of Biocryst drug (BCX4430) against Zika virus.	599,666
Boston University Medical Campus	Study effects of pre-existing dengue virus immunity on Zika virus infection.	246,750
Boston University Medical Campus	Study innate placental defense against Zika infection.	258,196
Colorado State University	Study how different cells contribute to sexual and mosquito transmission of Zika.	227,250
Colorado State University	Predicting genetic determinants of Zika virus emergence.	227,875
Colorado State University	Support the study of Zika virus urogenital tropism, pathogenesis and sexual transmission.	211,838
Colorado State University	Support the development of a rapid assay for Zika virus in biofluids and insect vectors.	222,546
Colorado State University	Study virus-host interactions and mechanisms of viral pathogenesis which will provide insights to identify novel targets for antiviral drug development or virus attenuation for vaccine production.	222,436
Columbia University Health Sciences	Support the development of point of care molecular diagnostics differentiating Zika virus from other arbovirus.	434,850
Duke University	Support the Generation of Zika virus-specific recombinant antibodies for the development of Zika Assays.	198,750
Duke University	Study Zika virus infections related birth defects in pregnant rabbit models.	235,406
Emory University	Continue study of Dengue-Zika cross reactivity in vaccine development.	286,546
Emory University	Support the repurposing of drugs to prevent and inhibit Zika virus inflections.	234,000
Fred Hutchinson Cancer Research Center	Supplement to develop novel designs and methods of analysis for upcoming Zika vaccine trials.	99,635
Fundacao Oswaldo Cruz	Continue support natural history study (ZIP) study in pregnant women in Brazil.	1,322,941
George Washington University	Examine genes participating in innate immune response to ZIKV and identify and characterize effector mechanisms involved in controlling ZIKV.	8,576
Georgia Institute of Technology	To develop Zika Virus Vaccines based on Nanoscale Constructs Presenting the Envelope Protein.	250,187
Harvard Medical School	Development of small molecule inhibitors against enveloped virus entry as potential Zika therapeutics.	500,867
Harvard Medical School	Manufacture a VSV vaccine for efficacy studies in mice and NHPs. Conduct efficacy studies in mice against lethal challenge and congenital disease.	299,999
Icahn School of Medicine at Mount Sinai	To study the infection mechanism of Zika virus.	254,250
Icahn School of Medicine at Mount Sinai	Study host determinants in resistance to Zika virus infection.	254,250
Infectious Disease Research Institute	Development of an Innovative, Effective, RNA-based Vaccine for Zika Virus.	178,600

Awardee	Activity description	Award (in dollars)
JHU	To construct a protein-protein interaction (PPI) network between the Zika virus (ZIKV) and the human proteome in order to identify host proteins that play roles in ZIKV life cycle.	245,282
Johns Hopkins University	Methods for Reducing Spatial Uncertainty and Bias in Zika Disease Surveillance.	938,706
Johns Hopkins University	Development of novel Zika vaccine platform using virus-derived chemokine-like molecules.	286,125
Mayo Clinic Rochester	Development of mucosal Single-Cycle Vaccines against Zika Virus.	198,750
Mount Sinai School of Medicine	Study the enhancement of Zika virus infection caused by antibodies to West Nile virus.	252,993
Mount Sinai School of Medicine	Study Zika virus envelop protein mutations.	274,277
New York State Univ	Support Structure-based Design of Zika Virus Inhibitors Targeting Envelope Glycoprotein.	199,089
New York State University, Stony Brook	Study of Zika virus pathogenesis in endothelial cells.	235,543
NirmidasBiotech, Inc.	Develop a Nanoscale Plasmonic-Gold diagnostic platform to differentiate Zika virus infection from other Flavivirus infections.	190,525
Ohio State University	Develop plant-derived, resistance-breaking mosquitocides.	193,125
Oregon Health & Science University	Determining the role of host lipids in Zika virus infection.	231,000
Pennsylvania State University-Univ Park	To investigate the potential role of native and introduced mosquito taxa in the United States to mediate Zika virus invasion and transmission.	235,800
Purdue University	To Study the structure of the Zika virus epitope involved in virus neutralization, which will improve the design of Zika vaccines.	373,831
Research Triangle Institute	Continue clinical data center support for the ZIP studies.	400,000
Rockefeller University	Continued development of a therapeutic mAb for Zika virus.This supplement focuses on developing an expression cell line and evaluating mAb in NHPs.	699,999
South Dakota State	Develop a Zika virus capsid dimerization assay that will be the platform to screen libraries for inhibitors of Zika virus infection.	179,239
Stanford University	Support Nucleotide library (Roche) screening for potential antiviral activity against Zika.	305,080
Stanford University	Study the diagnostic signatures of Zika virus infection.	219,762
State University of New York at Albany	Study the role of Post-transcription RNA Modifications on Zika Virus Gene Expression.	226,813
Texas A&M Agrilife Research	Study social-ecological factors influencing receptivity to Zika virus and the efficacy of interventions in communities along the Texas-Mexico border.	222,750
Texas Tech University Health SCIS Center	To study Zika virus infection in individuals previously exposed to West Nile Virus.	191,250
Texas Tech University Health SCIS Center	Identify ZIKV host factors with an improved CRISPR-based genome-wide knockout screen.	191,250

Table 24. (Continued)

Awardee	Activity description	Award (in dollars)
UC Davis	Develop a novel platform for rapid generation of therapeutic and prophylactic antibody against Zika virus, by site-specific ligation of the virus-capturing ligands to clinical grade intravenous-immunoglobulins.	196,250
University of Alabama at Birmingham	Support the development of high throughput screening (HTS) against ZIKV, using approach developed for screening Dengue.	157,657
University of Alabama at Birmingham	Support the study of Zika virus in semen, as part of ZIP study in Brazil.	457,241
University of California at Davis	Imaging and study of trafficking of Neurotropic Virus in Maternal/Fetal Nonhuman Primates.	193,000
University of California San Diego	To study Zika Virus Pathogenesis and Selective Autophagy Induction to Inhibit Virus Production.	232,500
University of California, Berkeley	Continue operations of the Zika in Infants and Pregnancy (ZIP) study in Nicaragua.	830,000
University of California, Davis	Supplement Zika natural history study in Peru, including simulation models to systematic assess different strategies for controlling and mitigating ZIKV disease burden.	356,436
University of California, Davis	Develop a nonhuman primate model of fetal Zika virus infection and disease.	308,800
University of California, Davis	Support the development of Zika fetal infection models in non-human primate (Rhesus macaque) for therapeutic testing.	1,478,154
University of California, Davis	To study the potential of Culex quinquefasciatus as a vector of the Zika virus.	171,750
University of California, Los Angel	Study the viral kinetics, immunity and transmission of Zika Virus.	201,907
University of California, San Francisco	Support the identification of diagnostic and prognostic biomarkers for Zika infection.	198,125
University of California, San Francisco	Study the role of Zika infection in human pregnancy.	197,523
University of California, San Francisco	Support the study of maternal and fetal cell receptors susceptible to Zika infection and geographical virulence.	397,293
University of California, San Francisco	To study antiviral immunity in the Zika virus mosquito vector.	237,750
University of Colorado, Denver[a]	To continue support the Zika in Infants and Pregnancy (ZIP) study in Guatemala.	589,999
University of Colorado, Denver	Study noncoding RNA production in Zika virus infection.	229,125
University of Connecticut Storrs	To support the rapid development and testing of Zika virus vaccine candidates.	192,254
University of Hawaii at Manoa	Study the modulation of the blood-testis barrier by Zika virus.	231,000
University of Kentucky	Develop novel formulations of double-stranded RNA molecules as tool to further study RNA interference (RNAi) as potential vector control.	210,000
University of Maryland Baltimore	Rapid Phenotyping of the ZIKV Genome.	231,750
University of Miami School of Medicine	Continue support effort to develop point-of-care Zika diagnostic.	167,617

Awardee	Activity description	Award (in dollars)
University of Michigan	To elucidate the molecular mechanisms of the flaviviral nonstructural protein 1 (NS1), a multi-functional virulence protein.	673,901
University of North Carolina Chapel Hill	Support the development and testing of nanoparticle planform for vaccine and adjuvant delivery.	529,300
University of North Carolina Chapel Hill	Study Zika virus in the human genital tract and implications for transmission.	207,868
University of North Carolina Chapel Hill	Study viral and host determinants of Zika virus tissue tropism.	228,000
University of North Carolina Chapel Hill	Structure based design of recombinant Zika virus antigens for serodiagnosis.	233,250
University of North Texas Hlth Sci Ctr	Prevention of Zika transmission with novel Aedes personal protective measures.	276,530
University of Oklahoma Hlth Sciences Ctr	Support development of olive baboon animal model for the study of Zika virus biology and pathogenesis.	222,000
University of Pennsylvania	Support the study of host factors impacting Zika infection via genetic screening.	235,388
University of Pennsylvania	To study mechanisms of Zika virus infection and anti-viral innate immunity.	40,240
University of Pittsburgh at Pittsburgh	Support the development of a Novel, Sensitive ZIKV-Specific Sero-diagnostic Assay Utilizing Biologically Inspired Synthetic Molecules.	703,978
University of Pittsburgh at Pittsburgh	Pre-clinical evaluation of a Zika virus vaccine.	193,332
University of Puerto Rico Med Sciences	To continue support the Zika in Infants and Pregnancy (ZIP) study in Puerto Rico.	830,284
University of Rochester	Support the study of Single-cycle infectious Zika viruses for the development of a live-attenuated vaccine.	180,457
University of Southern California	To study the role autophagy for Zika virus lifecycle.	247,500
University of Texas	To understand the mechanisms that mediate Zika virus replication in specific tissues by manipulating the host ubiquitin system, and identify host factors that can potentially be targeted for therapeutic intervention.	193,750
University of Texas Med Br Galveston	Preclinical development of candidate Zika virus vaccines using mouse models.	196,250
University of Texas Med Br Galveston	To study microbial interplay between ZIKA virus and the native microbiome in mosquitoes.	235,500
University of Texas Medical Br Galveston	Develop a novel system using human fetal brain neural stem cell to model ZIKV infection.	228,650
University of Texas Medical Br Galveston	Develop second generation platforms to deliver zikavaccines, and characterize newly collected zika virus strains in tissue culture, mosquito vectors and animal models for transmission and pathogenesis.	163,282
University of Washington	Support the development of a rapid and specific diagnostic for immunoglobulin response to Zika Virus exposure.	188,696
University of Washington	Study mechanisms of sexual Zika virus transmission and early immunopathogenesis.	232,063
University of Washington	Targeting Zika Virus infection with Chloroquine and related Drugs.	232,625
University of Wisconsin	To support the study of Zika virus using systems biology to better understand the host-pathogen response.	190,106

Table 24. (Continued)

Awardee	Activity description	Award (in dollars)
University of Wisconsin	To study evolution of biological transmission for ZIKV including determining whether or not Wolbachia biocontrol is a sustainable method for ZIKV control and prevention	229,500
University of Wisconsin	Examine the impact of DENV immunity on pregnancy in ZIKV infected rhesus macaques.	753,026
University of Wisconsin	Define South American Zika virus susceptibility and pathogenicity in adult and neonatal nonhuman primates, and testing of hyperimmune sera as potential Zika therapeutic.	1,569,399
University of Wisconsin-Madison	To perform functional analysis of Zika virus induced birth defects.	229,500
University of Wisconsin-Madison	Development of nonhuman Primate Model to Assess Fetal Zika Virus Infection Complications.	221,550
UTMB	Accelerate developmentand acquisition of reagents (cDNA clone, serum, antibodies), small animal model development and characterization of virus and mosquito vectors for Zika research.	499,999
Vanderbilt University[a]	Support efforts to establish a stable cell line for the optimized production of human monoclonal antibody-based prophylaxis.	1,327,897
Wadsworth Center	Study the efficiency of repurposed therapeutics against Flavivirus in mouse models.	238,240
Wadsworth Center	Study the efficiency of repurposed therapeutics against Zika.	235,470
Wadsworth Center	Develop a high throughput screen assay for the identification of orthosteric inhibitors of the critical viral protease consisting of NS2B and NS3 proteins of flaviviruses. As the NS2B-NS3 interactive segments are conserved, an inhibitor would have a broad spectrum of antiviral activity.	523,552
Wadsworth Center	Identifying genetic correlates of Zika virus infection and transmission in U.S. mosquitoes.	181,504
Washington University in St. Louis	Development of Zika vaccine in gorilla adenovirus platform.	190,625
Washington University in St. Louis	Support the development of mAb that can discriminate between Zika and Dengue virus.	530,000
Weill Medical Coll of Cornell Univ	Mapping the RNA modification N6-methyladenosine during Zika virus infection.	263,750
Yale University	Continue studies of Aedes aegyptiand Aedes albopictusas Zika virus vector.	252,460
Yale University	Study mechanisms of innate host defense against sexual Zika virus transmission.	251,250
Yale University	Support the Zika in Infants and Pregnancy (ZIP) study in Brazil.	891,134
Yale University	Support neurological evaluation in adults in Salvador, Brazil as part of the ZIP study.	315,063

Source: National Institutes of Health. | GAO-18-389.

[a] These awardees received more than one award and funding amounts for awards for the same awardee and activity were added together in this table.

Table 25. National institutes of health's Zika supplemental funding intramural awards

Awardee	Activity description	Award (in dollars)
Battelle	To perform PCR testing of clinical studies to evaluate vaccine efficacy.	8,135,441.00
Bioqual	Conduct preclinical studies of Zika vaccine in nonhuman primate models.	1,464,000.00
Johns Hopkins University	Conduct clinical evaluation and data management of NIAID DIR developed Dengue-Zika Chimera Vaccine studies in normal and immunocompromised adults.	4,099,000.00
Leidos Biomedical Research, Inc.	To conduct clinical trials for NIAID VRC developed DNA Vaccine.	48,635,750.00
Leidos Biomedical Research, Inc.	Manufacturing and clinical evaluation of NIAID DIR developed live attenuated Dengue-Zika Chimera Vaccine in Brazil.	11,664,304.09
The Emmes Corporation	To provide clinical data management and monitoring support for phase 2 DNA Vaccine studies.	11,390,893.00
Various	Labor, material, and supplies to support the preclinical development and testing of Zika vaccines at NIAID intramural laboratories.	9,593,809.09

Source: National Institutes of Health. | GAO-18-389.

Table 26. Other national institutes of health Zika supplemental funding awards

Awardee	Activity description	Award (in dollars)
AI Biosciences, Inc.	Support the development of rapid and low-cost point-of-care assay for Zika virus diagnosis.	224,955
Crosslife Technologies, Inc.	Development of a rapid paper strip nucleic acid test for the point-of-care detection of Zika virus.	299,574
L2 Diagnostics, LLC	Support the development of rapid, low-cost point of care diagnostic for detection of Zika virus RNA.	225,000
Springstar, Inc.	To modify the CDC autocidal gravid ovitrap (AGO) into a design amenable to large-scale, low cost production for development of improved vector control strategies.	618, 531
United States Dept. of Agriculture	Zika workshop support in collaboration with USDA-Scientific consultation on Zika Virus Vaccine Development.	75,000
United States Dept. of Agriculture	Zika workshop support in collaboration with USDA-Consultation on the Ethics of ZikV Human Challenge Trials.	75,000
University of Oxford, The	Printing of Zika-specific supplement in the JOURNAL OF INFECTIOUS DISEASES to disseminate research findings.	83,250

Source: National Institutes of Health. | GAO-18-389.

In: Infectious Diseases
Editor: Philippe Georges
ISBN: 978-1-53616-401-5

Chapter 4

EMERGENCY ASSISTANCE FOR ZIKA: USAID SUPPORTED ACTIVITIES OVERSEAS BUT COULD IMPROVE FUNDS TRACKING AND RESPONSE PLANNING*

United States Government Accountability Office

ABBREVIATIONS

ASSIST	Applying Science to Strengthen and Improve Systems
CAZ	Community Action on Zika
CDC	Centers for Disease Control and Prevention
State	Department of State
UNICEF	United Nations Children's Fund
USAID	U.S. Agency for International Development
WHO	World Health Organization
ZAP	Zika AIRS Project

WHY GAO DID THIS STUDY

The World Health Organization (WHO) declared the Zika virus a public health emergency of international concern in February 2016. According to WHO, as of March 2017, 79 countries and territories—including 48 in the Western Hemisphere—reported

* This is an edited, reformatted and augmented version of United States Government Accountability Office; Report to Congressional Requesters, Publication No. GAO-19-356, dated May 2019.

evidence of ongoing Zika transmission. In April 2016, USAID and State repurposed $215 million for Zika from funds appropriated for Ebola. Subsequently, the Zika Response and Preparedness Appropriations Act, 2016, provided over $175 million in supplemental funding to USAID and State to support Zika response efforts overseas. The act also included a provision for GAO to review the status of USAID and State actions to respond to Zika. In March 2019, the Centers for Disease Control and Prevention downgraded its international travel warning for Zika.

This chapter examines (1) the status of USAID and State funding for U.S. Zika response overseas, (2) activities supported by these funds, and (3) implementation challenges, if any, and responses to any challenges. GAO reviewed information from U.S. agencies and met with U.S. and host country officials in Washington, D.C. GAO also conducted fieldwork in a nongeneralizable sample of countries in Latin America and the Caribbean where agencies implemented key response activities.

WHAT GAO RECOMMENDS

USAID should (1) take steps to ensure it is able to compile funding information by country for future infectious disease emergency responses and (2) take steps to improve its infectious disease response planning. USAID concurred with GAO's recommendations.

WHAT GAO FOUND

The U.S. Agency for International Development (USAID) and the Department of State (State) obligated $385 million of the total $390 million available for international Zika response and disbursed $264 million as of September 2018. USAID obligated 95 percent of the total funding. USAID and State provided some country information to Congress but did not provide, or take steps to track, funding on a country basis. According to USAID officials, tracking funding information by country would be helpful in the future. The ability to compile funding by country when responding to future infectious disease outbreaks would enable USAID to provide additional information to key decision makers to better support spending oversight and inform budgetary and planning decisions.

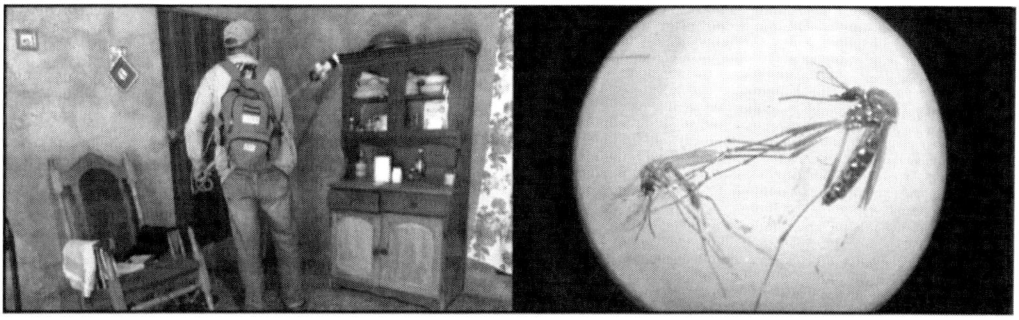

Source: GAO. | GAO-19-356

USAID-Supported Worker Collects Insects for Monitoring Purposes in a Home in Honduras (left), and Mosquito That Carries the Zika Virus Viewed under a Microscope (right).

In response to the Zika outbreak, USAID and State supported a broad range of activities overseas, including mosquito control, research efforts, and medical evacuations. In one activity, USAID implementing partners monitored mosquito populations; in another, they researched methods to reduce Zika virus transmission rates. USAID implementing partners reported various outputs from selected activities. For example, an implementing partner reported that its awareness campaign on Zika prevention reached more than 5 million people.

USAID faced sustainability and timeliness challenges in implementing its Zika response. According to agency and other officials, one-time funding and a short time frame posed a challenge related to sustainability of Zika response activities. In response, USAID worked to align activities with those of host governments and other organizations so they could continue in the long term. However, USAID's emergency response planning did not fully address the challenge of timely implementation of response activities in countries without bilateral USAID health programs. Twenty-two of 26 countries with Zika response activities did not have bilateral USAID health programs when the Zika outbreak began. As a result, response activities took additional time to deploy in some countries where USAID first had to establish relationships with key host country officials. Although USAID developed an infectious disease response plan in 2018, the plan does not provide guidance on how to address the timely implementation challenge in countries without bilateral health programs. By improving its planning, such as by adding such guidance in its 2018 plan, USAID would be better positioned to respond quickly to future disease outbreaks.

May 13, 2019

The Honorable Lindsey Graham
Chairman

The Honorable Patrick Leahy
Ranking Member
Committee on Appropriations
Subcommittee on State, Foreign Operations, and Related Programs
United States Senate

The Honorable Nita Lowey
Chairwoman

The Honorable Hal Rogers
Ranking Member
Committee on Appropriations
Subcommittee on State, Foreign Operations, and Related Programs
House of Representatives

Zika is a virus that is primarily transmitted through mosquito bites and causes symptoms that include fever, rash, conjunctivitis, and joint and muscle pain, though many infected individuals do not have symptoms or only experience mild symptoms. The Zika infection in pregnant women has been linked to adverse pregnancy and birth outcomes: The virus can be passed to the fetus and cause microcephaly and other severe brain defects and may be associated with miscarriage and stillbirth, according to the Centers for Disease Control and Prevention (CDC).[207] The Zika virus is also linked to other problems such as Guillain-Barré syndrome, an uncommon condition of the nervous system. In the Western Hemisphere, the first cases of locally transmitted Zika virus disease were confirmed in Brazil in May 2015. The World Health Organization (WHO) declared the Zika virus a public health emergency of international concern in February 2016. While WHO declared an end to the public health emergency in November 2016, it subsequently reported that 48 countries and territories in the Western Hemisphere reported evidence of ongoing Zika transmission, as of March 2017.[208]

To address the epidemic, according to U.S. Agency for International Development (USAID) documentation, $215 million of fiscal year 2015 supplemental Economic Support Fund funding initially appropriated to respond to the Ebola virus was repurposed for the U.S. Zika response overseas. The Zika Response and Preparedness Appropriations Act, 2016, also provided over $175 million in supplemental funding to USAID and the Department of State (State) through the end of fiscal year 2017 to support the U.S. Zika

[207] Microcephaly is a rare birth defect that causes a baby's head to be smaller than expected and not fully developed, which can lead to impaired thought processes, delayed development of motor skills, and other adverse outcomes.

[208] In March 2019, CDC downgraded its international travel warning for Zika, which had recommended that pregnant women not travel to Zika-affected countries in Latin America. The March 2019 travel warning recommended that pregnant women consult a health care provider before traveling to Zika-affected countries in Latin America.

response efforts overseas.[209] The act required USAID and State to submit a consolidated report to Congress on the anticipated uses of the funds appropriated in the act on a country and project basis and to submit updates every 60 days until September 30, 2017.[210] The act also included a provision for us to review the status of USAID and State actions to respond to Zika. This chapter examines (1) the status of USAID and State funding for the U.S. Zika response overseas, (2) activities supported by these funds, and (3) challenges, if any, to implementing Zika response activities and actions taken to address any challenges.

To examine the status of USAID and State funding for the U.S. Zika response overseas, we reviewed obligations and disbursements that the agencies reported as supporting international Zika response activities, as of September 30, 2018. We also reviewed USAID and State's consolidated reports to the Senate and House Committees on Appropriations mandated by the Zika Response and Preparedness Appropriations Act, 2016, and interviewed agency officials to discuss the status of the agencies' obligations and disbursements for Zika response activities. We determined that the data we used were sufficiently reliable for the purposes of determining the status of USAID and State funding for the U.S. Zika response overseas. We assessed USAID's tracking of funding data against federal internal control standards related to using quality information.[211]

To examine activities that USAID and State implemented in response to Zika overseas, we conducted fieldwork, analyzed agency documents, and interviewed officials. We examined the status and progress of Zika response activities. We conducted fieldwork in a nongeneralizable sample of countries: Barbados, Colombia, Dominican Republic, Guatemala, Honduras, Peru, and Trinidad and Tobago. We selected these countries based on criteria including, among others, geographic diversity to include the Caribbean, Central America, and South America and the presence of activities under way that accounted for a significant portion of total USAID and State Zika funding. During our fieldwork, we interviewed agency officials, host government officials, implementing partners, health care workers, community volunteers, and researchers to get their perspectives on the progress of Zika response activities. We analyzed agency documents describing the plans and goals of activities. We also analyzed progress reports of a sample of six activities to provide illustrative examples of results from these activities as reported by implementing partners. For this sample, we selected activities that had among the highest amounts of funding and that together represented a range of countries, lines of effort, and types of implementing partners. Our sample is not generalizable to all activities.

---

[209] Pub. L. No. 114-223, Div. B, Zika Response and Preparedness Appropriations Act, 2016, (Sept. 29, 2016).

[210] The agencies submitted their initial report on October 28, 2016.

[211] GAO, *Standards for Internal Control in the Federal Government,* GAO-14-704G (Washington, D.C.: September 2014).

To examine challenges, if any, to implementing Zika response activities and actions taken to address any challenges, we interviewed USAID officials, USAID implementing partners, and host government officials, and we analyzed progress reports from selected USAID-funded Zika response activities. We analyzed the information collected in the interviews and document reviews to identify the themes, or key challenges and responses to those challenges. We assessed USAID's infectious disease response plan against relevant federal internal control standards.[212] See appendix I for more information on our objectives, scope, and methodology.

We conducted this performance audit from December 2017 to May 2019 in accordance with generally accepted government auditing standards. Those standards require that we plan and perform the audit to obtain sufficient, appropriate evidence to provide a reasonable basis for our findings and conclusions based on our audit objectives. We believe that the evidence obtained provides a reasonable basis for our findings and conclusions based on our audit objectives.

BACKGROUND

Zika Transmission and Effects

Zika is spread to people primarily through the bite of an infected mosquito but can also be transmitted from mother to child during pregnancy or from person to person through sexual contact or blood transfusion.[213] The disease can cause symptoms that include fever, rash, conjunctivitis ("pink eye" where the eyes appear red or pink), and joint and muscle pain. Although most people with Zika have only mild symptoms or none at all, Zika in pregnant women has been linked to adverse pregnancy outcomes, such as miscarriage and stillbirth, and severe birth defects. Zika can be passed to the fetus and cause a birth defect of the brain called microcephaly and other severe brain defects, according to CDC.[214] Zika is also linked to other problems such as Guillain-Barré syndrome, an uncommon condition of the nervous system.[215] Although at present no vaccine has been approved by the U.S. Food and Drug Administration to prevent Zika, several vaccines are in different phases of development.

---

[212] GAO-14-704G.

[213] The *Aedes aegypti* is reportedly the primary mosquito spreading the Zika virus, while the *Aedes albopictus* mosquito, which shares many of the same traits as *Aedes aegypti*, also has the ability to spread the virus.

[214] Babies with microcephaly can have a range of other health problems, depending on the severity of their condition. These health problems can range from mild to severe, may be life-threatening in some cases, and are often lifelong issues.

[215] Guillain-Barré syndrome is a rare disorder in which the body's immune system attacks the nervous system outside the brain and spinal cord, causing muscle weakness and in some cases paralysis, although most people recover.

The Zika Epidemic

Zika was first identified in the Zika Forest in Uganda in 1947 and caused only sporadic human disease until 2007. In 2007, Zika was detected in Yap State, Federated States of Micronesia, and subsequent outbreaks occurred in Southeast Asia and the Western Pacific. In 2014, Zika spread east across the Pacific Ocean to French Polynesia, then to Easter Island. In May 2015, Brazil documented the first case of locally acquired Zika transmission in the Americas. See Figure 1 for a timeline of the Zika outbreak and the U.S. Zika response overseas. According to WHO, in November 2015, Suriname, El Salvador, Guatemala, Mexico, Paraguay, and Venezuela reported cases of locally acquired Zika, followed by Panama, Honduras, French Guiana, Martinique, and Puerto Rico in December 2015. Zika continued to spread throughout the region, and on February 1, 2016, WHO declared that the recent association of Zika with clusters of microcephaly and other neurological disorders constituted a public health emergency of international concern. In November 2016, WHO declared an end of the public health emergency of international concern regarding microcephaly, other neurological disorders, and Zika. However, WHO announced that Zika and the associated health outcomes remained a significant public health challenge requiring intense action.

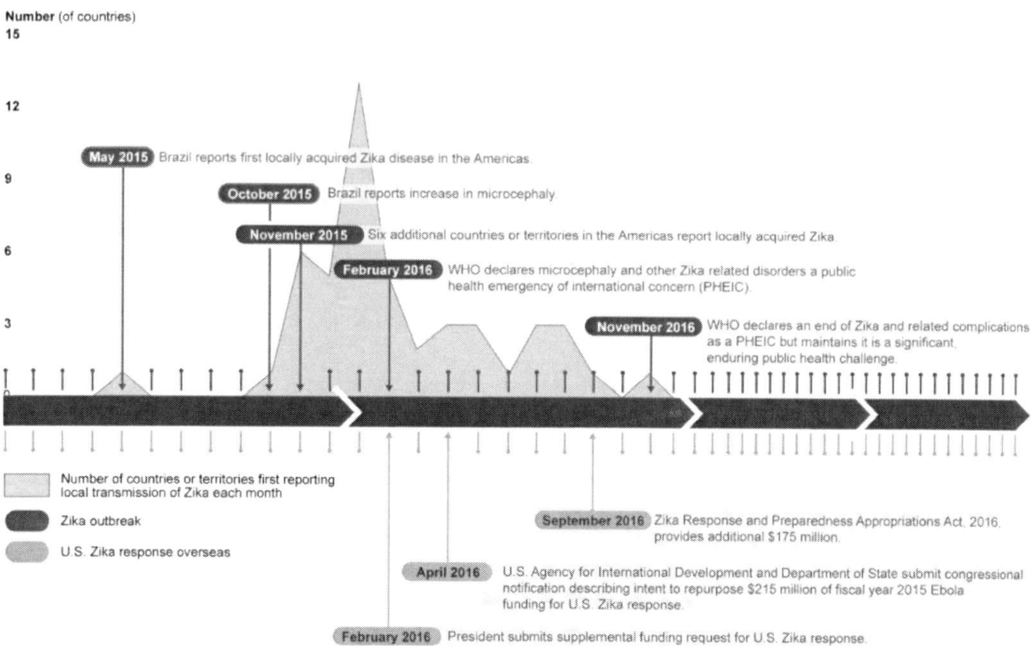

Source: GAO analysis of Pan American Health Organization, Word Health Orgnization (WHO) and U.S. government document. | GAO-19-356

Figure 1. Timeline of Zika Outbreak and the U.S. Zika Response Overseas, 2015–2018.

Zika spread to multiple countries throughout the globe but primarily affected countries in Latin America and the Caribbean region. According to WHO, as of March 2017, transmission of the Zika virus was occurring in 79 countries or territories, most of which are located in the Western Hemisphere.[216] According to WHO, from 2015 to 2017, there were approximately 583,000 suspected and 223,000 confirmed cases of Zika virus transmission in the Western Hemisphere. See Figure 2 for the cumulative Zika incidence rates in each country in Latin America and the Caribbean from 2015 to 2017.

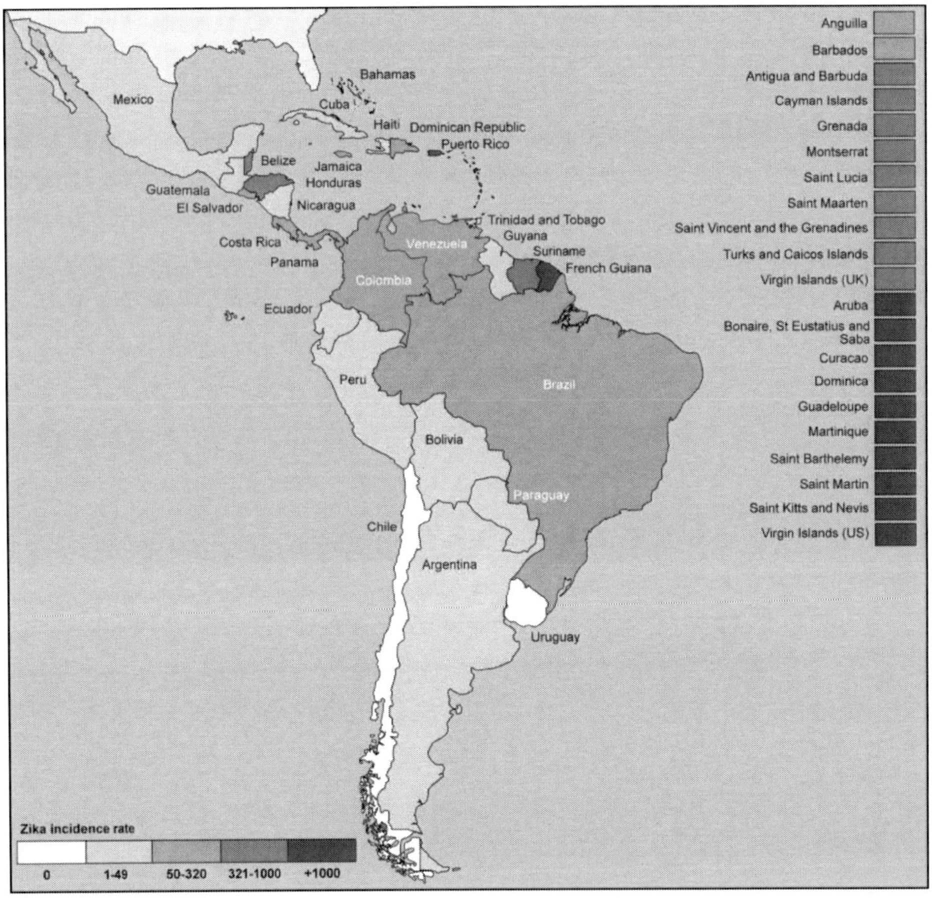

Source: GAO analysis of Pan American Health Organization data. | GAO-19-356

Notes: The incidence rate is the number of reported suspected and confirmed locally acquired Zika cases in a country or territory per 100,000 population from 2015 through 2017. The cases were those reported to the World Health Organization through the countries' ministry of health websites as of January 4, 2018.

Figure 2. Zika Incidence Rates in Latin America and the Caribbean, 2015–2017.

---

[216] Of the 79 countries or territories, 61 (including 47 in the Western Hemisphere) were classified by WHO in the most severe category: areas with new introduction or reintroduction with ongoing transmission of Zika. The other 18 countries or territories (including one in the Western Hemisphere) were classified by WHO in a less severe category: areas with either evidence of virus circulation before 2015 or ongoing transmission that was no longer in the new or reintroduction phase, but where there was no evidence of interruption.

U.S. Response to Zika Overseas

In February 2016, the President submitted a request to Congress for emergency funding to enhance ongoing U.S. efforts to prepare for and respond to Zika, including a request for funding for USAID and State to respond to the outbreak overseas. In addition, in April 2016, USAID and State notified Congress of their intent to repurpose $215 million of fiscal year 2015 supplemental Economic Support Fund Ebola funding for the U.S. Zika response overseas, which included $78 million for CDC international Zika activities.[217] In September 2016, Congress appropriated about $175.1 million in supplemental funding to USAID and State in the Zika Response and Preparedness Appropriations Act, 2016, for the U.S. Zika response overseas. USAID activities initially began in five countries—Haiti, Honduras, Guatemala, El Salvador, and Dominican Republic—based on an assessment of their Zika risk and limited host government capacity to prevent the spread and respond to the impact of the virus. USAID ultimately supported activities in 26 countries in the Latin America and Caribbean region.

USAID and State Obligated Almost All Funding Available for the Zika Response but Did Not Report Funding by Country

USAID and State Obligated Almost All Funding Available for the Zika Response and Disbursed Approximately Two-Thirds

As of September 30, 2018, USAID and State had obligated about $385 million (99 percent) of the total $390 million available for the U.S. Zika response overseas and had disbursed approximately $264 million (68 percent). Specifically, USAID had obligated all of its funds available for the Zika response and disbursed about two-thirds, and State had obligated and disbursed more than three-quarters of its funding for Zika. USAID and State had disbursed a higher proportion of the repurposed Ebola funds than the funds appropriated in the Zika Response and Preparedness Appropriations Act, 2016.[218] See Figure 3 for USAID and State Zika response funding appropriations, obligations, and disbursements as of September 30, 2018. Of the $215 million in repurposed Ebola funds, USAID and State had obligated $215 million (100 percent) and had disbursed almost $201 million (93 percent) as of September 30, 2018. Of the approximately $175 million

---

[217] According to State documentation, the funds, which were provided by the Department of State, Foreign Operations, and Related Programs Appropriations Act, 2015, Pub. L. No. 113-235, Div. J, (Dec. 16, 2014), were repurposed pursuant to section 7058(c) of the act.

[218] USAID and State have two sources of funding for Zika response activities: $215 million in fiscal year 2015 supplemental Economic Support Fund Ebola funding that was repurposed to the Zika response and about $175 million through a supplemental appropriation provided under the Zika Response and Preparedness Appropriations Act, 2016, for a total of $390 million.

appropriated in the Zika Response and Preparedness Appropriations Act, 2016, USAID and State had obligated about $170 million (about 97 percent) and had disbursed about $63 million (36 percent) as of September 30, 2018.

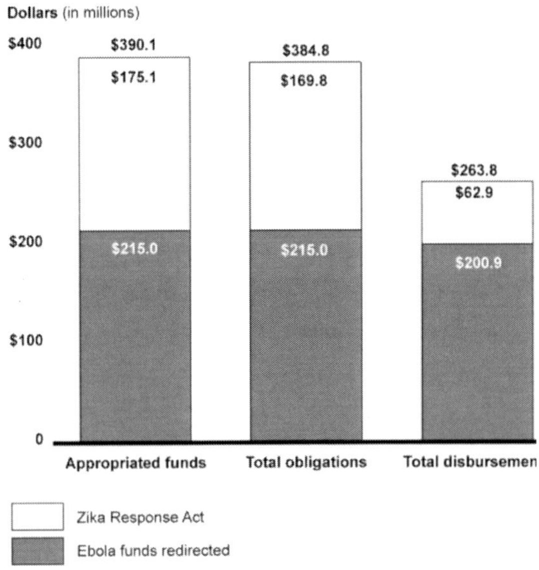

Source: GAO analysis of USAID and State data. | GAO-19-356

Notes: USAID and State have two sources of funding for Zika response activities: $215 million in fiscal year 2015 supplemental Economic Support Fund Ebola funding that was repurposed for the Zika response and about $175 million through a supplemental appropriation provided under the Zika Response and Preparedness Appropriations Act, 2016, for a total of $390 million.

Figure 3. U.S. Agency for International Development (USAID) and Department of State (State) Zika Response Appropriations, Obligations, and Disbursements, as of September 30, 2018.

USAID and State Track Zika Funding by Account and Activity

As of September 30, 2018, USAID had obligated all funds available for the Zika response and had disbursed about two-thirds, from three accounts. USAID has two sources of funding for Zika response activities: $211 million of fiscal year 2015 supplemental Economic Support Fund Ebola funding repurposed for the Zika response and about $155.5 million provided in the Zika Response and Preparedness Appropriations Act, 2016—including $145.5 million and $10.0 million through the Global Health Programs and Operating Expenses accounts, respectively—for a total of $366.5 million. As of September 30, 2018, USAID had obligated approximately $366.5 million (100 percent) and had disbursed approximately $245 million (67 percent), from the Economic Support Fund, Global Health Programs, and Operating Expenses appropriations accounts. See Figure 4 for USAID Zika response funding obligations and disbursements by account. USAID obligated all funding for Zika response activities within a year after it was repurposed or appropriated.[219] As of September 30, 2018, USAID had disbursed a higher proportion of repurposed fiscal year 2015 supplemental Economic Support Fund Ebola funding (93 percent) compared with Global Health Programs and Operating Expenses funding (28 percent and 72 percent, respectively), which was appropriated in the Zika Response and Preparedness Appropriations Act, 2016, in September 2016.

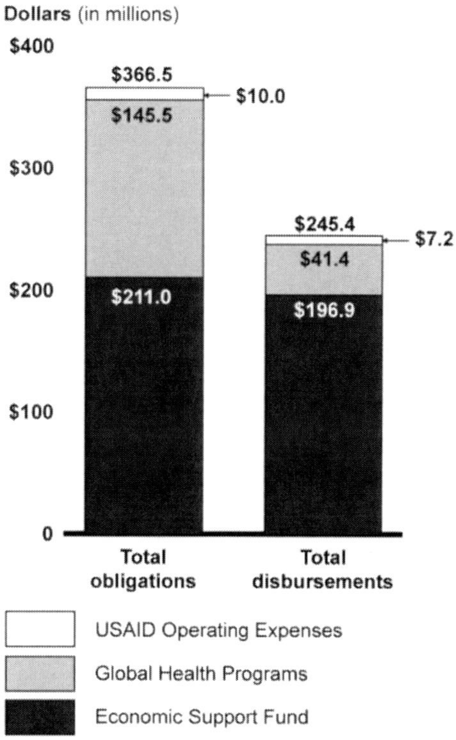

Source: GAO analysis of USAID data. | GAO-19-356

Note: USAID has two sources of funding for Zika response activities: $211 million of fiscal year 2015 supplemental Economic Support Fund Ebola funding that was repurposed for the Zika response and about $155.5 million provided in the Zika Response and Preparedness Appropriations Act, 2016, through the Global Health Programs and Operating Expenses accounts, for a total of $366.5 million.

Figure 4. U.S. Agency for International Development (USAID) Obligations and Disbursements by Account for Zika Response Activities, as of September 30, 2018.

The $211 million in Economic Support Fund obligations supported 56 USAID activities, as well as a $78 million interagency transfer to CDC. The $145.5 million in

[219] By November 2016, USAID had obligated all $211 million of the repurposed fiscal year 2015 Ebola funds. By September 2017, USAID had obligated all $155.5 million of the USAID Zika funds appropriated in September 2016.

Global Health Programs obligations supported 25 activities and program support.[220] Obligations for USAID-supported activities ranged from $12,000 to $37 million and included support for activities such as the procurement of insect repellent to assist pregnant women in avoiding Zika infection and strengthening the ability of civil society and community networks to disseminate information related to Zika. CDC supported 25 activities that ranged from $276,000 to $13.6 million, including activities such as collecting and analyzing public health data, conducting epidemiological studies to better understand the prevalence of Zika and related risk factors, building laboratory capacity, and providing training to conduct Zika virus testing.

As of September 30, 2018, State had obligated and disbursed more than three-quarters of funding available for the Zika response, from two accounts. State has two sources of funding for Zika response activities: $4 million from a fiscal year 2015 supplemental Economic Support Fund appropriation for the Ebola response that was repurposed for the Zika response and about $19.6 million provided in the Zika Response and Preparedness Appropriations Act, 2016, the majority of which was provided through the Diplomatic and Consular Programs account, for a total of about $23.6 million.[221] As of September 30, 2018, State had obligated and disbursed about $18.3 million (almost 78 percent) from the Economic Support Fund and Diplomatic and Consular Programs accounts. See Figure 5 for State Zika response funding obligations and disbursements by account.

Under the Zika Response and Preparedness Appropriations Act, 2016, State was provided almost $14.6 million through the Diplomatic and Consular Programs account, $4 million through the Emergencies in Diplomatic and Consular Services account, and $1 million through the Repatriation Loans Program account, for a total of almost $19.6 million. In September 2017, State notified Congress of its intent to transfer the $4 million from the Emergencies in Diplomatic and Consular Services account and $870,000 from the Repatriation Loans Program account to the Diplomatic and Consular Programs account. These transfers resulted in a total of $19.5 million available under the Diplomatic and Consular Programs account and $130,000 under the Repatriation Loans Program account.

[220] As of September 30, 2018, USAID had also obligated almost $10 million from the Operating Expenses account to support activities. For example, Operating Expenses funds covered some expenses related to the procurement of mosquito repellents and condoms for Zika prevention. The funds were also used to help build and strengthen USAID staff capacity to effectively plan, implement, and monitor malaria and vector-borne disease control in countries where USAID operates.

[221] Under the Zika Response and Preparedness Appropriations Act, 2016, State was provided almost $14.6 million through the Diplomatic and Consular Programs account, $4 million through the Emergencies in Diplomatic and Consular Services account, and $1 million through the Repatriation Loans Program account, for a total of almost $19.6 million. In September 2017, State notified Congress of its intent to transfer the $4 million from the Emergencies in Diplomatic and Consular Services account and $870,000 from the Repatriation Loans Program account to the Diplomatic and Consular Programs account, to support an additional $4,870,000 in Zika-related public diplomacy initiatives to be conducted by the Bureau of Oceans and International Environmental and Scientific Affairs.

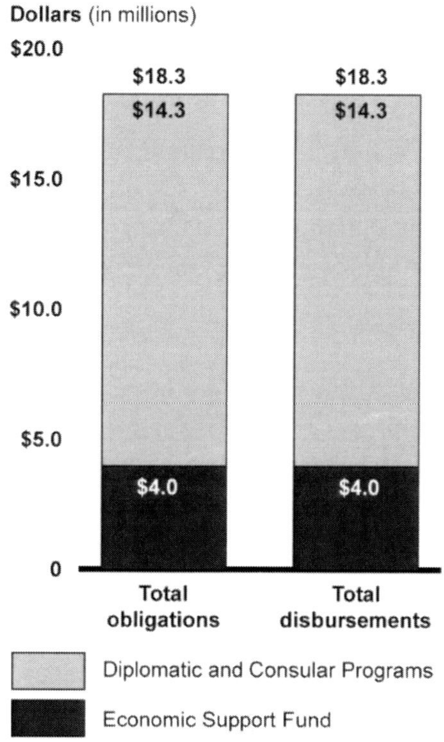

Source: GAO analysis of State data. | GAO-19-356

Notes: State has two sources of funding for Zika response activities: $4 million of fiscal year 2015 supplemental Economic Support Fund Ebola funding that was repurposed for the Zika response, and about $19.5 million under the Diplomatic and Consular Programs account and $130,000 under the Repatriation Loans Program account provided in the Zika Response and Preparedness Appropriations Act, 2016, for a total of $23.6 million. State has not made any obligations or disbursements under the Repatriation Loans Program account, and therefore this account does not appear in the figure above.

Figure 5. Department of State (State) Obligations and Disbursements by Account for Zika Response Activities, as of September 30, 2018.

The $4 million in Economic Support Fund obligations supported research and development activities by the International Atomic Energy Agency to control disease-carrying mosquito populations. The $14.3 million in Diplomatic and Consular Programs obligations supported activities including medical evacuations to protect the health of pregnant U.S. government personnel and eligible family members, mosquito abatement training and other measures to reduce Zika risk to overseas staff, as well as public diplomacy efforts to further inform journalists and the public about the U.S. response to Zika.

Agencies Did Not Track or Report Zika Funding by Country

In their reporting to Congress on the uses of Zika funds, USAID and State included some country information but did not track or provide information on funding uses broken down on a country basis. In October 2016, USAID and State submitted a consolidated report to the appropriations committees on the anticipated uses of funds made available to USAID and State by the Zika Response and Preparedness Appropriations Act, 2016, in response to a reporting requirement in Section 203 of the act.[222] After the initial submission, the act required the agencies to update and submit the report to the committees on appropriations every 60 days until September 30, 2017. The initial report described ongoing Zika response activities in five countries as well as planned activities in additional countries. Subsequent reports listed specific countries where USAID and State supported Zika response activities. However, USAID and State did not provide information to Congress on the uses of funding appropriated by the Zika Response and Preparedness Appropriations Act, 2016, broken down by country. The reports also included obligation and disbursement information for the fiscal year 2015 supplemental Economic Support Fund Ebola funding that was repurposed for the international Zika response; however, similar to the information provided regarding the funds appropriated by the Zika Response and Preparedness Appropriations Act, 2016, the reports' information on the use of the repurposed Ebola funds was also not broken down by country.[223]

USAID officials told us that Zika activities were designed to be implemented on a regional and multicountry basis. While over 95 percent of all U.S. government funds available for the Zika response overseas were obligated by USAID, and the agency had a number of financial tracking systems in place, the agency did not take steps to record its funding by country at the outset of Zika response programming. Specifically, USAID officials noted that the contracts and grants the agency had signed with its implementing partners did not include provisions requiring partners to provide information to USAID that broke down their use of funds by country. Consequently, USAID was unable to track the uses of Zika funds on a country basis.

---

[222] Pub. L. No. 114-223, Div. B, Zika Response and Preparedness Appropriations Act, 2016, § 203, (Sept. 29, 2016).

[223] While USAID and State provided information about the repurposed Ebola funds in the Zika reports, the reports indicated that the inclusion of that information was not required by the Zika Response and Preparedness Appropriations Act, 2016, which specifically required reporting on the use of funds made available by that act. The Zika reports noted that information about the repurposed Ebola funds could also be found in the agencies' Ebola reports; however, the information in the Ebola reports regarding the funds repurposed for the Zika response also did not include a breakdown of the use of those funds by country. The Ebola reports were created in response to a reporting requirement in the Department of State, Foreign Operations, and Related Programs Appropriations Act, 2015, which appropriated funds to USAID and State for necessary expenses to assist countries affected by, or at risk of being affected by, the Ebola outbreak, among other things. See Pub. L. No. 113-235, Div. J, Title IX, § 9004 (Dec. 16, 2014).

Federal internal control standards state that management should use and communicate the necessary quality information both internally and externally to achieve the entity's objectives and address related risks.[224] According to USAID officials, tracking information on the uses of Zika response funding broken down by country would be helpful in the future for mission directors, chiefs of missions, and partner-country ministries of health, some of whom have requested this information. Moreover, data on USAID funding to address future infectious disease outbreaks if broken down by uses in each country could provide additional useful information to decision makers in assessing risks and planning responses. The ability to compile funding by country when responding to future infectious disease outbreaks would enable USAID to provide key decision makers, including Congress and agency officials, with additional information to better support spending oversight and inform budgetary and planning decisions.

USAID and State Supported a Broad Range of Activities in Response to Zika

USAID Supported Mosquito Control, Public Awareness, Capacity Building, and Research Activities

As part of the U.S. Zika response overseas, USAID provided assistance to several countries in the Caribbean, Central America, and South America and conducted a variety of activities related to mosquito control, public awareness, capacity building, and research.

Mosquito Control

In support of mosquito control, USAID's Zika AIRS Project (ZAP) conducted activities that included

- Entomological monitoring: collecting and reporting information on the location and population of mosquitoes;
- Larviciding: placing agents that kill mosquito eggs in likely breeding sites, such as water receptacles;
- Source reduction interventions: facilitating the removal or mitigation of likely breeding sites, such as tires, pots, barrels, or anything that may allow for standing water; and
- Indoor residual spraying: spraying insecticide that has a lasting effect in houses.

[224] GAO-14-704G.

We observed mosquito control activities during our fieldwork. For example, in Honduras we followed a team as they went house to house to implement and facilitate mosquito control activities. They collected information from mosquito egg traps, which serve as indicator of breeding activity, and recorded it for monitoring purposes. They also examined the premises for potential mosquito breeding sites, treated susceptible areas such as wash basins with larvicide, and spoke with residents about picking up trash and covering outdoor plant pots to reduce potential breeding sites.

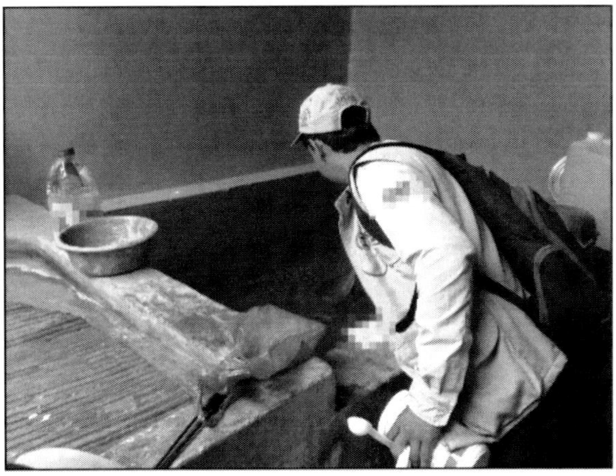

Source: GAO. | GAO-19-356

Figure 6. A Worker for a U.S. Agency for International Development Implementing Partner Puts Mosquito Larvicide in a Wash Basin in a House in Honduras.

Public Awareness

To support raising public awareness of the risk of Zika virus and to promote behavior change to reduce the spread of the disease, USAID implementing partners such as the Red Cross and CARE told us that they collaborated with communities, local government, and schools to communicate information about Zika. For example, in Trinidad, the Red Cross conducted educational campaigns at schools to improve students' awareness. During our fieldwork, we observed a session led by adult volunteers during which children played games and engaged in discussions designed to teach Zika prevention and response methods. Implementing partners told us that the impact of such efforts extends beyond those reached directly; for example, they said the children who learned about Zika risks and prevention also conveyed the knowledge to their families, who in turn may pass it on to friends or others in the community.

In Peru, CARE worked with schools to develop written education guides for application in the classroom and conducted communication campaigns. During our fieldwork, we went to schools and observed students delivering oral presentations on Zika risks and prevention. In addition, we witnessed other student activities, such as classroom discussions and art projects focused on Zika, designed to demonstrate understanding, raise awareness, and promote behavior change.

Capacity Building

To support capacity building, the Applying Science to Strengthen and Improve Systems (ASSIST) activity, which USAID funding supported, focused on improving Zika-related health services. Specific efforts included conducting a baseline assessment of the quality of care, improving clinical guidelines, training health care providers, and implementing a quality improvement program. During our fieldwork in Honduras, we visited a hospital and met with ASSIST-supported health workers who told us that they applied new guidance in their practice, and as a result, improved care in areas including counseling, screening, diagnosis, and follow-up of those affected by Zika. We also visited a hospital in Dominican Republic, where health care workers stated that they collaborated with ASSIST in responding to Zika by training staff and producing guidance materials. These activities raised awareness, increased prevention efforts, and improved care, according to health care workers.

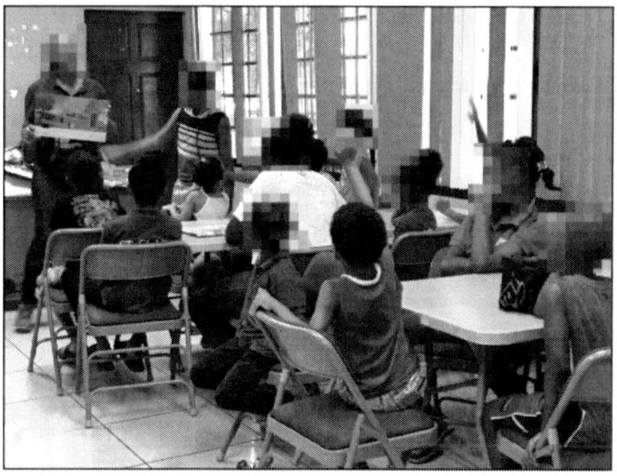

Source: GAO. | GAO-19-356

Figure 7. School Children Participate in a Learning Activity Aimed at Promoting Awareness of Zika Risks and Prevention in Trinidad.

Research

USAID supported research, training, and innovation activities through its "Grand Challenge" program as well as its interagency agreement with CDC. USAID launched a series of Grand Challenge efforts, providing $30 million in grants to foster innovation on new methods and technologies to respond to Zika. One grant, for example, supported the World Mosquito Program's research into the feasibility and effectiveness of infecting mosquitoes with bacteria to hinder transmission of the Zika virus. We visited the program's operations in Colombia, met with scientists, and observed the breeding lab.

Program scientists told us that initial efforts have been promising and that if more tests prove successful, the potential for reducing Zika transmission could be significant. Another USAID Grand Challenge grant supports research into the possible use of genetically modified yeast to prevent mosquito eggs from hatching. We spoke with scientists, lab technicians, and viewed facilities supported by this grant in Trinidad during our field work. Scientists stated that yeast attracts mosquitoes and is inexpensive, commonly available, and environmentally friendly. Testing is ongoing, but if successful, the approach could help reduce populations of mosquitoes in critical areas, according to the scientists.

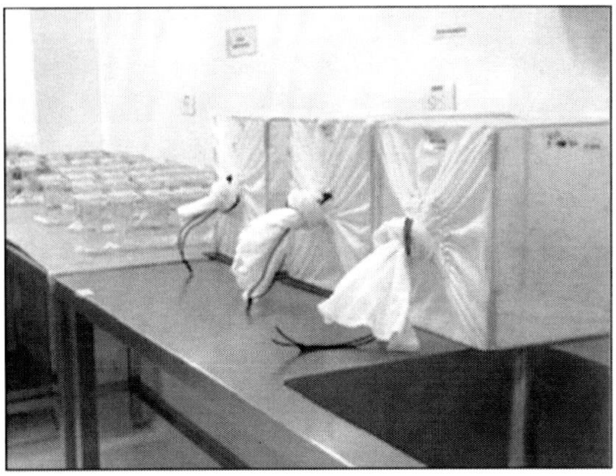

Source: GAO. | GAO-19-356

Figure 8. The World Mosquito Program Breeds Mosquitoes Harboring Bacteria to Test the Feasibility of Hindering Transmission of the Zika Virus.

The USAID–CDC interagency agreement identifies a range of activities that involve technical assistance to help strengthen surveillance, emergency operations and management, and epidemiological investigations and research. One CDC activity, for example, focuses on supporting public health surveillance and epidemiological studies to better understand the prevalence and risk factors for severe health outcomes related to Zika. Another activity aims to build laboratory capacity in areas such as Zika diagnostic test production and distribution. In addition, the objectives of CDC's Field Epidemiology Training Program are to train qualified professionals, build sustainable capacity for detecting and responding to health threats, and develop in-country expertise so that disease outbreaks can be detected locally and prevented from spreading. In Dominican Republic, CDC officials told us that this program delivers 3 months of classroom and field project training, and that as of August 2018, four cohorts of approximately 80 students each had completed the training. CDC officials told us that in addition to implementing various activities, CDC's Central America Regional Office in Guatemala played an important role in facilitating U.S. government cooperation with Colombia, which had the second largest outbreak of Zika after Brazil.

Implementing Partners Reported Various Results from Selected Activities

We reviewed status reports for six USAID activities that received among the highest amounts of funding, and each identified various results. Below, we describe the activities and examples of reported results. For more information, see appendix II.

- ASSIST: This activity sought to strengthen Zika-related health services and systems in Latin America and the Caribbean with a focus on pregnant women, newborns, and women of reproductive age. ASSIST reported that it conducted virtual and in-person training, courses, and workshops on Zika prevention, diagnosis, and care. ASSIST also reported that 8,133 health care workers had been trained as of March 2017, and that its efforts had supported the development of Zika care protocols and guidelines with a new emphasis on clinical care and support for affected infants and families. ASSIST further reported that through March 2018, 75 percent of children affected by Zika in Dominican Republic received specialized care at Hospital Infantil Robert Reid Cabral, an ASSIST-supported hospital in the capital, Santo Domingo.
- Red Cross: This activity aimed to reduce risks associated with Zika infection through community involvement, sharing lessons learned, and improving practices. The Red Cross reported that its communication efforts reached approximately 3,000 students, 29 communities, and almost 140,000 people via TV, radio, and social media engagement, providing them with information on risk and protection methods.
- Zika AIRS Project (ZAP): This is a mosquito control activity focused on reducing Zika transmission in Latin America and the Caribbean. Specific activities supported by USAID funding included entomological monitoring, larviciding, source reduction interventions, and indoor residual spraying. ZAP reported that five countries (El Salvador, Guatemala, Haiti, Honduras, and Jamaica) implemented comprehensive mosquito control activities.
- Population Services International: The purpose of this activity was to improve the capacity and raise awareness of people in countries affected by and at risk of Zika and other vector-borne diseases. Population Services International reported that through March 2018, 35 health providers in Dominican Republic, El Salvador, and Guatemala had been trained in raising awareness about Zika prevention and the use of printed educational materials. In addition, 1,006 pregnant women received counseling on Zika prevention, and 967 received prevention kits containing condoms, mosquito repellent, and printed educational materials. Additionally, 227 pharmacy attendants from 195 pharmacies received information on Zika prevention.

- Save the Children's Community Action on Zika (CAZ): The goal of this project was to reduce Zika transmission and minimize the risk of Zika-related microcephaly and other neurological disorders. The project focused on helping the most vulnerable through community- based prevention strategies in Colombia, Dominican Republic, and three Central American countries. CAZ reported that it had reached approximately 65,000 students and trained 3,838 community agents and volunteers who supported efforts to strengthen the capacity to prevent Zika in 921 communities.
- United Nations Children's Fund (UNICEF): This activity focused primarily on four countries: Guatemala, El Salvador, Honduras, and Dominican Republic. UNICEF worked to promote the adoption of prevention behaviors among at-risk populations through actions to raise awareness at multiple levels: individual, interpersonal, community, institutional, and national policy levels. UNICEF reported that these efforts reached more than 5.5 million people with key risk-communication messages and more than 150,000 people through coordinated social mobilization and person-to-person communication. For example, in Guatemala, UNICEF worked with a local partner to train young people and adolescents in schools and social groups to lead prevention activities in their communities. Moreover, around 25,000 pregnant women benefited from counseling sessions on Zika-prevention behaviors.

State Conducted Public Awareness Initiatives and Medical Evacuations

In response to Zika, State conducted public awareness and communication initiatives, medical evacuations for overseas staff, and other activities. According to a State official, State conducted Zika-related public outreach to U.S. citizens abroad through social media and the Smart Traveler Enrollment Program, a service that provides information from U.S. embassies about local safety conditions. According to a State official, State also implemented public diplomacy activities related to Zika awareness and communication. For example, one activity aimed to raise awareness of vector-borne diseases such as Zika and collect information on insect breeding grounds. Another supported the addition of a science envoy who focused specifically on Zika and mosquito-borne diseases. In addition, according to a State official, State conducted Zika-related medical evacuations as part of those normally offered to female staff who became pregnant while serving abroad. State's medical services division also supported overseas posts by purchasing and distributing mosquito repellent. State officials also told us that they coordinated Zika response efforts internally and externally. For example, State participated in a U.S. government interagency group led by CDC to exchange information on Zika and coordinated with other agencies on the response effort.

USAID Took Steps to Address Sustainability Challenge but Only Partially Mitigated Challenge to Timely Implementation

Over the course of our fieldwork, USAID and implementing partner officials identified two key challenges to the implementation of Zika response activities. The first was the long-term sustainability of Zika response activities. The second was the timely implementation of Zika response activities in countries without bilateral USAID health programs. While USAID took steps to address the challenge related to sustainability, it only partially mitigated the challenge to timely implementation of Zika response activities in countries without bilateral USAID health programs.

USAID Implementing Partners Aligned their Activities with Host Governments and Involved Local Communities to Address Sustainability Challenge

Agency and implementing partner officials identified the sustainability of Zika response efforts as a key challenge. While USAID did not intend to continue U.S. Zika response activities after the one-time emergency funding, sustainability was a consideration and posed a challenge due to the short implementation time frame, according to agency and implementing partner officials. One official further elaborated that Zika funding efforts occurred during the acute phase of the outbreak, which made it difficult to focus on long-term needs. For example, an implementing partner said that Zika-affected children require long-term care that host country governments may not be able to support after U.S. assistance ends. In addition, host country government officials, U.S. government officials, and implementing partners said that some Zika activities may not be sustainable after U.S. assistance is finished due to a lack of funds and limited capacity to continue the work.

To address this challenge and support the long-term continuation of Zika response activities, implementing partners aligned their activities with those of host country governments and other organizations. Implementing partners reported working with governments and other organizations to incorporate Zika activities into their plans and practices so they could continue over the long term. One implementing partner and the Dominican Republic's Ministry of Health, for example, planned mosquito control efforts together, and a Ministry of Health official said they intend to continue those control efforts after the end of Zika funding. Implementing partners in various countries also stated that Zika activities brought broader benefits to mosquito control, disability services, maternal health care, surveillance efforts, and emergency preparedness, which facilitated partners' efforts to align their Zika response activities. For example, an implementing partner reported using Zika funding to develop organizational guidelines for treating Zika-affected children, which will be used by the health care system in Dominican Republic to treat children with related disabilities in the long term. According to some implementing partners in countries we visited, they developed Zika protocols and guidelines in response to new scientific information, trained government and other personnel on the protocols, and worked with officials of host country governments and other organizations to encourage adoption of Zika activities. For example, according to an agency official, an implementing partner in Peru developed a curriculum for epidemiologists and trained them on how to detect and contain mosquito-borne diseases, such as Zika. The agency official said that the implementing partner shared the training curriculum and materials with Peru's Ministry of Health so it could continue the trainings after the end of Zika funding.

According to implementing partners, they also involved local communities in activities to increase community ownership and address sustainability. For example, an implementing partner official said they trained a cadre of community volunteers in Guatemala and El Salvador on behavior change practices so that they can continue activities after the end of Zika funding. In addition, implementing partner officials said that engaging with communities to learn about needs and resources is important to continued community interest in activities. For example, an implementing partner that works with communities on health priorities developed an approach that includes a toolkit for identifying a community's specific risks for Zika and the efforts best suited to helping the community eradicate mosquito breeding sites. In places affected by violence, some implementing partners engaged with communities to better understand how to prioritize community worker and volunteer safety to enable the continuation of activities. For example, an implementing partner in Guatemala engaged with local communities to understand areas they recommended health workers avoid due to safety concerns.

USAID Only Partially Mitigated the Challenge to Timely Implementation in Some Countries Where It Did Not Have Health Programs

Agency and implementing partner officials described timely implementation of activities in some countries without bilateral USAID health programs as a second key challenge.[225] Twenty-two out of the 26 countries where USAID implemented its Zika response activities were countries without bilateral USAID health programs. USAID officials stated that, as a result, there were no USAID health program officials present in these countries to build on relationships with host country health officials and help

[225] Over the last several years, USAID has transitioned out of providing assistance in the health sector when it determines that a country can sustain health progress without depending on foreign aid. For the purposes of this chapter, we refer to this transition as "countries without bilateral health programs."

facilitate the start of implementing partners' activities during the Zika response. USAID officials noted two reasons that working with host country governments took time. First, some U.S. Zika response activities started after a decline in Zika cases, when some host country governments were no longer as focused on countering the disease. Implementing partners responded to this situation by identifying related health service improvements that could stem from implementing a Zika response and were of interest to the host country governments. Second, agency and implementing partner officials said that in some countries without bilateral USAID health programs it also took time to identify the appropriate points of contact and establish relationships—preliminary steps needed to obtain approval from the host country government before activities could get underway. According to USAID officials, these relationships are critical to navigating bureaucratic systems and assist in designing activities that meet the needs of host country governments and communities, which are needed for timely implementation.

USAID took some steps to address the timely implementation challenge in countries without bilateral health programs. For example, according to USAID officials, USAID worked with multilateral partners that had a health presence in those countries and relied on regional field-based Zika coordinators to build relationships with in-country points of contact. As noted above, however, agency officials indicated that Zika response activities took additional time to deploy in some of the countries without bilateral USAID health programs. Further, implementing partners reported it took additional time to start up activities in those countries because of the time it took to obtain approval for them from the ministries of health. For example, one implementing partner reported that activity startup was postponed for nearly 3 months until it received approval from the host country government. Another implementing partner said it was a challenge to get information on Zika from the host country government or establish dialogue until USAID officials became involved. USAID officials also said that efforts to start and integrate Zika response activities in countries with ongoing USAID health programs did not face a number of the obstacles to timely implementation experienced in countries without bilateral USAID health programs.

According to federal internal control standards, agencies should design control activities, such as a plan, to achieve their objectives and address related risks, such as the challenge related to timely implementation.[226] In an effort to enhance its planning for outbreaks, USAID developed an infectious disease response plan in July 2018 during the time frame of our review. However, the plan does not provide specific guidance on how to address the challenge of initiating emergency response activities in countries without bilateral USAID health programs, such as by noting particular practices that implementing partners and other officials can use to address that challenge. For example,

[226] GAO-14-704G.

our fieldwork and interviews with USAID officials indicate that the following may be helpful practices for infectious disease response:

- Immediately establish an in-country working group that includes implementing partners, host country government officials, and U.S. government officials to help initiate and coordinate outbreak response.
- Communicate a current list of health ministry and other relevant government officials to implementing partners and other officials so they can quickly identify the appropriate points of contact.

According to USAID officials, USAID missions maintain regular contact with host country governments, maintain contact lists, and participate in coordination meetings. However, in the case of overseas Zika response, some implementing partner officials in the field told us that they did not initially know who to contact in the host country government. Likewise, a host country government official told us that a working group on Zika outbreak response was not established until after officials recognized that implementing partner and host country government officials did not have regular channels of communication. By taking steps to improve planning for countries without bilateral USAID health programs—such as by adding specific guidance for initiating emergency response activities in such countries to its July 2018 plan—USAID would be better positioned to quickly build relationships with health ministry and other key government officials in host countries and thus be better able to provide a timely infectious disease response to future outbreaks.

CONCLUSION

The Zika virus quickly spread to dozens of countries in 2015 and 2016, prompting WHO to declare the virus and associated health risks an international public health emergency. As future infectious disease outbreaks arise, Congress will be called on to fund overseas response efforts, as it did with the Zika outbreak, and USAID is likely once again to play a vital role in those efforts. Because USAID did not provide key decision makers with information on how Zika funding was distributed across the various countries where it conducted response activities, decision makers lack visibility into a key aspect of the overall U.S. Zika response overseas. The ability to compile this information by country when responding to future infectious disease outbreaks would enable USAID to provide key decision makers, including Congress and agency officials, with additional information to better support spending oversight and inform budgetary and planning decisions.

Further, while USAID took steps to address the challenge of sustaining Zika response activities over the long term, it did not fully mitigate the challenge of timely implementation of activities in countries without bilateral USAID health programs. As a result, the agency's response to Zika took additional time in some countries without bilateral USAID health programs. Infectious disease response planning that addresses countries without bilateral USAID health programs would better position USAID to quickly respond to infectious disease outbreaks, such as Zika, whenever the need arises.

Recommendations for Executive Action

We are making the following two recommendations to USAID:

- The Administrator of USAID should take steps to ensure that, in responding to future public health emergencies of international concern, the agency is able to compile funding information broken down by country. (Recommendation 1)
- The Administrator of USAID should take steps to improve its infectious disease response planning to address the challenge of initiating response activities in countries without bilateral USAID health programs in a timely manner. (Recommendation 2)

Agency Comments and Our Evaluation

We provided a draft of this chapter to USAID, State, and CDC for review and comment. USAID provided written comments, which we have reproduced in appendix III. In its comments, USAID agreed with our findings and recommendations and identified a number of actions it plans to take in response. Specifically, USAID stated that in responding to future public health emergencies of international concern, it plans to compile and report on funding by country. USAID also outlined the steps it plans to take to develop additional guidance for USAID officials in countries without bilateral health programs. State and CDC did not provide formal responses. CDC provided technical comments, which we incorporated throughout the report, as appropriate.

We are sending copies of this chapter to the appropriate congressional committees, the Administrator of USAID, the Secretaries of State and of Health and Human Services, and to other interested parties.

David B. Gootnick, Director

APPENDIX I: OBJECTIVES, SCOPE, AND METHODOLOGY

The Zika Response and Preparedness Appropriations Act, 2016, included a provision for us to review the status of U.S. Agency for International Development (USAID) and Department of State (State) actions to respond to Zika.[227] In this chapter, we examine (1) the status of USAID and State funding for the U.S. Zika response overseas, (2) activities supported by these funds, and (3) challenges, if any, to implementing Zika response activities and actions taken to address any challenges.

To examine the status of funding for U.S. Zika response overseas, we reviewed USAID and State's reports to the Senate and House Committees on Appropriations mandated by Section 203 of the Zika Response and Preparedness Appropriations Act, 2016.[228] We reviewed agency reporting submitted to Congress and discussed the reports with agency officials. We also reviewed USAID and State's reports to the Senate and House Committees on Appropriations mandated by the Department of State, Foreign Operations, and Related Programs Appropriations Act, 2015.[229] We obtained additional funding and activity information from USAID covering a period beyond that included in the reports to Congress.[230] We reviewed the interagency agreement between USAID and the Centers for Disease Control and Prevention (CDC), outlining the CDC's Zika response activities supported by $78 million in funds USAID obligated to CDC. We also obtained additional funding data from CDC and interviewed CDC officials to discuss the status of the agencies' obligations and disbursements for Zika response activities. We analyzed USAID's and State's obligations and disbursements that the agencies reported as supporting the U.S. Zika response overseas, as of September 30, 2018. We analyzed agency obligations and disbursements across agency bureaus, funding accounts, and activities for the Zika response.

Additionally, we interviewed officials from USAID and State to discuss the agencies' obligations and disbursements for Zika response activities. We then reviewed the funding data and related documentation and consulted with USAID and State officials on the accuracy and completeness of the data. In the small number of instances where we identified potential issues or inconsistencies in the data, we contacted relevant agency officials and obtained information from them necessary to resolve the discrepancies. We

---

[227] Pub. L. No. 114-223, Div. B, Zika Response and Preparedness Appropriations Act, 2016, §204, (Sept. 29, 2016).

[228] On October 28, 2016, USAID and State submitted a consolidated report to the appropriations committees on the anticipated uses of funds appropriated in the Zika Response and Preparedness Appropriations Act, 2016, as required by the act. USAID and State also submitted periodic updates to this chapter.

[229] While USAID and State provided information about repurposed Ebola funds in the Zika reports, the reports indicated that the inclusion of that information was not required by the Zika Response and Preparedness Appropriations Act, 2016, and noted that information about the repurposed Ebola funds could also be found in the agencies' Ebola reports. We reviewed USAID and State's Ebola reports submitted to Congress from April 2016 to September 2017 and discussed the contents of subsequent reports with agency officials.

[230] USAID and State's consolidated reports to Congress contained funding and activity information through September 30, 2017. We obtained additional data directly from USAID and State covering funding information through September 2018.

assessed USAID's tracking of funding data against federal internal control standards related to using quality information.[231] We also utilized information from data reliability assessments for two recent GAO reports that utilized funding data from the same USAID and State systems.[232] We determined that the data we used were sufficiently reliable for our purposes of examining USAID's and State's obligations and disbursements of the funds.

To examine activities that USAID and State implemented in response to Zika overseas, we conducted fieldwork, analyzed agency documents, and interviewed officials. We examined the status and progress related to Zika response activities. We conducted a teleconference with officials in Haiti and El Salvador and conducted fieldwork in Barbados, Colombia, Dominican Republic, Guatemala, Honduras, Peru, and Trinidad and Tobago. We selected these countries based on the following criteria: (1) geographic diversity to include the Caribbean, Central America, and South America; (2) coverage of the main lines of effort (mosquito control, public awareness, capacity building, and research); and (3) the presence of activities under way that accounted for a significant portion of funding. During our fieldwork, we interviewed agency officials who played a role in Zika response activities, which included officials from State, USAID, and CDC. We also interviewed host government officials, implementing
partners, health care workers, community volunteers, and researchers. In addition, we visited offices, toured facilities, and observed operations. We also attended a conference in Guatemala that addressed topics including status, successes, challenges, and lessons learned related to USAID's Zika response. We reviewed agency documents describing the plans and goals of activities. We also analyzed progress reports of six activities to provide illustrative examples of results. We selected activities from those with among with the highest amounts of funding and that together represented approximately 33 percent of all USAID funding for Zika response and a range of countries, lines of effort, and types of implementing partners (such as nongovernmental organizations and international organizations). The sample is not generalizable to all of USAID's Zika response activities.

To examine challenges, if any, to implementing Zika response activities and actions taken to address any challenges, we interviewed U.S. government officials, USAID implementing partners, and host government officials, and we analyzed progress reports from selected USAID-funded Zika response activities. We identified key challenges based on the nature of the description and the degree to which a diversity of interviewees

[231] GAO, *Standards for Internal Control in the Federal Government,* GAO-14-704G (Washington, D.C.: September 2014).

[232] GAO, *Ebola Recovery: USAID Has Initiated or Completed Most Projects, but a Complete Project Inventory Is Still Needed for Evaluating Its Efforts,* GAO-18-350 (Washington, D.C.: Mar. 28, 2018) and *Emergency Funding for Ebola Response: Some USAID Reimbursements Did Not Comply with Legislative Requirements and Need to Be Reversed,* GAO-17-35 (Washington, D.C.: Nov. 2, 2016).

and documents made mention of them. We reviewed USAID policy, USAID's infectious disease response plan, federal internal controls, implementing partner progress reports, and interviews with officials to determine what agencies did to address these challenges. We assessed USAID's infectious disease response plan against relevant federal internal control standards.[233]

We conducted this performance audit from December 2017 to May 2019 in accordance with generally accepted government auditing standards. Those standards require that we plan and perform the audit to obtain sufficient, appropriate, evidence to provide a reasonable basis for our findings and conclusions based on our audit objectives. We believe that the evidence obtained provides a reasonable basis for our findings and conclusions based on our audit objectives.

APPENDIX II: ILLUSTRATIVE EXAMPLES OF RESULTS FOR SELECTED ZIKA RESPONSE ACTIVITIES

To provide illustrative examples of the results of Zika response activities funded by the U.S. Agency for International Development (USAID), we analyzed implementing partners' progress reports for a sample of six activities. We selected activities from those with among the highest amounts of funding and that together represented approximately 33 percent of all USAID funding for Zika response and a range of countries, lines of effort, and types of implementing partners (such as nongovernmental organizations and international organizations). Quantitative figures related to individual indicators listed below reflect the targeted population of the activity. Start dates and funding information provided below reflect the date of the report to Congress in which the activity first appeared and the associated funds obligated. The sample is not generalizable to all USAID's Zika response activities.

Applying Science to Strengthen and Improve Systems

Table 1 presents the progress on key indicators as of March 2018 reported to USAID by the Applying Science to Strengthen and Improve Systems activity. The aim of the activity was to strengthen Zika-related health services and systems in Latin America and the Caribbean with a focus on pregnant women, newborns, and women of reproductive age.

[233] GAO-14-704G.

Table 1. Indicators Reported to USAID by the Applying Science to Strengthen and Improve Systems Activity, as of March 2018

Key indicator	Number or Percentage
Number of health care providers who treat family planning users, pregnant women, and mothers of newborns who are trained to provide Zika counseling	3,351
Number of affected individuals referred to psychosocial support services	Data not available
Number of babies born with suspected or confirmed microcephaly or Congenital Syndrome associated with Zika who are referred to appropriate clinical care services according to national norms	Data not available
Percentage of pregnant women who are given condoms for Zika protection during antenatal care sessions	79
Percentage of pregnant women who receive counseling on prevention of Zika virus transmission during antenatal care sessions	91
Percentage of completion of counseling criteria during family planning, antenatal care, and postpartum consultations, as set forth in the Zika Counseling Guide	87
Percentage of women (pregnant women, mothers of newborns, women of reproductive age) who can identify both the risk of Zika sexual transmission and the use of condoms as a preventative measure	85
Percentage of pregnant women who are screened properly for Zika signs and symptoms during antenatal care sessions	83
Percentage of newborns who are properly evaluated for microcephaly	77
Percentage of infants with suspected or confirmed microcephaly or congenital syndrome associated with Zika who receive appropriate clinical care according to age milestones in accordance with the national norms	Data not available
Percentage of affected individuals, including pregnant women with suspected Zika virus infection and mothers of infants with microcephaly or congenital syndrome associated with Zika, who are attended to by a provider trained in psycho-emotional support during each visit to the health care facility	Data not available

Source: GAO analysis of U.S. Agency for International Development (USAID) implementing partner progress report. | GAO-19-356

International Federation of Red Cross and Red Crescent Societies Global Health

Table 2 presents the progress on key indicators as of May 2018 reported to USAID by the International Federation of Red Cross and Red Crescent Societies Global Health activity. The activity aimed to reduce risks associated with Zika infection through promoting community involvement, sharing lessons learned, and improving practices.

United Nations International Children's Emergency Fund

Table 3 presents the progress on key indicators as of March 2018 reported to USAID by the United Nations International Children's Emergency Fund activity. The activity aimed to promote the adoption of prevention behaviors among at-risk populations through actions targeting multiple levels of their environment: individual, interpersonal, community, institutional, and national policy levels.

Table 2. Indicators Reported to USAID by the International Federation of Red Cross and Red Crescent Societies Global Health Activity, as of May 2018

Indicator	Number
Communities with improved information about risks	67
Communities accessing educational materials	54
Students reached via school activities including Zika clubs, awareness campaigns	14,123
Individuals of reproductive age who identify preventative measures	8,362
Individuals of reproductive age who received messaging through TV, radio, and social media engagement	109,570
Community clean-up campaigns	43
Communities with reduced breeding sites	24
Households that have taken one action within the last month to prevent Zika infection	6,011
Pregnant women in targeted facilities who receive Zika counseling or information	3,665

Source: GAO analysis of U.S. Agency for International Development (USAID) implementing partner progress report. | GAO-19-356

Table 3. Indicators Reported to USAID by the United Nations International Children's Emergency Fund Activity, as of March 2018

Indicator	Number
Number of pregnant women benefited with quality counselling sessions to prevent Zika virus infection	24,475
Number of territories (departments/municipalities) in the region reporting the implementation of plans with Zika response components	45
Number of target population reached with key risk communication messages through multiple communication channels	5,577,085
Number of target population reached with social mobilization and interpersonal communication at Zika virus prevention sessions	155,113
Number of children and adolescents trained in Zika virus transmission, prevention measures, and consequences	50,479
Number of families with children affected by Zika Congenital Syndrome benefiting with nonclinical care and support interventions	301
Number of providers trained in family-focused early intervention services for young children affected by Zika syndrome	1,661

Source: GAO analysis of U.S. Agency for International Development (USAID) implementing partner progress report. | GAO-19-356

Save the Children Community Action on Zika

Table 4 presents the progress on key indicators as of September 2017 reported to USAID by the Save the Children Community Action on Zika project. The goal of the project was to reduce Zika transmission and minimize the risk of Zika-related microcephaly and other neurological disorders among the most vulnerable through community-based prevention strategies.

Population Services International

Table 5 presents the progress on an illustrative selection of key indicators, by objective, as of March 2018 reported to USAID by the Population Services International activity. The purpose of the activity was to improve the capacity and raise awareness of people in countries affected by and at risk of Zika and other vector-borne diseases.

Table 4. Indicators Reported to USAID by the Save the Children Community Action on Zika Project, as of September 2017

Indicator	Percentage or number
Percentage of women of reproductive age who report applying key Zika protective practices	48.70
Percentage of communities that show capacity for surveillance, prevention, and control of Zika virus disease and care and support of affected infants	47
Percentage of communities that show capacity for surveillance of Zika virus disease and vector	71
Percentage of communities that show capacity for prevention and control of Zika virus disease	48
Percentage of communities that show capacity for care and support of affected infants	52
Percentage of women of reproductive age who report implementing personal preventive measures to avoid Zika virus infection	15.80
Percentage women of reproductive age who recognize Zika risk, prevention, and transmission	49.90
Percentage and number of women of reproductive age reporting that condoms & other contraceptives are available at their local health facilities	62.50
Number of volunteers trained in community-based vector control	4,331
Number of students informed about Zika prevention and control	64,898
Number of community members participating in clean-up campaigns	76,448
Number of target population provided with Zika key risk communication messages	342,082
Number of pregnant women informed on Zika	2,870
Number of communities with community plans for the prevention and control of Zika	599
Number of communities with members actively participating in vector and/or case surveillance activities	558
Number of children and adolescents participating as agents of social mobilization at community level	7,103
Number of community volunteers with community-based surveillance reporting cases and suspected cases of Zika	1,073
Number of community volunteers with community-based surveillance reporting vector positive breeding sites	2,612
Number Zika events that involve families, schools, local governments, or community organizations	2,346
Percentage and number of communities engaged in vector control activities	62 (percentage) 568 communities
Percentage and number of schools which have implemented breeding site elimination campaigns with participation from school children	60 (percentage) 252 schools
Percentage and number of communities which have implemented breeding site elimination campaigns	65 (percentage) 597 communities
Percentage and number of communities with a Zika risk communication strategy	53 (percentage) 479 communities
Percentage and number of communities with a Zika implementation plan	62 (percentage) 569 communities

Source: GAO analysis of U.S. Agency for International Development (USAID) implementing partner progress report. | GAO-19-356

Table 5. Illustrative Selection of Indicators, by Objective, Reported to USAID by the Population Services International Activity, as of March 2018

Objective and illustrative indicator	Number
Objective 1.1: Increased use of personal safeguards, including the voluntary use of family planning and condoms to prevent unintended pregnancy and sexual transmission of Zika among women of reproductive age, pregnant women, and their sexual partners Number of users who participated in online outreach for Zika prevention	3,956
Objective 1.2: Developed body of evidence regarding target communities' knowledge about Zika transmission and prevention seeking behavior to strengthen social and behavior change communication messaging and program responses at the community, regional, and national levels Total sample of participants in study to measure recall and affinity for key messages from Zika campaign	1,254
Objective 2.1: Increased provider knowledge about Zika and increased number of private health service providers who incorporate Zika counseling into integrated sexual and reproductive health services Pregnant women who received counseling on Zika prevention	1,006
Objective 2.2: Increased youth and adolescent knowledge about Zika and increased number of public educational institutions that incorporate Zika counseling into integrated sexual and reproductive health services. Teachers and health ministry authorities participating in meeting in Honduras to share experiences from the first year of project implementation and learn updated information about Zika prevention	145

Source: GAO analysis of U.S. Agency for International Development (USAID) implementing partner progress report. | GAO-19-356

Note: Because the set of key indicators is long and varied for this activity, we list an illustrative selection.

Zika AIRS Project (ZAP)

Table 6 presents illustrative examples of accomplishments as of March 2018 reported to USAID by the Zika AIRS Project (ZAP). This was a mosquito control project focused on reducing Zika transmission in Latin America and the Caribbean. Specific activities included entomological monitoring, larviciding, source reduction interventions, and indoor residual spraying.

Table 6. Illustrative Examples of Accomplishments Reported to USAID by the Zika AIRS Project (ZAP), as of March 2018

Example of accomplishment
ZAP country teams collaborated extensively with Ministry of Health counterparts in each country, not only in planning and implementing ZAP activities, but also in exploring ways in which the project could support sustained efforts.
Five countries implemented comprehensive vector control activities, combining source reduction through environmental management and routine larviciding with Bacillus thuringiensis israelensis.
Six countries conducted routine entomological monitoring, including adult mosquito collection, egg collection, and larvae/pupae surveys.
New and innovative vector control methods were piloted in selected ZAP countries, including a pilot in Dominican Republic on the use of lethal ovitraps as a method of both entomological monitoring and vector control.
ZAP has reinforced a focus on learning across the project during this reporting period, and cross-country learning through several south-to-south technical assistance trips during which ZAP staff have shared best practices and innovations.

Source: GAO analysis of U.S. Agency for International Development (USAID) implementing partner progress report. | GAO-19-356

Note: Because accomplishments reported varied for this activity, we list an illustrative selection.

APPENDIX III: COMMENTS FROM THE U.S. AGENCY FOR INTERNATIONAL DEVELOPMENT

USAID
FROM THE AMERICAN PEOPLE

David B. Gootnick
U.S. Government Accountability Office
441 G Street, N.W.
Washington, D.C. 20226

Re: EMERGENCY ASSISTANCE FOR ZIKA: USAID Supported Activities Overseas but Could Improve Funds Tracking and Response Planning (GAO-19-356)

Dear Mr. Gootnick:

I am pleased to provide the formal response from the U.S. Agency for International Development (USAID) to the draft report produced by the U.S. Government Accountability Office (GAO) titled, "*EMERGENCY ASSISTANCE FOR ZIKA: USAID Supported Activities Overseas but Could Improve Funds Tracking and Response Planning,*" (GAO-19-356).

The International Health Regulations (2005) (IHRs) define a "Public Health Emergency of International Concern" (PHEIC) as "an extraordinary event which is determined ... to constitute a public health risk to other States through the international spread of disease and to potentially require a coordinated international response." The Director-General of the World Health Organization (WHO) has only declared four PHEICs since the IHRs entered into force on June 15, 2007: H1N1 Influenza, in 2009; Poliomyelitis, in 2014; Ebola, in 2014; and Zika Virus, in 2016. USAID has gained extraordinary knowledge as a result of the unprecedented battle to contain Ebola and Zika, and is committed to strengthening the aspects of reporting and coordination highlighted by the GAO, particularly the Agency's policies and practices to prepare for, respond to, and learn from public health crises around the globe, including PHEICs.

USAID must point out, however, that some challenges identified by the GAO in the draft report depend on international actions beyond the Agency's control. Responding to a PHEIC is not the purview of USAID or the U.S. Government alone, but is a shared global responsibility. USAID is committed to strengthening our emergency-response coordination by institutionalizing the Agency's logistical support for temporary Task Forces through the creation of a new Task-Force Readiness Unit (TFRU) within the Bureau for Management (M), as outlined in the Congressional Notification for the M Bureau under our Transformation. We hope for Congress's support in establishing this new Unit to respond even more efficiently to emergencies across the world.

I am transmitting this letter and the enclosed USAID comments for incorporation as an appendix to the GAO's final report. Thank you for the opportunity to respond to the draft report, and for the courtesies extended by your staff while conducting this engagement. We appreciate the opportunity to participate in the complete and thorough review of our programs. As an Agency, we believe the GAO's engagements provide a valuable opportunity to assess and improve upon our policies, procedures, and programs.

Sincerely,

Angelique M. Crumbly
Acting Assistant Administrator
Bureau for Management

COMMENTS BY THE U.S. AGENCY FOR INTERNATIONAL DEVELOPMENT ON THE DRAFT REPORT PRODUCED BY THE U.S. GOVERNMENT ACCOUNTABILITY OFFICE (GAO) TITLED: "EMERGENCY ASSISTANCE FOR ZIKA: USAID Supported Activities Overseas but Could Improve Funds Tracking and Response Planning" (GAO-19-356)

The U.S. Agency for International Development (USAID) would like to thank the GAO for the opportunity to respond to this draft report. We appreciate the extensive work of the GAO engagement team and the specific findings that will help USAID achieve greater effectiveness in future public health emergencies.

USAID worked closely with partners across the U.S. Government to implement a collective response to the outbreak of Zika outbreak that aimed to minimize the number of pregnancies affected by the virus. Together, U.S. Government Departments and Agencies undertook surveillance efforts to identify the progression of Zika, diagnose infections when they occurred, provide care and support for pregnant women identified as having contracted the Zika virus and their affected babies, and take efforts to prevent further infections.

The base of scientific knowledge regarding the Zika virus was evolving as USAID partners were implementing their programs. For example, when the Director-General of the World Health Organization (WHO) declared Zika a Public Health Emergency of International Concern (PHEIC) in 2016, the scientific community was unaware of the relative risk of sexual transmission of the virus. As that knowledge emerged, USAID worked with our implementers to adjust programs to target efforts toward both pregnant women and their partners.

USAID has a long history of funding health programs in countries in Latin America and the Caribbean, which allowed the Agency to provide technical assistance to Ministries of Health and health providers to ensure they could respond to changing circumstances when Zika arrived in this Hemisphere. We know that in many of these countries, social, demographic, and geographic inequities exist, and infectious-disease outbreaks, economic shocks, or political crises can easily damage hard-wrought gains.

USAID's response to Zika sought to support and strengthen local institutions, including those responsible for ensuring pregnant women have access to high-quality prenatal care. We ensured that our short-term focus on minimizing the negative pregnancy outcomes associated with Zika infection strengthened, rather than undermined, training, curricula, and the delivery of broader health care. The Agency improved the quality of Zika-related prevention and care through both public- and private-sector delivery channels, and also by engaging vulnerable communities to reduce the risk of Zika infection in pregnant women. USAID's response focused on four interconnected lines of effort: Innovation; Vector-Control; Social and Behavior-Change Communication; and Service-Delivery related to voluntary family planning, antenatal and postnatal care, and early-childhood development and care for families with infants affected by Zika.

USAID designed its Zika program to implement it strategically through regional programs managed from Washington. This was both expedient, because it allowed for the rapid mobilization of funds across all the key lines of technical effort, and provided the necessary operational and programmatic flexibility needed to address a rapidly expanding outbreak across multiple countries in Latin America and the Caribbean.

To design the response to Zika, USAID adapted lessons learned in mobilizing and managing resources for the outbreak of Ebola in West Africa in 2013 and 2014. However, detailed, country-level financial data from previous outbreaks have limited utility in planning for future responses to future outbreaks, as each will have distinct scale, spread, and engagement from other donors. For example, in a subsequent outbreak of the same disease in the same country, such as sequential Ebola outbreaks in the Democratic Republic of Congo (DRC), each outbreak has its own particularities that influence investment priorities and plans. While USAID did not require its implementers to provide as much country-level funding detail as the GAO would have preferred, the rapid placement of country and regional Zika advisors facilitated in-country knowledge and accountability, and the coordination of the programs with local stakeholders. The Zika advisors helped adapt the programs to local contexts and priorities, in line with Ministries of Health and community strategies.

By responding effectively to the spread of Zika throughout Latin America and the Caribbean, USAID helped reduce the outbreak's impact on at-risk countries, and prevented its potential spread to the United States. The Agency's investments focused on protecting individuals, particularly pregnant women, from Zika by controlling the spread of the virus, increasing awareness of how the virus is transmitted and how to prevent infection, improving disease-detection and the surveillance of transmission, and supporting affected people. In addition, USAID catalyzed the development of innovative tools to combat mosquito-borne diseases like Zika so the world is better prepared for the next outbreak. USAID's efforts support the ability of governments and civil-society to respond to Zika, as well as to future disease threats, because we know that strength abroad means safety at home.

USAID concurs with both recommendations made in the GAO's report. Please find below our responses and mitigation plan.

Recommendation 1: The USAID Administrator should ensure that, in responding to future Public Health Emergencies of International Concern, the Agency is able to compile funding information broken down by country.

Section 203 of the Zika Response and Preparedness Appropriations Act, 2016, states that the Department of State and USAID, "Shall submit a consolidated report to the Committees on Appropriations on the anticipated uses of such funds on a country and project basis." Consistent with the Act, USAID's initial report on the anticipated uses of Zika supplemental funds included information on the types of activities the Agency would undertake in priority countries. The subsequent Zika report updates identified changes to assumptions and estimates in the original report, as appropriate. Further, USAID's Zika financial-management practices met the policies and requirements of the 600 series of Chapters (Financial-Management Principles and Standards) of USAID's Automated Directives System.

- USAID will ensure that in responding to future PHEICs, the Agency will compile and report on funding obligated and disbursed to implementers by country. The Agency will incorporate this requirement into the programming process prior to the obligation of funds, and into the terms of awards.

Recommendation 2: The USAID Administrator should improve the Agency's infectious-disease response planning to address the challenge of initiating response activities in a timely manner in countries without bilateral USAID health programs.

USAID recognizes that the experiences with Ebola in West Africa and the DRC and Zika throughout the Western Hemisphere demonstrate that the United States must be prepared to respond quickly to infectious-disease outbreaks that could pose a global danger, in some cases before an official PHEIC declaration by the WHO. USAID and the rest of the U.S. Government gained extraordinary knowledge as a result of the unprecedented, multi-sectoral battle to contain Ebola in West Africa, which now is influencing the response to the virus in DRC, and is committed to the continual strengthening of the Agency's policies, practices, structures, and systems to prepare for, respond to, and learn from global infectious-disease outbreaks.

On July 31, 2018, USAID issued an internal Agency Notice titled, "USAID Response to Global Infectious Disease Outbreaks," which included three outbreak-response scenarios that clarified the level of operational and programmatic response by the Agency. USAID updated the Agency Notice for Fiscal Year (FY) 2019 to include four outbreak-response scenarios, and reissued it on October 31, 2018. The Agency Notice outlines the roles and responsibilities of USAID staff when preparing for, and responding to, outbreaks of infectious-diseases, instructs USAID Missions and overseas offices to be vigilant for local outbreaks, and a requirement to notify outbreak@usaid.gov when an outbreak occurs that could require international or additional assistance. The Agency Notice also asks Missions and overseas offices to be prepared to participate in coordination meetings with host governments and other donors related to such outbreaks.

USAID's broad-based and multisectoral approach allows the Agency to collaborate across the U.S. Government to leverage our technical expertise to strengthen local capacity around the world to prevent, detect, and respond to infectious diseases. USAID has established partnerships with the U.S. Departments of Agriculture, Defense, Health and Human Services, and State, and with relevant international, non-governmental, and other organizations, to strengthen preparedness for, and response to, potential disease outbreaks that could require an international emergency response.

- By June 30, 2019, USAID will develop and provide specific guidance for USAID Desk Officers in Washington and Program Officers in countries without bilateral USAID health programs to ensure they are aware of the Agency's process and resources to respond to outbreaks of infectious disease and remind them of the outbreak@usaid.gov e-mail address. This guidance will also request that Desk Officers reach out to their Mission counterparts and regularly engage with counterparts in Ministries of Health, as well as remind them that USAID can provide support and funding in an outbreak, in coordination with the WHO and other U.S. Government partners, including the Centers for Disease Control (CDC) within HHS.

- By September 30, 2019, USAID Missions without bilateral health programs will develop lists of country-level point-of-contacts with their respective Ministries of Health, and will provide the information to the USAID Desk Officers; the Bureau for Global Health (GH); and the Office of U.S. Foreign Disaster Assistance (OFDA) within the Bureau for Democracy, Conflict, and Humanitarian Assistance (DCHA). The Agency will update the information annually.
- By December 30, 2019, GH will pilot the development of a roster of former USAID Foreign Service Nationals and third-country nationals with expertise in global health for rapid, temporary surge support during an infectious-disease outbreak. The surge support will complement USAID/Washington personnel from GH, DCHA/OFDA, and other Bureaus and Independent Offices that might have to work with the affected Missions to support the international response. USAID will continually assess and establish, as needed, internal coordination structures that bring together relevant Agency Bureaus, Independent Offices, and Missions, and other U.S. Government Departments and Agencies, to coordinate response-related efforts and investments.

APPENDIX IV: ACCESSIBLE DATA

Data Tables

Accessible Data for Figure 1: Timeline of Zika Outbreak and the U.S. Zika Response Overseas, 2015–2018

Month	Total number of countries with new Zika transmission
15-Jan	0
15-Feb	0
15-Mar	0
15-Apr	0
15-May	1
15-Jun	0
15-Jul	0
15-Aug	0
15-Sep	0
15-Oct	1
15-Nov	6
15-Dec	5
16-Jan	13
16-Feb	5
16-Mar	2
16-Apr	3
16-May	3
16-Jun	1
16-Jul	3
16-Aug	3
16-Sep	1
16-Oct	0
16-Nov	1
16-Dec	0
17-Jan	0
17-Feb	0

Accessible Data for Figure 1: (Continued)

Month	Total number of countries with new Zika transmission
17-Mar	0
17-Apr	0
17-May	0
17-Jun	0
17-Jul	0
17-Aug	0

Accessible Data for Figure 2: Zika Incidence Rates in Latin America and the Caribbean, 2015–2017

Country/Territory	Zika incidence rate group
Chile	zero
Uruguay	zero
United States of America	0 < 49
Cuba	0 < 49
Argentina	0 < 49
Guyana	0 < 49
Mexico	0 < 49
Paraguay	0 < 49
Haiti	0 < 49
Peru	0 < 49
Guatemala	0 < 49
Bolivia (Plurinational State of)	0 < 49
Ecuador	0 < 49
Nicaragua	0 < 49
Dominican Republic	49 - 320
Trinidad and Tobago	49 - 320
Bahamas	49 - 320
Panama	49 - 320
Brazil	49 - 320
El Salvador	49 - 320
Venezuela (Bolivarian Republic of)	49 - 320
Costa Rica	49 - 320
Colombia	49 - 320
Jamaica	49 - 320
Barbados	49 - 320
Anguilla	49 - 320
Virgin Islands (UK)	320 - 1000
Honduras	320 - 1000
Grenada	320 - 1000
Turks and Caicos Islands	320 - 1000
Montserrat	320 -1000
Cayman Islands	320 - 1000
Saint Lucia	320 - 1000
Saint Vincent and the Grenadines	320 - 1000
Antigua and Barbuda	320 - 1000
Belize	320 - 1000
Suriname	320 - 1000
Sint Maarten (Dutch part)	320 - 1000
Puerto Rico	> 1000

Country/Territory	Zika incidence rate group
Saint Kitts and Nevis	> 1000
Dominica	> 1000
Aruba	> 1000
Virgin Islands (US)	> 1000
Bonaire, St Eustatius and Saba	> 1000
French Guiana	> 1000
Curacao	> 1000
Guadeloupe	> 1000
Martinique	> 1000
Saint Martin	> 1000
Saint Barthelemy	> 1000

Accessible Data for Figure 3: U.S. Agency for International Development (USAID) and Department of State (State) Zika Response Appropriations, Obligations, and Disbursements, as of September 30, 2018

Dollars in billions	Appropriated funds	Total Obligations	Total Disbursements
Total Zika funding	$390.1	$384.8	$263.8
Zika Response and Preparedness Appropriations Act, 2016	$175.1	$169.8	$62.9
Ebola funds redirected	$215.0	$215.0	$200.9

Accessible Data for Figure 4: U.S. Agency for International Development (USAID) Obligations and Disbursements by Account for Zika Response Activities, as of September 30, 2018

Category	Total Obligations	Total Disbursements
Total	$366.5	$245.4
USAID Operating Expenses	$10.0	$7.2
Global Health Programs	$145.5	$41.4
Economic Support Fund	$211.0	$196.9

Accessible Data for Figure 5: Department of State (State) Obligations and Disbursements by Account for Zika Response Activities, as of September 30, 2018

Dollars in billions	Total Obligations	Total Disbursements
Total	$18.3	$18.3
Diplomatic & Consular Programs	$14.3	$14.3
Economic Support Fund	$4.0	$4.0

In: Infectious Diseases
Editor: Philippe Georges
ISBN: 978-1-53616-401-5

Chapter 5

EBOLA RECOVERY: USAID HAS INITIATED OR COMPLETED MOST PROJECTS, BUT A COMPLETE PROJECT INVENTORY IS STILL NEEDED FOR EVALUATING ITS EFFORTS*

United States Government Accountability Office

ABBREVIATIONS

ADS	Automated Directives System
CDC	Centers for Disease Control and Prevention
CIO	Contributions to International Organizations
ESF	Economic Support Fund
FFP	Office of Food for Peace
GDP	gross domestic product
GHP	Global Health Programs
IDA	International Disaster Assistance
INCLE	International Narcotics and Law Enforcement
Lab	Global Development Lab
PKO	Peacekeeping Operations
State	Department of State
UNICEF	United Nations Children's Fund
USAID	U.S. Agency for International Development
WHO	World Health Organization

* This is an edited, reformatted and augmented version of United States Government Accountability Office; Report to Congressional Committees, Publication No. GAO-18-350, dated March 2018.

Why GAO Did This Study

The 2014-2015 Ebola outbreak in West Africa caused long-term second-order impacts, including disruptions to health systems, job loss, and food insecurity. Congress appropriated about $2.5 billion for USAID and the Department of State (State), in part, for international efforts to prevent, prepare for, and respond to an Ebola outbreak and mandated that the agencies report to congressional committees on the use of the funds. As of September 2017, USAID had allocated almost all of the appropriated Ebola funds. In 2016, USAID contracted for an evaluation of Ebola recovery activities.

The fiscal year 2015 appropriations act included a provision for GAO to conduct oversight of USAID and State activities supported with funds from the Ebola response and preparedness appropriations. GAO's 2016 report (GAO-17-35) focused on USAID and State funding for Ebola response and preparedness. This chapter examines (1) obligations for USAID's Ebola recovery projects, (2) the status of USAID's implementation of these projects, and (3) USAID's evaluation of Ebola recovery efforts. GAO analyzed USAID funding data as of September 30, 2017, which are the latest data provided to Congress, reviewed project documents and evaluation plans, interviewed agency officials, and conducted fieldwork in Guinea, Liberia, and Sierra Leone.

What GAO Recommends

The Administrator of USAID should ensure that a complete and accurate inventory of Ebola recovery projects is compiled for the ongoing evaluation. USAID concurred with GAO's recommendation.

What GAO Found

As of September 30, 2017, of the $1.6 billion that the U.S. Agency for International Development (USAID) had obligated for the Ebola outbreak, $411.6 million was obligated for 131 Ebola recovery projects. Of the $411.6 million, USAID obligated the largest amount—about $247.6 million (60 percent)—from the Economic Support Fund account for recovery projects to support health systems recovery, governance and economic crisis mitigation, and Ebola survivors, among others. USAID obligated about $118.5 million from the International Disaster Assistance account for food security projects, such as food assistance and agricultural market support, and $45.5 million from the Global Health Programs account for Ebola survivor and world health reform projects.

As of September 2017, USAID had completed 62 of its 131 planned Ebola recovery projects, had 65 projects that were ongoing, and had 4 planned projects that it had not yet started. Of the 62 completed projects, USAID had completed 39 within original time frames and budgeted costs and extended 23. Of the 65 ongoing projects, USAID expected to implement 46 within original time frames and costs, but had extended 19. USAID extended projects, in part, to complete host-government actions, hire staff, finalize project activities, and continue and expand food assistance.

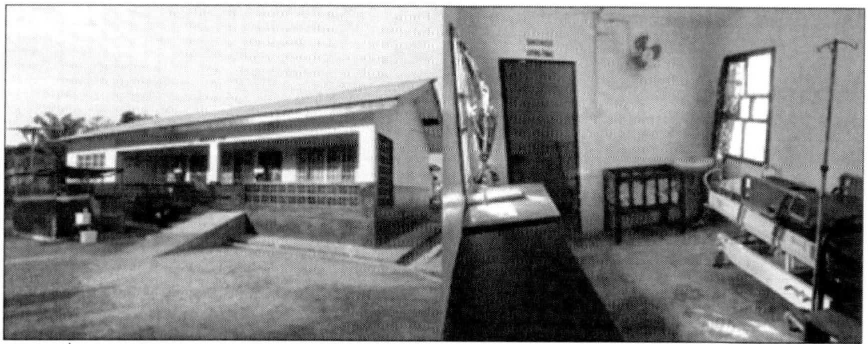

Source: GAO. | GAO-18-350.

Health Facilities Rehabilitated in Sierra Leone by a USAID Ebola Recovery Project.

In 2016, USAID contracted for an evaluation of its Ebola recovery activities. Although the contractor has completed some design elements for the evaluation, USAID had not ensured that a complete and accurate inventory of USAID's Ebola recovery projects had been compiled for the evaluation as of December 2017. USAID intends to use the information and lessons learned from this evaluation to inform and improve its ability to respond to future global health emergencies. GAO's comparison of the contractor's inventory with USAID data provided to Congress found a number of discrepancies that USAID officials could not explain with certainty. USAID policy states that information collected should be of sufficient quality to be useful for the intended users. Until USAID ensures that the contractor develops a complete and accurate inventory of USAID's Ebola recovery projects, USAID will not have assurance that the resulting evaluation will be of sufficient quality.

March 28, 2018

The Honorable Lindsey Graham
Chairman

The Honorable Patrick J. Leahy
Ranking Member
Subcommittee on State, Foreign Operations, and Related Programs
Committee on Appropriations
United States Senate

The Honorable Hal Rogers
Chairman

The Honorable Nita M. Lowey
Ranking Member
Subcommittee on State, Foreign Operations, and Related Programs
Committee on Appropriations
House of Representatives

The 2014-2015 Ebola outbreak led to an estimated 28,600 Ebola cases and more than 11,300 deaths. It also caused long-term disruptions to health systems, adverse economic effects, and other second-order impacts in the three primarily affected countries in West Africa—Guinea, Liberia, and Sierra Leone.[1] Specifically, the outbreak resulted in a redirection of these countries' scarce health-care resources to Ebola response efforts, job loss, disruptions to trade, reduced agricultural production, decreased household purchasing power, and increased food insecurity.

In September 2014, the President announced a four-pillar U.S. government strategy to address the impacts of the Ebola outbreak.[2] The second pillar of the strategy focuses on mitigating the second-order impacts of the outbreak, including efforts to assist in the primarily affected countries' recovery. In November 2014, the President submitted a request to Congress for additional funds to enable the U.S. government to implement the strategy, including a request for funding to support Ebola recovery projects to address the second-order impacts in the three primarily affected countries. In December 2014, Congress enacted the Department of State, Foreign Operations, and Related Programs Appropriations Act, 2015 (the Act), which appropriated about $2.5 billion to the U.S. Agency for International Development (USAID) and the Department of State (State) for necessary expenses to assist countries affected by, or at risk of being affected by, the Ebola outbreak, among other things.[3] The Act also required State, in consultation with USAID, to periodically submit reports to congressional committees on the proposed uses of the funds on a country and project basis.[4] USAID and, to a lesser extent, State have

1 The direct impacts of the Ebola outbreak in West Africa were increased morbidity and mortality. As of June 2016—the most recent date for which the World Health Organization (WHO) has reported data—the outbreak had resulted in more than 28,600 confirmed, probable, and suspected cases of Ebola and more than 11,300 deaths in the three primarily affected countries.

2 The four pillars of the *U.S. Government Strategy for Reducing Transmission of the Ebola Virus Disease in West Africa* are (1) controlling the outbreak, (2) mitigating the second-order impacts of the crisis, (3) building coherent leadership and operations, and (4) strengthening global health security.

3 Pub. L. No. 113-235, Div. J, Title IX, 128 Stat 2130, 2692 (Dec. 16, 2014). In addition, the Act appropriated funding for efforts to mitigate the risk of illicit acquisition of the Ebola virus and to promote biosecurity practices associated with Ebola response efforts.

4 The Act requires State, in consultation with USAID, to submit a report to the Senate and House Committees on Appropriations on the proposed uses of the funds on a country and project basis, for which the obligation of funds is anticipated, no later than 30 days after enactment. It further requires State, in consultation with USAID, to update and submit these reports every 30 days until September 30, 2016, and every 180 days

allocated portions of funding from that appropriation for Ebola recovery projects to address the second-order impacts and assist the three primarily affected countries' recovery.

The Act also includes a provision for GAO to conduct oversight of USAID and State activities supported with funds from the Ebola response and preparedness appropriation. In November 2016, we reported on USAID's and State's funding for Ebola response and preparedness activities.[5] This chapter examines (1) obligations for USAID's Ebola recovery projects, (2) the status of USAID's implementation of these projects, and (3) USAID's evaluation of Ebola recovery efforts.

To examine obligations for USAID's Ebola recovery projects, we reviewed USAID's and State's reports to congressional committees mandated by the Act and USAID's strategic framework for Ebola recovery. We focus this chapter on USAID because it has allocated more than $2.3 billion (91 percent) of the approximately $2.5 billion appropriated and has implemented most of the Ebola recovery projects funded from the appropriation. We conducted interviews with USAID and State officials to determine the projects that they identified as supporting Ebola recovery. We analyzed USAID's obligations data and information that USAID reported as supporting Ebola recovery as of September 30, 2017, the most recent data and information that USAID and State have reported for congressional committees.[6] To examine the status of USAID's implementation of Ebola recovery projects, we analyzed agency data on the implementation of Ebola recovery projects and the amounts of funding that USAID had obligated for these projects in its most recent report to Congress. To gain more in-depth information and context on the implementation of Ebola recovery projects, we selected a non-generalizable sample of 10 Ebola recovery projects that USAID had reported in Pillar 2 as of July 1, 2016.[7] We selected projects such that the sample would achieve a mix of projects by country; USAID office, bureau, and mission; and category of USAID's strategic framework for Ebola recovery.[8] We reviewed documents for our sample of projects and, where possible, conducted site visits in Guinea, Liberia, and

---

thereafter, until all funds have been fully expended. In the reports, USAID and State are required to include (1) information detailing how the estimates and assumptions contained in the previous reports have changed, and (2) obligations and expenditures on a country and project basis. The most recent report is as of September 30, 2017.

[5] GAO, Emergency Funding for Ebola Response: Some USAID Reimbursements Did Not Comply with Legislative Requirements and Need to Be Reversed, GAO-17-35 (Washington, D.C.: Nov. 2, 2016).

[6] In a draft of this chapter that we provided to USAID and State for comment, we reported funding data that were current, as of March 31, 2017. State subsequently provided updated data, as of September 30, 2017. We updated our report accordingly.

[7] We selected our sample of projects from among those that USAID had reported as of July 1, 2016 because we had assessed the reliability of the project data and information that USAID had reported as of that date during our prior work. In addition, to allow for an assessment of the implementation, we sought to select projects that had either begun implementation or had been completed. For more information about our 10 selected projects, see appendix II.

[8] The categories of USAID's strategic framework for Ebola recovery are (1) health systems recovery, (2) emergency non-Ebola health services, (3) governance and economic crisis mitigation, (4) innovation and communications technology, and (5) food security.

Sierra Leone to examine project implementation. To identify the numbers and types of Ebola recovery projects that USAID had planned and implemented, we also analyzed funding data from USAID's reports to Congress. We assessed the reliability of the data that USAID reported for its implementation of Ebola recovery projects and its obligations for such projects. We requested and reviewed information from agency officials regarding the underlying financial data systems and the checks and reviews used to generate the data to ensure its accuracy and reliability. We also compared the data to USAID's documentation from selected projects to assess the reliability of USAID funding and project data. When we found discrepancies, we contacted agency officials and obtained information from them necessary to resolve the discrepancies. Based on these steps, we determined that the data we used were sufficiently reliable for the purposes of reporting the numbers of recovery projects and obligations. We also conducted fieldwork in Guinea, Liberia, and Sierra Leone, interviewing USAID officials, implementing partners, and host country officials about the planning and implementation of projects. To examine USAID's evaluation of Ebola recovery efforts, we compared the evaluation plan prepared by USAID's contracted evaluator (contractor) to criteria for designing effective evaluations.[9] We also interviewed USAID officials and contractor staff in Washington, D.C. to discuss the evaluation plan details, including the methods, measures, and analysis plans for each objective. See appendix I for more details on our scope and methodology.

We conducted this performance audit from November 2016 to March 2018 in accordance with generally accepted government auditing standards. Those standards require that we plan and perform the audit to obtain sufficient, appropriate, evidence to provide a reasonable basis for our findings and conclusions based on our audit objectives. We believe that the evidence obtained provides a reasonable basis for our findings and conclusions based on our audit objectives.

BACKGROUND

Second-Order Impacts of the Ebola Outbreak in Guinea, Liberia, and Sierra Leone

In addition to its direct impacts of increased morbidity and mortality, the Ebola outbreak also caused longer-term second-order impacts in all three primarily affected countries, including impacts on health systems, economies, governance, and food security.

---

[9] GAO, *Designing Evaluations: 2012 Revision*, GAO-12-208G (January 2012); Centers for Disease Control and Prevention, *Framework for Program Evaluation in Public Health* (Atlanta, GA: Sept. 17, 1999).

Impact on Health Systems

The Ebola outbreak overwhelmed the health systems and affected the quality and availability of health-care services in Guinea, Liberia, and Sierra Leone, which already had limited numbers of health-care workers and weak health-care infrastructure, according to WHO. Before the outbreak, the World Health Organization (WHO) estimated that there were 1 or 2 doctors per 100,000 people in the three countries; for example, WHO estimated that there were approximately 50 doctors in Liberia for a population of about 4.5 million. The quality and availability of care deteriorated as health-care workers succumbed to Ebola, and patients and health-care workers avoided health facilities for fear of contracting the disease. Health-care workers in the three primarily affected countries were 21 to 32 times more likely to be infected with Ebola than the general population. According to WHO, as of May 2015 health-care workers constituted about 4 percent of those infected in the three countries and, of those health-care workers infected, about two-thirds died.

The outbreak also caused health resources to be diverted from other basic health services. For example, the United Nations Children's Fund (UNICEF) reported that the outbreak contributed to a drop in vaccination coverage, resulting in a significant number of children being exposed to the risks of contracting vaccine-preventable diseases. The number of children in Sierra Leone receiving basic immunizations declined by 21 percent in 2014, following the outbreak, according to UNICEF.

Impact on Economies, Governance, and Food Security

All three countries experienced serious economic consequences from the Ebola outbreak, according to USAID. The closure of international borders in response to the outbreak hampered economic activity by limiting and restricting the movement of people, goods, and services. As a result, USAID noted that Guinea, Liberia, and Sierra Leone experienced market disruption, reduced agricultural production, and decreased household purchasing power. The gross domestic product (GDP) growth in all three countries declined in 2015 following the outbreak, most markedly in Sierra Leone (see Figure 1).

All three countries' governance and public management was already generally weak before the outbreak, according to World Bank indicators, and during the outbreak, their governments faced challenges in providing basic public services. As Ebola spread in West Africa in 2014 and early 2015, food security became a concern in the three primarily affected countries, according to USAID. Travel bans created market disruptions and shortfalls in agricultural production. Food prices increased while household incomes and purchasing power decreased, resulting in food insecurity, according to USAID. Additionally, the outbreak occurred at the beginning of the planting season, which further affected agricultural markets and food supplies.

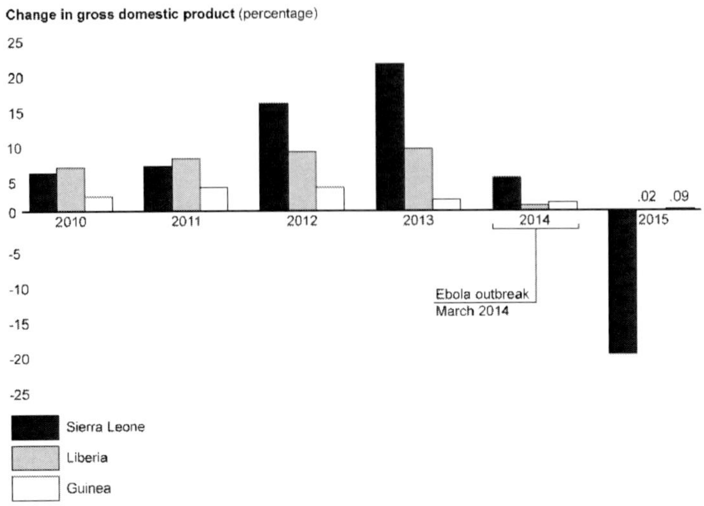

Source: GAO analysis of International Monetaru Fund data. | GAO-18-350.

Figure 1: Percent Change in Gross Domestic Product for Sierra Leone, Liberia, and Guinea, 2010-2015.

USAID's Strategic Framework for Ebola Recovery and Number and Status of Projects

In June 2015, USAID designed a strategic framework in part to explain the objectives of its Ebola projects to internal and external stakeholders, such as agency officials, Congress, and implementing partners, according to USAID officials. USAID derived the Ebola recovery portion of its strategic framework from Pillar 2 of the U.S. government strategy for Reducing Transmission of the Ebola Virus Disease in West Africa. Specifically, the overall objective of Pillar 2 of USAID's strategic framework is to address the second-order impacts of the outbreak by preventing the loss of development gains and strengthening key institutions and infrastructure whose weaknesses enabled the rapid spread of Ebola or slowed the response.

USAID's strategic framework for Ebola recovery consists of five project categories, which have the following goals:

- Health systems recovery. Improve the delivery of services and health-care commodities, enhance the management of health crises through revised protocols and response capabilities, and address health-care workforce issues.
- Emergency non-Ebola health services. Restart health services to pre-Ebola outbreak levels and communicate the risks of Ebola to mobilize the population to change its behaviors.
- Governance and economic crisis mitigation. Improve public services, governance, elections processes, water and sanitation, and social protection systems.

- Innovation, technology, and partnership. Attract innovations, new technologies, and partnerships to address response and recovery challenges, as well as improve health information systems.
- Food security. Increase food access for groups impacted by Ebola and increase food availability through the recovery of local food production and agricultural markets.

According to USAID, after developing the strategic framework in June 2015, it programmed Ebola funds for Ebola survivor and world health reform projects, which have the following goals:

- Ebola survivors. Support the procurement of medicines and supplies for Ebola survivors and build the capacity of health-care services to monitor and treat Ebola survivors.
- World health reform. Strengthen WHO's ability to lead and coordinate an effective response to ongoing and future health emergencies.

As of September 2017, USAID had implemented the largest number of recovery projects in Liberia.[10] Table 1 shows the numbers of completed, ongoing, and planned USAID recovery projects by geographic area.

Table 1. Total Numbers of USAID Ebola Recovery Projects by Implementation Status and Geographic Area, as of September 2017

Geographic area	Number of completed projects	Number of ongoing projects	Number of planned projects not yet initiated	Total
Liberia	20	29	2	51
Regional	25	13	0	38
Sierra Leone	8	14	0	22
Guinea	9	9	2	20
Total	62	65	4	131

Source: GAO analysis of U.S. Agency for International Development (USAID) data. | GAO-18-350.

Note: Geographic areas are shown in order of the total numbers of completed, ongoing, and planned USAID Ebola recovery projects.

USAID Obligated $412 Million for 131 Projects Across 7 Categories of Ebola Recovery Assistance

USAID had obligated approximately $411.6 million for 131 Ebola recovery projects as of September 30, 2017, from three different appropriations accounts: the Economic

[10] Regional Ebola recovery projects encompass multiple countries.

Support Fund (ESF) account, the International Disaster Assistance (IDA) account, and the Global Health Programs (GHP) account.[11] USAID obligated the largest amount of funding from the ESF account. USAID's funding for Ebola recovery projects supported seven categories of assistance: health systems recovery, emergency non-Ebola health services, governance and economic crisis mitigation, innovation and communications technology, food security, world health reform, and Ebola survivors. Food security projects received the largest share of Ebola recovery funds.

USAID Has Funded Ebola Recovery Projects through Three Appropriations Accounts

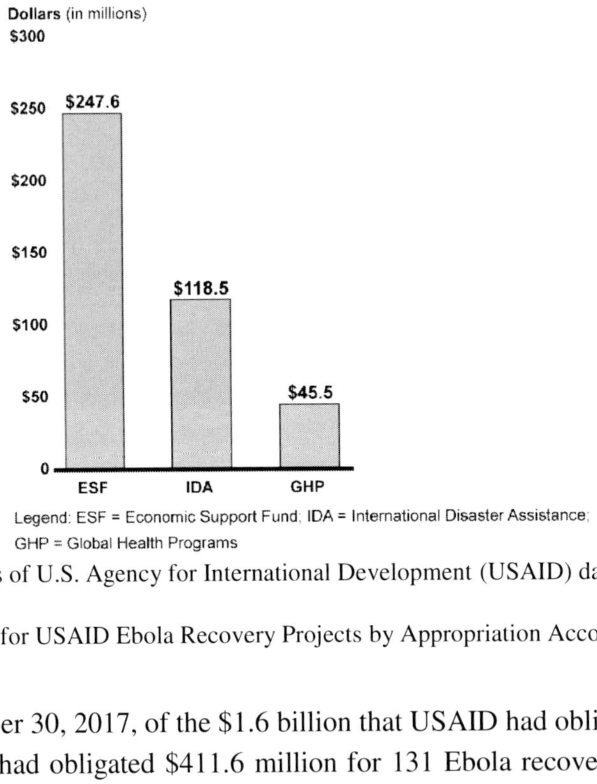

Source: GAO analysis of U.S. Agency for International Development (USAID) data. | GAO-18-350.

Figure 2. Obligations for USAID Ebola Recovery Projects by Appropriation Account, as of September 30, 2017.

As of September 30, 2017, of the $1.6 billion that USAID had obligated for the Ebola outbreak, USAID had obligated $411.6 million for 131 Ebola recovery projects that we identified.[12] Of the $411.6 million, USAID obligated the largest amount—$247.6 million (60 percent)—from the ESF account. Figure 2 shows USAID's obligations for its recovery projects by account.

---

[11] We report obligations from the Act in accordance with USAID's and State's reporting to Congress because the reports are the source of our data. The obligations data in this chapter are as of September 30, 2017 because USAID's and State's most recent report for Congress is as of that date.

[12] State and the Centers for Disease Control and Prevention (CDC) have also implemented Ebola recovery projects funded from the Act, as of September 30, 2017. For more information about State and CDC Ebola recovery projects, see appendix III. For additional information about the status of USAID's and State's reported allocations from the Act by appropriation account, see appendix IV.

ESF Account

USAID obligated funding from the ESF account for recovery projects to support health systems recovery, emergency non-Ebola health services, governance and economic crisis mitigation, innovation and communications technology, and Ebola survivors. For example, USAID obligated

- $2.0 million for a project to provide routine immunizations to more than 130,000 children under 5 years of age and more than 130,000 pregnant women in Liberia;
- $17.0 million for a project to restore routine health services in Sierra Leone by (a) installing water and sanitation and solar power infrastructure at more than 300 health facilities, (b) providing medical equipment, and (c) training more than 900 health-care professionals on reproductive, maternal, newborn, and child health and infection prevention and control practices (see Figure 3);

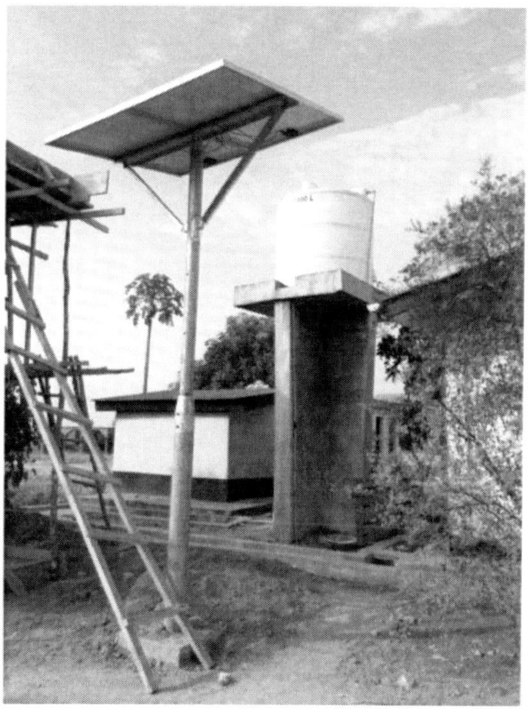

Source: GAO. | GAO-18-350.

Figure 3: Solar Panel at a Health Facility in Sierra Leone Installed as Part of a USAID Ebola Recovery Project.

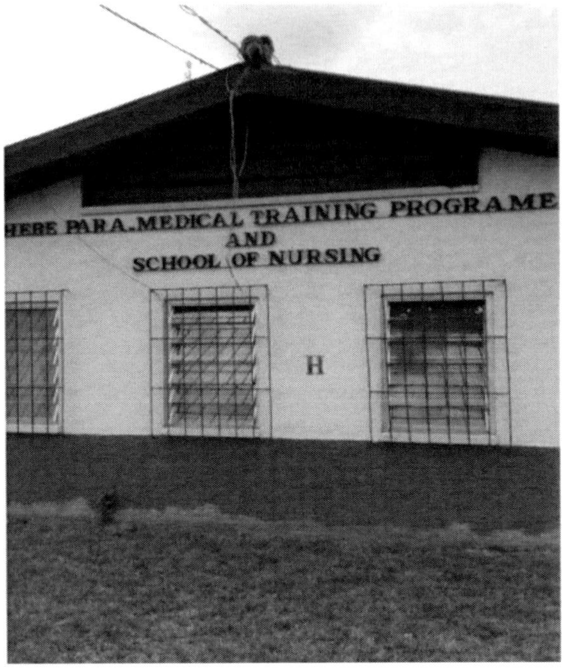

Source: GAO. GAO-18-350.

Figure 4. Health Facility in Liberia at Which a USAID Ebola Recovery Project Funds Trainings for Midwives and Laboratory Technicians.

- $10.0 million for a project to improve the quality of pre-service education for midwives and laboratory personnel in Liberia (see Figure 4);
- $6.0 million for a project to support health finance and governance in Guinea, which assessed the financial management of the Ministry of Health and updated the ministry's administrative and financial procedures, and provided management trainings to 65 senior health officials;
- $1.5 million for projects to develop health information system strategies in Guinea, Liberia, and Sierra Leone, including embedding expert advisors in each country's Ministry of Health; and
- $1 million for an Ebola survivor and transmission prevention project in Liberia to build the capacity of specialty care services to treat and monitor survivors.

IDA Account

USAID obligated $118.5 million from the IDA account for food security projects, such as food assistance and agricultural market support. For example, USAID obligated approximately $4.6 million in IDA funding for an emergency food security project in Liberia that increased 5,000 Ebolaaffected households' access to food through unconditional cash transfers delivered by a mobile money service provider. The project also provided seed kits for six crop varieties to 4,000 of these households. In addition, USAID obligated approximately $9.9 million for an emergency food security project in

Sierra Leone that provided unconditional cash transfers to more than 10,300 households and conditional cash transfers to 400 small-scale agricultural traders to support the restocking of food supplies in areas affected by the Ebola outbreak. As a condition for receiving assistance, the small-scale agricultural traders participated in business trainings.

GHP Account

USAID obligated $45.5 million from the GHP account for Ebola survivor and world health reform projects. The Ebola survivor project provides training to local medical staff to ensure long-term care for Ebola survivors in Liberia. USAID intends the world health reform project to guide WHO to reform its structures and processes to support its capacity to respond to future disease outbreaks and health emergencies.

Food Security Projects Received the Largest Share of Ebola Recovery Obligations

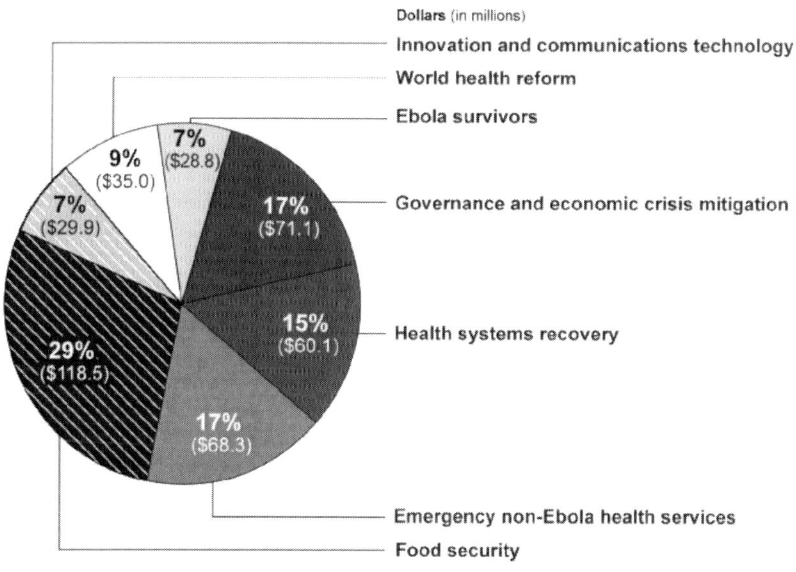

Source: GAO analysis of U.S. Agency for International Development (USAID) data. GAO-18-350.

Note: This figure does not include Ebola recovery projects that the Centers for Disease Control and Prevention are implementing through an interagency agreement with USAID. The interagency agreement contains $80 million in obligations for Ebola, including obligations for Ebola recovery projects.

Figure 5. USAID's Obligations for Ebola Recovery Projects, as of September 30, 2017.

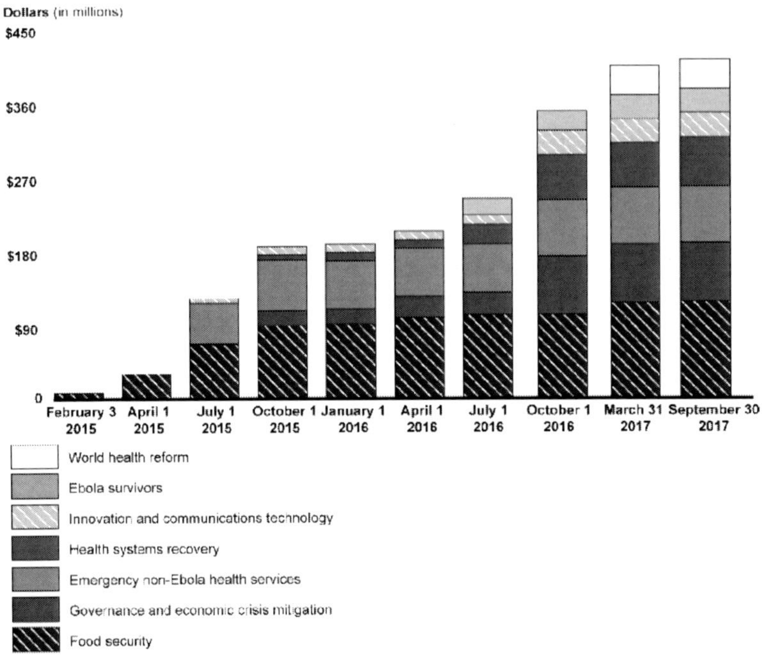

Source: GAO analysis of U.S. Agency for International Development (USAID) data. GAO-18-350.

Figure 6. USAID's Obligations for Ebola Recovery Projects, February 2015— September 2017.

As of September 2017, USAID had obligated the greatest amount of funding for food security projects, followed by projects supporting governance and economic crisis mitigation, and emergency non-Ebola health services. Figure 5 depicts Ebola recovery project categories as a percentage of total obligations.

As shown in Figure 6, USAID began obligating funds for food security in early 2015 in order to meet immediate food security needs and began obligating funds for other types of Ebola recovery activities in May 2015.

USAID obligated funds for Ebola survivor projects in May 2016 after identifying the level of need for survivor care.

Appendix II provides additional information on USAID Ebola recovery projects, including detailed information on our sample of 10 selected recovery projects.

Almost Half of USAID's Ebola Recovery Projects Had Been Completed; the Remaining Were Ongoing, or Not Yet Started, as of September 2017

As of September 2017, USAID had completed 62 of its 131 planned Ebola recovery projects, had 65 projects that were ongoing, and had 4 planned projects that it had not yet started.[13] Of the 62 completed projects, USAID completed 39 within originally planned time frames and budgeted costs and extended the remaining 23. Of the 65 ongoing projects, USAID expected to implement 46 within original time frames and costs, but extended 19. USAID extended projects, in part, to complete host-government actions, hire staff, finalize project activities, and continue and expand food assistance.

USAID Had Completed 62 Ebola Recovery Projects as of September 2017, Most within Originally Planned Time Frames and Budgeted Costs

USAID had completed more than half of its 62 completed Ebola recovery projects within originally planned time frames and budgeted costs, as of September 2017. Table 2 shows the numbers of recovery projects that each USAID bureau, office, or mission had completed within original time frames and the obligations for such projects, as of that date.

Table 2. Ebola Recovery Projects That USAID Had Completed within Originally Planned Time Frames and Budgeted Costs, as of September 2017 (Dollars in thousands)

USAID bureau, office, or mission	Number of projects	Types of projects	Total obligations
Global Development Lab	21	Governance and economic crisis mitigation Innovation and communications technology	4,430
Bureau for Global Health	11	Innovation and communications technology Health systems recovery Emergency non-Ebola health services	25,818
Office of Food for Peace	4	Food security	30,145
USAID/Liberia	2	Emergency non-Ebola health services Governance and economic crisis mitigation	5,600
USAID/Guinea	1	Governance and economic crisis mitigation	500
Total	39	—	66,493

Source: GAO analysis of U.S. Agency for International Development (USAID) data and information. | GAO-18-350.

Note: We report obligations for funding appropriated in the Department of State, Foreign Operations, and Related Programs Appropriations Act, 2015 in accordance with USAID's and State's reporting to Congress because the reports are the source of our data. The obligations data are as of September 30, 2017 because USAID's and State's most recent report for Congress is as of that date. Amounts shown may not sum to totals because of rounding.

[13] We report project time frame data as of September 2017 because we obtained data on the implementation status of Ebola recovery projects from USAID bureaus, offices, and missions as of that date.

Table 3 shows the 23 completed projects that USAID bureaus and offices had extended beyond original time frames and the obligations for such projects, as of September 2017. On average, the length of time originally planned for these projects was 12 months. USAID had extended these projects by an average of about 6 months and added a total of $6.6 million to 4 of the projects, as of September 2017.

Table 3. Completed Ebola Recovery Projects That USAID Had Extended beyond Originally Planned Time Frames and Budgeted Costs, as of September 2017 (Dollars in thousands)

USAID bureau, office, or mission	Number of projects	Types of projects	Initial obligations	Additional obligations for cost extensions	Total obligations
Bureau for Global Health	16	Innovation and communications technology Emergency non-Ebola health services	33,774	81	33,855
Office of Food for Peace	6	Food security	33,894	6,451	40,345
Global Development Lab	1	Innovation and communications technology	100	43	143
Total	23	—	67,768	6,574[a]	74,343

Source: GAO analysis of U.S. Agency for International Development (USAID) data and information. | GAO-18-350.

Notes: We report obligations for funding appropriated in the Department of State, Foreign Operations, and Related Programs Appropriations Act, 2015 in accordance with USAID's and State's reporting to Congress because the reports are the source of our data. The obligations data are as of September 30, 2017 because USAID's and State's most recent report for Congress is as of that date. Amounts shown may not sum to totals because of rounding.

[a]USAID added a total of approximately $6.6 million in obligations for 4 of the 23 completed projects, as of September 30, 2017.

As of September 2017, USAID's Bureau for Global Health had approved time frame extensions for 16 completed projects to allow time to develop innovations, complete host-government actions, and finalize project activities. The bureau approved these extensions for 10 of these projects to allow additional time to develop, test, or modify innovations to help health-care workers provide better care and stop the spread of Ebola. For example, the bureau approved an extension of approximately 4 months for one project to develop a modular Ebola treatment unit to complete required tests of the unit's performance at testing facilities that were not readily available to conduct such tests, according to USAID officials. In addition, the bureau approved time frame extensions for 2 projects to obtain host-government approvals and complete actions needed to implement project activities. For example, the bureau approved an extension for a selected recovery project that supported immunization services of Liberia's Ministry of Health by 7 months because of delays in the ministry's implementation of the project's activities. According to project staff, the project required additional time to engage with the ministry to develop and disseminate materials and messages about the importance of immunization, and to conduct vaccine distribution and waste management at local health facilities. Figure 7 shows a poster displayed at a health facility supported by the project to inform mothers about the importance of child immunizations. In addition, the bureau approved an extension of 3 months for a project to refurbish health facilities and improve access to maternal and child health services in Sierra Leone. Figure 8 shows a refurbished health facility supported by the selected project. According to project staff, the project had experienced delays in completing renovation activities—such as installing water towers and pumps and drilling boreholes to meet the health facilities' water needs for infection prevention—because of challenges in locating suitable sites for drilling at health facilities and the rainy season. Figure 9 shows a water well installed at a health facility supported by the selected project.

USAID's Office of Food for Peace (FFP) had approved time frame extensions for 6 completed projects and obligated an additional $6.5 million for 2 of the 6 projects, as of September 2017. Specifically, FFP approved these extensions for 4 projects to address ongoing food security needs in existing Ebola-affected areas, according to USAID officials. For example, FFP approved an extension of 3 months for a selected emergency food assistance project in Liberia to conduct an additional cash transfer to the project's existing 5,000 beneficiary households to address short-term food assistance needs during the lean period. In addition, FFP approved extensions of 12 and 15 months and obligated an additional $6.5 million for 2 projects to address continued food security needs of Ebola-affected populations currently receiving assistance and to expand assistance to additional beneficiaries, according to USAID officials.

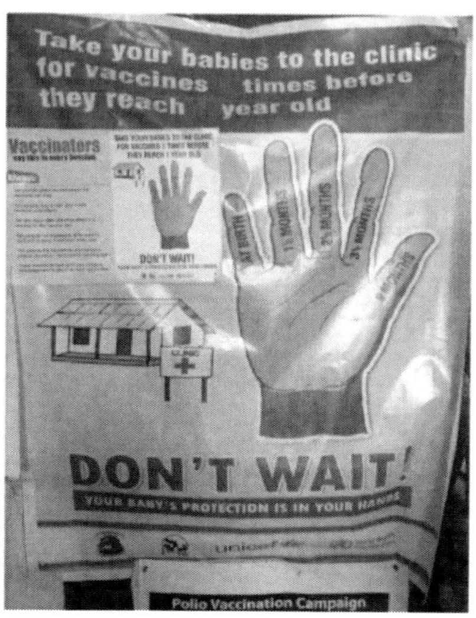

Source: GAO. GAO-18-350.

Figure 7. Vaccination Poster at Health Clinic in Liberia Provided by a USAID Ebola Recovery Project.

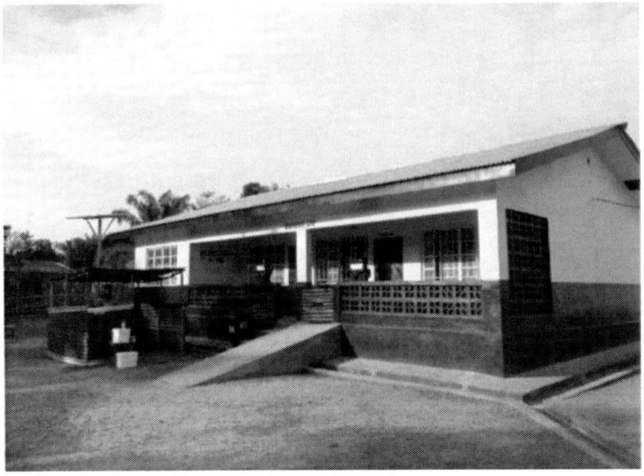

Source: GAO. GAO-18-350.

Figure 8. Community Health Center in Sierra Leone Rehabilitated by a USAID Ebola Recovery Project.

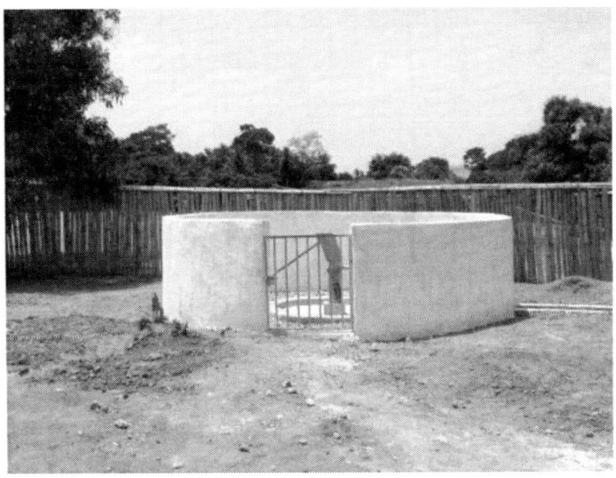

Source: GAO. GAO-18-350.

Figure 9. Water Well at a Maternal and Child Health Post in Sierra Leone Installed by a USAID Ebola Recovery Project.

USAID's Global Development Lab (Lab) had approved a time frame extension of 3 months for one completed project and obligated an additional $42,956 to complete the project's activities, as of September 2017. The project assessed the use of data and digital technologies in crisis response, resulting in the publication of a final report providing recommendations on the use of data and digital systems for future response efforts. The Lab approved the extension to provide time for editing and design of the published report, according to these officials.

USAID Had Started but Not Yet Completed 65 Ebola Recovery Projects as of September 2017, with Most Expected to Meet Original Time Frames and Costs

More than half of USAID's 65 ongoing projects were expected to meet originally planned time frames and budgeted costs, as of September 2017. Table 4 shows the number of ongoing recovery projects for each bureau, office, or mission that were on track for meeting original time frames and costs and the obligations for such projects, as of September 2017.

Table 4. Ongoing USAID Ebola Recovery Projects on Track for Meeting Originally Planned Time Frames and Budgeted Costs, as of September 2017 (Dollars in thousands)

USAID bureau, office, or mission	Number of projects	Types of projects	Total obligations
Global Development Lab	27	Governance and economic crisis mitigation Innovation and communications technology Ebola survivors	38,536
Bureau for Global Health	11	Innovation and communications technology Emergency non-Ebola health services Health systems recovery Ebola survivors	51,030
USAID/Liberia	4	Governance and economic crisis mitigation	29,911
USAID/Guinea	2	Governance and economic crisis mitigation	12,000
USAID/Sierra Leone	1	Governance and economic crisis mitigation	4,000
Office of U.S. Foreign Disaster Assistance	1	World health reform	35,000
Total	46	—	170,477

Source: GAO analysis of U.S. Agency for International Development (USAID) data and information. | GAO-18-350.

Note: We report obligations for funding appropriated in the Department of State, Foreign Operations, and Related Programs Appropriations Act, 2015 in accordance with USAID's and State's reporting to Congress because the reports are the source of our data. The obligations data are as of September 30, 2017 because USAID's and State's most recent report for Congress is as of that date. Amounts shown may not sum to totals because of rounding.

As of September 2017, USAID had extended 19 ongoing projects by an average of approximately 12 months beyond the projects' originally planned average time frames of about 15 months. USAID had obligated an additional $22.8 million to 6 of the 19 projects. Table 5 shows the numbers of ongoing projects that each bureau, office, or mission had extended beyond original time frames and costs and the additional obligations for such projects, as of September 2017.

Table 5. Ongoing Ebola Recovery Projects That USAID Had Extended beyond Originally Planned Time Frames and Budgeted Costs, as of September 2017 (Dollars in thousands)

USAID bureau, office, or mission	Number of projects	Types of projects	Initial obligations	Additional obligations for cost extensions	Total obligations
Bureau for Global Health	8	Emergency non-Ebola health services Health systems recovery	41,508	0	41,508
Office of Food for Peace	6	Food security	25,202	22,791	47,993
Global Development Lab	4	Innovation and communications technology Governance and economic crisis mitigation	2,362	0	2,362
USAID/Guinea	1	Governance and economic crisis mitigation	1,000	0	1,000
Total	19	—	70,072	22,791	92,863

Source: GAO analysis of U.S. Agency for International Development (USAID) data and information. | GAO-18-350.

Note: We report obligations for funding appropriated in the Department of State, Foreign Operations, and Related Programs Appropriations Act, 2015 in accordance with USAID's and State's reporting to Congress because the reports are the source of our data. The obligations data are as of September 30, 2017 because USAID's and State's most recent report for Congress is as of that date. Amounts shown may not sum to totals because of rounding.

As shown in Table 5, USAID's Bureau for Global Health had approved time frame extensions for 8 ongoing projects, as of September 2017. The bureau approved these extensions for 4 projects to allow time to obtain host-government approvals and actions needed to implement project activities. For example, the bureau approved an extension of 18 months for one project to restore routine health service delivery and strengthen infection prevention and control in Liberia. The extension allowed additional time to support the project's ongoing renovation work at health facilities, which had been delayed because of difficulty in obtaining approvals from the Ministry of Health, according to project staff. In addition, the bureau approved an extension of 9 months for a selected recovery project that supports the governance and financial management of the health system in Guinea to allow additional time to coordinate with Ministry of Health officials and other partners to implement project activities. The implementation of the project's activities requires host-government officials' approvals of draft plans and strategies to improve the capacity of institutions to conduct oversight and improve the Ministry of Health's internal and external communications; however, project staff noted that delays in officials' reviews of draft documents affected the timeliness of the approvals. The bureau extended the remaining 4 projects because of delays in procuring supplies and hiring staff with the skills to manage the project and to allow additional time to complete ongoing project activities, according to USAID officials.

FFP approved time frame extensions and obligated an additional $22.8 million for 6 ongoing food security projects to address continued needs of Ebola-affected populations currently receiving assistance and to expand assistance to additional beneficiaries. For example, FFP approved an extension of 23 months and obligated an additional $5.6 million for a selected food assistance project in Sierra Leone. The additional time and funding allowed the implementing partner to continue cash transfers to the project's 6,445 household beneficiaries and expand assistance to an additional 3,873 households whose ability to purchase food remained limited primarily because of the loss of employment and currency depreciation.

The Lab approved time frame extensions for 4 ongoing recovery projects because of delays in hiring staff to manage the project, and to allow additional time to implement project activities. For example, the Lab approved an extension of 4 months for a selected project in Liberia to develop a digital salary payment system for health-care workers to allow them to continue working in the hospitals and clinics without needing to be away from work for a lengthy period of time to receive payments. The project had experienced lower enrollment of health-care workers than expected, primarily because of a lack of understanding and trust in the system among health-care workers, according to project staff. The Lab approved the time frame extension so that the implementing partner and the Ministry of Health could collaborate on a more targeted approach to health-care worker enrollment, according to USAID officials.

USAID had planned 4 Ebola recovery projects that it had not yet started, as of September 2017. USAID had obligated $7.4 million to these 4 projects, as of September 30, 2017. Specifically, the mission in Guinea has planned one governance and economic crisis mitigation project and 1 health systems recovery project, and the Lab has planned 2 innovation and communications technology projects in Liberia.

USAID Has Initiated an Evaluation of Its Ebola Recovery Activities, but It Has Not Yet Ensured that Its Contractor Has Compiled a Complete and Accurate Inventory of Recovery Projects

USAID has initiated an evaluation of its recovery activities, but it has not yet ensured that its contracted evaluator (contractor) has compiled a complete and accurate inventory of USAID's recovery projects. In 2016, USAID contracted for an evaluation of its Ebola recovery efforts. USAID intends to use the information and lessons learned from this evaluation to inform and improve its ability to respond to future global health emergencies. The contractor has developed several key aspects of the study design.

However, as of December 2017, USAID had not ensured that the contractor compiled a complete and accurate inventory of USAID's recovery projects. USAID policy states that information collected should be of sufficient quality to be useful for the intended users. Without a complete and accurate inventory of USAID's Ebola recovery projects, USAID does not have assurance that the resulting evaluation will be of sufficient quality.

USAID Has Contracted for an Evaluation of Its Ebola Recovery Activities

The purpose of the evaluation[14] is to assess the overall performance of USAID's Ebola recovery activities in achieving Pillar 2's objective.[15] According to the contractor's evaluation design plan, the contractor plans to determine

- how the Pillar 2 activities in Guinea, Liberia, and Sierra Leone are contributing to the achievement of the mission and the Pillar 2 of USAID's Strategic Framework's objective;
- the extent to which Pillar 2 accomplishments are still observable after the projects are completed, and why;
- whether there were unanticipated barriers or consequences of Pillar 2 investments, and if opportunities were seized or missed; and
- any lessons that were learned regarding how to use the strengths of USAID's development mechanisms in a complex emergency.

USAID intends to use the information and lessons learned from the evaluation to inform and improve its ability to respond effectively and efficiently to future global health emergencies. The contractor plans to submit its first report on the evaluation's findings in March 2018.[16]

The contractor's evaluation design plan calls for the evaluation to be organized into three phases:

---

[14] The evaluation is part of the Ebola Pillar II Monitoring, Evaluation, and Learning Project. According to USAID guidance, a monitoring, evaluation, and learning project report is an essential step in managing USAID's process of assessing and reporting progress toward achieving project outputs and outcomes, and to identify what evaluation questions will be addressed through evaluation.

[15] As described in the contractor's evaluation design plan, this evaluation is a macro-level evaluation in that the overall performance of Pillar 2 activities is evaluated. It is not intended to measure performance at the individual project level. USAID's Bureau for Global Health and Global Development Lab are conducting separate evaluations that will include assessments of performance at the project level.

[16] A second performance evaluation report, due in 2019, would provide an assessment of overall summative outcome questions. As defined by USAID's *Glossary of Evaluation Terms*, a summative evaluation would assess the program in its later stages or after it has been completed to (1) assess its impact, (2) identify the factors that affected its performance, (3) assess the sustainability of its results, and (4) draw lessons that may inform other interventions.

- In the first phase, the contractor would conduct a review to summarize what activities had been implemented using Pillar 2 funds. Using categories of activities that the contractor and USAID agreed upon, the contractor would (1) identify project-level activities that were under way or completed, and were implemented between April 2015 and March 31, 2017, and (2) assign each project-level activity to a category.[17] To carry out these tasks, according to the design plan, the contractor is to compile an inventory of USAID's Ebola recovery projects, including detailed information on each project's stakeholders, locations, scale, and other descriptive information.
- In the second phase, the contractor would collect and analyze data from a variety of sources to assess the performance of selected main activities in achieving Pillar 2's objective.[18] The contractor told us that it has developed an initial inventory of projects through in-person interviews with USAID staff and stakeholders in Washington, D.C., and in the three countries, and by reviewing project documentation.
- In the third phase, the contractor would assess the overall combined effects of Pillar 2 activities on the objective of Pillar 2 recovery efforts.

USAID's Contractor Has Developed Several Key Aspects of the Evaluation Design, but USAID Has Not Ensured that the Contractor Compiled a Complete and Accurate Inventory of USAID's Pillar 2 Projects

Although USAID's contractor has developed several key evaluation design details, some over the course of our review, USAID has yet to ensure that the contractor compiled a complete and accurate inventory of USAID's Pillar 2 recovery projects. We compared the contractor's study design plan to criteria for developing effective evaluations (see app. I for criteria).[19] Based on this analysis, we identified elements that were incomplete or unclear in the contractor's evaluation design plan. When we brought these issues to USAID's and the contractor's attention, they took steps to further develop these design details and provided additional documentation to us to demonstrate the steps that they had taken. Specifically, the contractor provided an updated version of the evaluation plan that includes the sampling methodology for a survey and control group;

---

[17] The second and third phases of the contractor's work are to build on the results of the first phase. In the second phase, the contractor will focus on assessing the performance of selected main activities that are completed or under way. It will identify and describe accomplishments and lessons learned from Pillar 2 investments. In the third phase, the contractor plans to assess the overall combined effects of Pillar 2 activities on the objective of Pillar 2 recovery efforts.

[18] The contractor is selecting main activities based on geographic coverage, funding levels, and implementation status of the projects that comprise the categories of activities.

[19] USAID and the contractor refer to the evaluation design plan document as an "Inception Report."

the contractor also developed a data analysis plan that further identifies indicators for the outcome measures and data sources for the indicators.

However, as of December 2017, USAID had not ensured that the contractor compiled a complete and accurate inventory of Pillar 2 projects that was to be completed as part of the evaluation's first phase. When we compared the contractor's most recent inventory, as of December 2017, to the inventory of Pillar 2 projects that USAID had included in its reports to congressional committees, we found major differences in terms of the nature and number of projects included. For example, we identified at least 10 projects in the contractor's inventory that USAID had not included in the lists of recovery projects it reported to congressional committees, including projects related to solid waste management and malaria control. We also found that the contractor's inventory omitted projects that USAID had identified as Pillar 2 projects in those reports, including Ebola innovation projects implemented by the Lab and by the Bureau for Global Health.

As of December 2017, USAID officials were uncertain as to why the contractor's most recent inventory differed from the inventory that USAID had provided in the congressional reports. USAID and contractor officials subsequently told us that the contractor was continuing to finalize the inventory. USAID guidance for monitoring and reporting criteria cites the importance of ensuring that the information collected is of sufficient quality to be useful for intended users and of ensuring that the evaluation design, measures, and analysis plans are appropriate for the evaluation questions. Unless this inventory is complete and accurate, the contractor's evaluation may not be able to reliably assess the extent to which Pillar 2 activities are on track to achieve the Pillar 2 objective. Thus, USAID does not have assurance of the quality of the evaluation findings.

CONCLUSION

As the Ebola outbreak in West Africa subsided, USAID initiated more than 130 projects aimed at helping three West African countries recover from the outbreak's devastating second-order effects on their economies, health care systems, and food security. When the scope and nature of recovery needs grew to include greater support for Ebola survivors, USAID initiated projects to meet those needs. To inform its response to any future Ebola outbreak or similar global health emergency, USAID has contracted for an evaluation of its Ebola recovery activities to assess whether those activities contributed to its efforts to achieve its Ebola recovery objective. This evaluation relies on an inventory of USAID's Ebola recovery projects. However, to date, USAID has not ensured that the contractor compiled a complete and accurate inventory of USAID's Ebola recovery projects. Without such an inventory, USAID does not have assuranc of the quality of the evaluation's findings.

Recommendation for Executive Action

The Administrator of USAID should take steps to ensure that USAID's contractor compiles a complete and accurate inventory of Ebola recovery projects prior to finalizing its analysis. (Recommendation 1)

Agency Comments and Our Evaluation

We provided a draft of this chapter to USAID, State, and CDC for comment. In its formal comments, provided in appendix V, USAID agreed with our findings and recommendation. USAID noted that all Ebola recovery projects should be included in the evaluation. USAID further noted that it is collaborating with the contractor to help ensure that the contractor will compile a complete and accurate inventory of Ebola recovery projects prior to finalizing its analysis. State and CDC did not provide formal comments. USAID, State, and CDC provided technical comments, which we incorporated throughout the report, as appropriate.

We are sending copies of this chapter to the appropriate congressional committees, the Administrator of the U.S. Agency for International Development, the Secretary of State, and other interested parties.

David B. Gootnick
Director, International Affairs and Trade

Appendix I: Objectives, Scope, and Methodology

The Department of State, Foreign Operations, and Related Programs Appropriations Act, 2015 (the Act) included a provision for us to conduct oversight of the U.S. Agency for International Development's (USAID) and the Department of State's (State) activities to prevent, prepare for, and respond to the 2014 Ebola outbreak.[20] We examined (1) obligations for USAID'S Ebola recovery projects, (2) the status of USAID's implementation of these projects, and (3) USAID's evaluation of Ebola recovery efforts.

To examine obligations for USAID's Ebola recovery projects, we reviewed USAID's and State's reports to the Senate and House Committees on Appropriations mandated by the Act from February 3, 2015 to September 30, 2017.[21] We analyzed USAID's obligations data and project information that it reported as supporting Ebola recovery, as

---

[20] Pub. L. No. 113-235, Div. J, Title IX, 128 Stat. 2130, 2692 (Dec. 16, 2014).

[21] We report funding from the Act for Ebola in accordance with USAID's and State's reporting to Congress. USAID and State have reported to Congress on Ebola funding from February 3, 2015 to September 30, 2017.

of September 30, 2017, the most recent data and information that USAID and State have reported for congressional committees.[22] We focused this chapter on USAID because it has allocated more than $2.3 billion (91 percent) of the approximately $2.5 billion appropriated and has implemented most of the Ebola recovery projects funded from the appropriation. We also reviewed U.S. government-wide and USAID strategy documents for Ebola response and recovery in order to determine the categories of Pillar 2 of the U.S. government strategy for Reducing Transmission of the Ebola Virus Disease in West Africa—mitigation of the second-order impacts of the crisis—and the projects that support these categories. Additionally, we interviewed USAID officials in Washington, D.C. from the Bureau for Africa, Office of Food for Peace, Office of U.S. Foreign Disaster Assistance, Global Development Lab, and Bureau for Global Health to identify each bureau's or office's Ebola recovery projects. We also interviewed State officials from the Bureau of International Narcotics and Law Enforcement Affairs, and the Office of U.S. Foreign Assistance Resources to identify each bureau's or office's Ebola recovery projects. We analyzed USAID's obligations data and information that USAID reported as supporting the categories of Pillar 2—health systems recovery, emergency non-Ebola health systems, governance and economic crisis mitigation, innovation and communications technology, and food security—as well as Ebola survivors and world health reform projects that agency officials had identified as supporting Ebola recovery. Our calculations of obligations for Ebola recovery projects do not include funding for program support or for monitoring and evaluation. We also reviewed Centers for Disease Control and Prevention (CDC) and State documents and interviewed USAID, CDC, and State officials in Guinea, Liberia, and Sierra Leone to identify each agency's Ebola recovery projects.

To examine the status of USAID's implementation of Ebola recovery projects, we analyzed agency data on the implementation of Ebola recovery projects and the amounts of funding that USAID had obligated for these projects. We also requested and obtained data and information from USAID on the progress of implementation of the Ebola recovery projects that USAID had reported as of September 2017. We analyzed the data and information from USAID to determine the extent to which recovery projects had met planned time frames and budgeted costs. We reviewed agency documentation of the agency's time frame and cost extensions for extended projects to determine the reasons for the extensions. We also analyzed USAID's obligations data in the report to the Senate and House Committees on Appropriations mandated by the Act to identify the numbers and types of Ebola recovery projects that USAID had planned and implemented and the amounts of funding obligated for these projects, as of September 30, 2017. In addition, to gain more in-depth information and context on the implementation of Ebola recovery

[22] In a draft of this chapter that we provided to USAID and State for comment, we reported funding data that were current as of March 31, 2017. State subsequently provided updated data as of September 30, 2017. We updated our report accordingly.

projects, we selected a non-generalizable sample of 10 USAID recovery projects. For the non-generalizable sample of projects, we reviewed project documents, including, among other things, implementing partners' annual and quarterly reports to determine project activities and examine project implementation. We selected our non-generalizable sample of 10 projects from the 84 Ebola recovery projects that USAID had reported in Pillar 2 as of July 1, 2016.[23] We selected projects to achieve a mix of projects by country; USAID office, bureau, and mission; and category of USAID's strategic framework for Ebola recovery.[24] In addition, we conducted fieldwork in Guinea, Liberia, and Sierra Leone. During our fieldwork in these countries, we met with USAID mission officials, USAID's implementing partners, host government officials, and project beneficiaries. Where possible, we conducted site visits to our selected projects in Guinea, Liberia, and Sierra Leone to examine implementation.

We assessed the reliability of the data that USAID reported for its implementation of Ebola recovery projects and its obligations for such projects. We requested and reviewed information from agency officials regarding the underlying financial data systems and the checks and reviews used to generate the data and ensure its accuracy and reliability. We also compared the data to USAID's documentation for selected projects to assess the reliability of USAID funding and project data. When we found data discrepancies, we contacted relevant agency officials in Washington, D.C., Guinea, Liberia, or Sierra Leone, and obtained information from them necessary to resolve the discrepancies.[25] In addition, we have assessed the reliability of these data in our prior work and have found them to be reliable for the purposes of examining USAID's and State's obligations and disbursements of the appropriated funds.[26] As a result of these steps, we determined that the data were sufficiently reliable for our purposes of reporting the numbers of Ebola recovery projects and obligations for these projects, as of September 30, 2017.

To examine USAID's evaluation of Ebola recovery efforts, we reviewed USAID's contracted evaluator's (contractor) evaluation design plan document and subsequent revisions and compared its contents to standards regarding key elements of evaluation design plans. We identified these standards in sources including USAID's policies and requirements for monitoring and evaluation in the *Automated Directives System* (ADS), Chapter 201; *Evaluation: Learning from Experience*,

---

[23] We selected our sample of projects from among those that USAID had reported as of July 1, 2016 because we had assessed the reliability of the project data and information that USAID had reported as of that date during our prior work. In addition, to allow for an assessment of the implementation, we sought to select projects that had either begun implementation or had been completed.

[24] The categories of USAID's strategic framework for Ebola recovery are (1) health systems recovery, (2) emergency non-Ebola health services, (3) governance and economic crisis mitigation, (4) innovation and communications technology, and (5) food security.

[25] As a result of our efforts to ensure data reliability, the data that we report for obligations may differ from the data that USAID has reported to congressional committees.

[26] GAO, *Emergency Funding for Ebola Response: Some USAID Reimbursements Did Not Comply with Legislative Requirements and Need to Be Reversed*, GAO-17-35 (Washington, D.C.: Nov. 2, 2016).

USAID Evaluation Policy, 2016 Update;[27] GAO's *Designing Evaluations: 2012 Revision*;[28] and the Centers for Disease Control and Prevention's *Framework for Program Evaluation in Public Health*.[29] We also interviewed USAID officials and contractor staff in Washington, D.C. to discuss the evaluation plan details, including the methods, measures, and analysis plan.

We conducted this performance audit from November 2016 to March 2018 in accordance with generally accepted government auditing standards. Those standards require that we plan and perform the audit to obtain sufficient, appropriate evidence to provide a reasonable basis for our findings and conclusions based on our audit objectives. We believe that the evidence obtained provides a reasonable basis for our findings and conclusions based on our audit objectives.

APPENDIX II: SUMMARIES OF SELECTED U.S. AGENCY FOR INTERNATIONAL DEVELOPMENT EBOLA RECOVERY PROJECTS

The following is a summary of information on U.S. Agency for International Development (USAID) Ebola recovery projects, including the project objectives and examples of project activities for the 10 projects that we selected by country; USAID office, bureau, and mission; and the components of USAID's strategic framework for Ebola recovery. USAID's Bureau for Global Health, Global Development Lab, Office of Food for Peace, Office of U.S. Foreign Disaster Assistance, and missions in Liberia, Guinea, and Sierra Leone obligated $411.6 million for the 131 recovery projects, as of September 2017. The recovery projects support health systems recovery, emergency non-Ebola health services, governance and economic crisis mitigation, innovation and communications technology, food security, Ebola survivor transmission prevention, and world health reform projects.

Health Systems Recovery

As of September 30, 2017, USAID had obligated approximately $60.1 million for 16 health system recovery projects to improve the ability of health systems in Ebola-affected countries to manage health crises, improve service delivery, and increase demand for health services within communities.

---

[27] U.S. Agency for International Development, *Evaluation: Learning From Experience. USAID Evaluation Policy, 2016 Update* (Washington, D.C.: October 2016).

[28] GAO, *Designing Evaluations: 2012 Revision*, GAO-12-208G (January 2012).

[29] Centers for Disease Control and Prevention, *Framework for Program Evaluation in Public Health* (Atlanta, GA: Sept. 17, 1999).

USAID's Bureau for Health obligated funding for projects to procure and deliver commodities to health facilities, train and strengthen the curriculum for community health-care workers and other health professionals in collaboration with the ministries of health; and support governance, finance, and human resources for health systems. For example, the overall goal of the Maternal and Child Survival Program: Human Resources for Health in Liberia is to improve the competency of midwives and laboratory technicians through the strengthening of pre-service training institutions. The project supports the development of a health and laboratory workforce that may address Liberia's maternal and child health needs and prevent future outbreaks of Ebola and other infectious diseases. As of September 30, 2017, the Bureau for Global Health had obligated $10.0 million for this project, which began in April 2016 and is scheduled to end in June 2018. Table 6 provides summary information about selected project activities.

Table 6. USAID Bureau for Global Health-Funded Ebola Recovery Project: Maternal and Child Survival Program: Human Resources for Health in Liberia Project

Project objectives	Selected project activities
Objective 1: Increase the quality of instruction at targeted pre-service training institutions by upgrading the technical competencies and teaching skills of faculty, including preceptors, and by strengthening curricula, course materials, and delivery of both didactic and clinical training. **Objective 2:** Strengthen the learning environment at targeted pre-service training institutions and clinical teaching sites in a comprehensive way through improved access to high-quality instructional resources, equipmen, and technology.	• Sponsored a 3-day interactive leadership management training for managers of midwifery and lab pre-service education institutions. • Conducted 4-day management training workshop for 12 laboratory preceptors and faculty from three supported pre-service training institutions to improve management and quality systems in laboratories and skills labs and to ensure continuous improvement of management and quality systems in laboratories. • Conducted a 3-day curriculum finalization workshop to confirm the adequacy of an updated curriculum for meeting pre-service education training needs. Fifty participants attended the workshop, representing six project-supported pre-service institutions for midwives and medical laboratory technicians. • Assisted faculty in the preparation of course schedules and lesson planning for courses, including emergency preparedness, teaching in midwifery, and pediatrics.

Source: GAO analysis of U.S. Agency for International Development's (USAID) implementing partner project documentation. | GAO-18-350.

Emergency Non-Ebola Health Services

Table 7. USAID Bureau for Global Health-Funded Ebola Recovery Project: Advancing Partners and Communities, Post Ebola Health Services Strengthening in Sierra Leone

Project objectives	Selected project activities
Objective 1: Improve regulatory and policy environment to enable increased service delivery at health posts and community levels. **Objective 2:** Increase capacity and effectiveness of the health workforce and community platforms to provide quality reproductive, maternal, neonatal, and child health services, including infection prevention control, and water and sanitation health guidelines. **Objective 3:** Improve physical and operational conditions of community, maternal, and child health posts to enhance quality, safety, and access to health services.	• Disseminated water, sanitation, and hygiene standards and guidelines approved by Sierra Leone's Ministry of Health and Sanitation nationwide. • Trained more than 900 health professionals and 1,500 community health workers on reproductive, maternal, newborn, and child health and infection prevention and control practices. • Conducted a data quality review on the completeness, consistency, and reliability of the Ministry of Health and Sanitation's Health Information Management System data for 305 health facilities. • Rehabilitated 110 health posts to enhance infection prevention and control, and water, sanitation, and hygiene standards. • Installed solar lighting systems in 108 health facilities, drilled 26 bore holes, and drilled or rehabilitated 62 wells to provide water to health facilities. • Distributed minor medical equipment and furniture to 305 health posts, including delivery kits, delivery beds, stethoscopes, resuscitators, instrument trays, and patient privacy screens.

Source: GAO analysis of U.S. Agency for International Development's (USAID) implementing partner project documentation. | GAO-18-350.

As of September 30, 2017, USAID's Bureau for Global Health and the USAID mission in Liberia had obligated $68.3 million for 12 recovery projects to restore regional emergency health services to ensure that basic health services are accessible to the populations most in need and to re-establish and sustain routine health service delivery. These recovery projects also focus on increasing the utilization of health services and expanding health worker capacity and capability, and providing technical assistance to rebuild sustainable capacity, including activities to address adverse effects on maternal and child health.

Table 8. USAID Bureau for Global Health-Funded Ebola Recovery Project: Strengthening Routine Immunization in Liberia

Project objective	Selected project activities
Attain and maintain national routine immunization coverage of 85 percent in the target population, including in hard-to-reach areas, as measured by the third dose of Pentavalent vaccine.	• Procured and installed 40 solar refrigerators for health facilities to maintain the vaccination cold chain. • Provided routine immunizations for approximately 160,840 children aged 0 to 11 months, including polio, bacillus calmette-guerin, penta, pneumococcal conjugate, yellow fever, and measles vaccines. • Trained 60 health facility vaccinators, 7 district supervisors, and 17 cold chain officers on solar refrigerator installation and maintenance. • • Conducted community outreach on the importance of routine vaccinations by distributing 1,000 posters and broadcasting on 30 radio stations across Liberia.

Source: GAO analysis of U.S. Agency for International Development's (USAID) implementing partner project documentation. | GAO-18-350.

For example, the overall goal of the Advancing Partners and Communities: Strengthening Health Services as Part of the Post-Ebola Transition in Sierra Leone project is to improve the access to and availability of quality routine health services at community levels. As of September 30, 2017, the Bureau for Global Health had obligated $17.0 million for the project, which began in August 2015 and was completed in September 2017 (see Table 7). In another example, the overall objective of the Strengthening Immunization in Liberia project is to contribute to the reduction of mortality rates for children under 5 in Liberia by restoring immunization services and addressing gaps in immunizations created as a result of the Ebola outbreak (see Table 8). As of September 30, 2017, the Bureau for Global Health had obligated $2.0 million for the project, which began in July 2015 and was completed in July 2017.

Governance and Economic Crisis Mitigation

As of September 30, 2017, USAID's Global Development Lab (Lab) and USAID missions in Guinea, Liberia, and Sierra Leone had obligated approximately $71.1 million for recovery projects to support economic, social, and governance programs and address the effects of immediate job loss and other income opportunities, and to strengthen infrastructure and critical institutions, including governance institutions. These recovery projects included private sector partnerships to support education and livelihood development for youths and women and provide financial and technical support to local small and medium enterprises in Ebola-affected communities by enabling them to access finance and technical assistance through small loans. In addition, these recovery projects support legitimate, participatory, transparent, and peaceful elections to help rebuild political trust and strengthen the practices of citizen participation in key political processes in support of Ebola recovery efforts. For example, the overall goal of the Health Finance and Governance project in Guinea is to strengthen Guinea's health system to enhance the functioning of institutions and programs and improve the country's capacity to deliver better health services to the population (see Table 9). As of September 30, 2017, the mission in Guinea had obligated $1.0 million for this project, which began in June 2016 and is scheduled to end in June 2018.

Table 9. USAID Mission in Guinea-Funded Ebola Recovery Project: Health Finance and Governance

Project objectives	Selected project activities
Objective 1: Improve institutional capacity of health governance across the health system. **Objective 2:** Enable a health financing environment and improve the Ministry of Health's capacity to efficiently mobilize and manage resources to foster greater coverage of quality health services. **Objective 3:** Improve the institutional capacity of the Ministry of Health to effectively manage human resources.	• Conducted an audit of the ability of central health units, regional and district health management teams, and the Ministry of Health to carry out core functions. Finalized audit findings and recommendations in October 2016 and began development of a roadmap to implement the audit recommendations. • Conducted a strategic planning workshop with 33 pre-service training institutions to develop a draft national plan for pre-service training institutions. • Completed an evaluation of the financial management of the Ministry of Health. The project included the development of a 3-year road map to strengthen the programmatic and financial management of the Ministry of Health. • Supported a forum between Guinea's Health Commission and officials of the Ministry of Health to assess the execution of the health budget and pharmaceutical industry reform, and other issues raised by civil society representatives.

Source: GAO analysis of U.S. Agency for International Development's (USAID) implementing partner project documentation. | GAO-18-350.

Innovation and Communications Technology

As of September 30, 2017, USAID's Bureau for Global Health and the Lab had obligated $29.9 million for 54 recovery projects to develop and test innovations and technologies to address the Ebola outbreak and to prepare for future outbreaks. These recovery projects supported innovations to redesign a protective suit to enable health-care workers to spend more time with patients and lessen exposure to contamination, develop rapidly deployable Ebola treatment units and easy-to-assemble decontamination chambers, and strengthen digital infrastructure, including mobile telephone networks, digital payment systems, and health data systems.

For example, the Bureau for Global Health obligated $500,000 for the Modula S Infection Isolation Containerized Living Unit Clinic recovery project, which began in May 2015 and was completed in December 2015. The overall objective of the project was to develop modular, rapidly deployable treatment units that used technology to moderate temperature and simplified decontamination for safer and more comfortable conditions for treating patients (see Table 10).

Table 10. USAID Bureau for Global Health-Funded Ebola Recovery Project: Modula S Infection Isolation Containerized Living Unit Clinic

Project objective	Selected project activities
Develop modular and rapidly deployable treatment units that use technology to moderate unit temperature and simplify decontamination efforts for safer, more comfortable conditions.	• Developed a modular Ebola treatment unit that allows the internal temperature to be cooler than outside air temperature in hot climates. • Tested the modular treatment unit and found it to have a lifespan of 25 years. • Constructed the surfaces of the treatment unit out of anti-bacterial and anti-viral materials to improve the overall safety of health-care workers and patients.

Source: GAO analysis of U.S. Agency for International Development's (USAID) implementing partner project documentation. | GAO-18-350.

Table 11. USAID Bureau for Global Health-Funded Ebola Recovery Project: Africa Stop Ebola Music and Media Campaign to Raise Public Health Awareness in Guinea

Project objective	Selected project activities
Use music to educate audiences about how to stop the spread of Ebola and reduce stigmatization of survivors and family members of Ebola victims.	• Sponsored a song contest in Guinea to engage local artists, health-care workers, and the media in educating community members about the transmission of Ebola. • More than 100 health-care workers participated in the project by educating song contest participants about Ebola or by attending the final song contest event. • The winning song from the Africa Stop Ebola competition was played on radio and broadcast on television more than 5,000 times.

Source: GAO analysis of U.S. Agency for International Development's (USAID) implementing partner project documentation. | GAO-18-350.

The Bureau for Global Health obligated $268,455 for another recovery project, Africa Stop Ebola Music and Media Campaign to Raise Public Health Awareness, which began in May 2015 and was completed in August 2015 (see Table 11).

The overall objective of the project was to conduct a music and media campaign to change behaviors about humanto-human transmission of Ebola in West Africa through the recording of a song in local languages to promote communities' adoption of behaviors that prevent Ebola transmission. In addition, as of September 30, 2017, the Lab had obligated $562,113 for the Mobile Solutions Technical Assistance and Research in Liberia recovery project, which began in June 2016 and is scheduled to end in March 2018 (see Table 12).

Table 12. USAID Global Development Lab-Funded Ebola Recovery Project: Mobile Solutions, Technical Assistance, and Research, Liberia

Project objectives	Selected project activities
Objective 1: Design and plan the conversion of health-care worker salary and stipend disbursements to mobile money payments. **Objective 2:** Support the establishment and implementation of a consolidated payment platform and processes for disbursement of Ministry of Health payroll through mobile money payments. **Objective 3:** Support the measured scale-up and adoption of digital payments by salaried and contract health-care workers, as well as other types of health-care worker payments, where opportunities exist.	• Contracted the services of a consultant to map salary, benefits, and stipend payment streams within the Ministry of Health and the broader health sector to develop a plan to introduce and scale up mobile money payments for health workers. • Conducted a technical assessment and feasibility study on linking Liberia's Ministry of Health functional system with mobile network operators. • Conducted research to inform the strategy and scale for mobile money payments for health-care workers in Liberia and disseminated the results of the research with the Ministry of Health for decision-making about payment streams and the targeting of geographic areas for mobile money payments to health-care workers. • Disbursed mobile money payments to more than 300 Ministry of Health staff, as of June 2017.

Source: GAO analysis of U.S. Agency for International Development's (USAID) implementing partner project documentation. | GAO-18-350.

The overall objective of the project is to assist the Government of Liberia in increasing the efficiency of government payments by enabling the use of mobile money payments for health-care worker salary and stipend disbursements. The Lab also obligated $399,986 for the Ebola Recovery Technical Assistance and Guidance Development for Health Information Systems Work for Reproductive Health recovery project, which began in October 2015 and was completed in September 2016. The overall objective of the project was to strengthen health information systems and facilitate the Sierra Leone Ministry of Health and Sanitation's application of digital tools for programmatic needs and health system challenges (see Table 13).

Table 13. USAID Global Development Lab-Funded Ebola Recovery Project: Ebola Recovery Technical Assistance and Guidance Development for Health Information Systems Work for Reproductive Health in Sierra Leone

Project objectives	Selected project activities
Objective 1: Establish a process to review digital information and communications technology assets that are high priority for health systems recovery. **Objective 2:** Establish a guidance tool for defining, reviewing, and operationalizing functional requirements based on identified health system constraints. **Objective 3:** Establish standards for health information systems minimum content to ensure value, and facilitate interoperability between systems. **Objective 4:** Develop and test processes and guidance tools to ensure their validity. **Objective 5:** Determine content functionality and interoperability requirements related to maternal and child health in development and deployment of routine health information system tools.	• Conducted an inventory of digital health projects implemented to determine the existing digital information communication and technology assets in Sierra Leone. • Developed a web platform—Digital Health Atlas—to enable the government to more efficiently monitor and manage the deployment of digital health systems in-country. • Initiated the mapping of different data elements that existed on government health management information systems to facilitate interoperability by identifying data points needed by the government and linking these data with those collected digitally by nongovernmental organizations. • Hosted a meeting of international experts to define and come to consensus on the parameters of digital strategies for a reproductive, maternal, newborn, and child health tool kit, which the project developed and tested in Sierra Leone. • Developed a report on opportunities for strategic investments in digital health for reproductive, maternal, newborn, child, and adolescent health in Sierra Leone to guide the Ministry of Health and Sanitation's planning and prioritization of investments in digital health systems.

Source: GAO analysis of U.S. Agency for International Development's (USAID) implementing partner project documentation. | GAO-18-350.

Food Security

As of September 30, 2017, USAID's Office of Food for Peace (FFP) had obligated approximately $118.5 million for 16 recovery projects to address decreases in agricultural production and sales and food availability as well as reductions in household incomes and income generation opportunities. These recovery projects support household and market recovery by stimulating local food production and market functions by providing cash transfers to vulnerable households and vouchers for agricultural inputs to support household food production. For example, the overall objective of the Emergency Food Assistance for Ebola Affected Families in Liberia was to increase access to food through unconditional cash transfers and increased agricultural production for households directly and indirectly affected by Ebola in two Liberian counties. FFP obligated approximately $4.6 million for the project, which began in August 2015 and was completed in February 2017 (see Table 14). Similarly, the overall objective of the Kailahun Food for Emergency

Ebola Virus Disease Support in Sierra Leone is to address reduced access to food caused by the Ebola outbreak by providing unconditional cash transfers to households directly and indirectly affected by the Ebola outbreak. The project also provides conditional cash transfers to small-scale traders to support the restocking and recapitalization of businesses for food supplies in the Kailahun District in northeast Sierra Leone. The project began in March 2015 and was completed in December 2017 (see Table 15).

Table 14. USAID Office of Food for Peace-Funded Ebola Recovery Project: Emergency Food Assistance for Ebola-Affected Families in Liberia— Margibi and Bong Counties

Project objective	Selected project activities
Increase household access to and availability of food.	• Assisted 5,000 Ebola-affected households, comprising more than 25,000 individuals, to increase access to food through monthly unconditional cash transfers using mobile money payments. • Provided 4,000 of the 5,000 Ebola-affected households with a seed kit containing maize, eggplant, okra, hot pepper, cucumber, and bitter ball seeds, as well as trainings on agronomic best practices.

Source: GAO analysis of U.S. Agency for International Development's (USAID) implementing partner project documentation. | GAO-18-350.

Table 15. USAID Office of Food for Peace-Funded Ebola Recovery Project: Kailahun Food for Emergency Ebola Virus Disease Support in Sierra Leone

Project objectives	Selected project activities
Objective 1: Improve ability of households to cope with shocks. **Objective 2:** Reestablish and expand market and trade engagement among small-scale female traders in Kailahun. **Objective 3**: Enhance human and institutional capacity development for increased agricultural sector productivity.	• Provided unconditional cash transfers to more than 10,300 households directly and indirectly affected by the Ebola outbreak to facilitate access to food for households with reduced agricultural production, earned income, and market access as a result of market disruptions stemming from the Ebola outbreak. • Provided conditional cash transfers to 400 predominantly female small-scale traders to support restocking and recapitalization of businesses for food supplies in target areas; as a condition for receiving assistance, traders participated in entrepreneurship and business training, including trainings on basic bookkeeping and sound business practices.

Source: GAO analysis of U.S. Agency for International Development's (USAID) implementing partner project documentation. | GAO-18-350.

Ebola Survivor

Transmission Prevention and World Health Reform

As of September 30, 2017, USAID's Bureau for Global Health and the Lab had obligated approximately $28.8 million for recovery projects to prevent further Ebola transmission, support clinical care, and ensure that research results around transmission are incorporated into new guidelines for health-care workers. For example, the Bureau for Global Health obligated funding for recovery projects to research stigmatization of survivors and establish systems to track survivors and facilitate their referral to professionals trained to identify and prevent retransmission when they need medical services. In addition, the Lab obligated funding Development Ebola Recovery Projects for recovery projects to train local clinicians and medical specialists capable of supporting disease surveillance activities and providing longterm care for Ebola survivors.

In addition, USAID's Office of U.S. Foreign Disaster Assistance obligated $35.0 million for the World Health Organization (WHO) Emergencies Program to strengthen WHO's ability to lead and coordinate an effective response to health emergencies. In collaboration with other donors, the project intends to guide WHO to reform structures and processes to effectively respond to global infectious disease outbreaks and other humanitarian emergencies. Specifically, the project will help support the establishment of the new WHO Outbreaks and Health Emergencies unit, develop coordination mechanisms and incident management systems within WHO's agencies, and reinforce WHO's leadership during humanitarian emergencies.

Appendix III: Department of State and Centers for Disease Control and Prevention Ebola Recovery Projects for West Africa

As of September 30, 2017, the Department of State (State) had obligated $32.9 million for recovery projects to support security sector emergency response capabilities in Guinea, Liberia, and Sierra Leone, and fund postEbola economic development and treatment programs in Sierra Leone.[30] In addition, as of September 30, 2017, the U.S. Agency for International Development (USAID) had obligated $80 million to the Centers for Disease Control and Prevention (CDC) for Ebola recovery projects for West Africa through an interagency agreement.

State Obligated $32.9 Million for Ebola Recovery Projects for West Africa

As of September 30, 2017, State had obligated $32.2 million that it transferred from the Economic Support Fund (ESF) account of the Department of State, Foreign

[30] We report funding from the Department of State, Foreign Operations, and Related Programs Appropriations Act, 2015, for Ebola in accordance with USAID and State's reporting to Congress because the reports are the source of our data. The most recent report for Congress is as of September 30, 2017.

Operations, and Related Programs Appropriations Act, 2015, to State's International Narcotics Control and Law Enforcement (INCLE) and Peacekeeping Operations (PKO) accounts for Ebola recovery projects.[31] State obligated $30.0 million in INCLE account funds for recovery projects to strengthen the capacity of the civilian security sector to respond to and prevent the reemergence of Ebola in Guinea and Liberia. Specifically, State obligated $10.0 million in INCLE account funds to document and teach lessons learned and best practices to civilian security personnel and develop guidance on how to respond to the reemergence of Ebola in Guinea. In addition, the project is intended to provide communications equipment to law enforcement agencies and supports coordination between public health authorities and the media through curriculum development, practical exercises and trainings. The project also facilitates improvement in collaboration among security services, the military, and civilian agencies for public health emergency response. State obligated $20.0 million in INCLE account funds for a project in Liberia to support security services' engagement with local communities to mitigate disputes and provide stability following epidemics and other crises, as well as another project in Liberia to establish a secure radio network that the government may use to communicate emergency response during crises, including health epidemics. State obligated $2.2 million in PKO account funding to support the construction of patrol bases with medical screening facilities along theinternational border of Sierra Leone and train military personnel controlling the border on how to conduct medical screenings.

State obligated $700,000 in ESF account funds for recovery projects in Sierra Leone that support economic stabilization and expand treatment for Ebola and other diseases. State obligated $500,000 for a recovery project that provides 26 small grants of approximately $10,000 to $50,000 to local organizations to implement small business initiatives in underserved areas of Sierra Leone. For example, the project provided grants to local organizations to implement projects to restart agricultural programs that were suspended or diminished during the Ebola outbreak. In addition, the project provides grants to small businesses to support employment opportunities to vulnerable populations, particularly Ebola survivors and family members of Ebola victims. Also, State obligated $200,000 for a recovery project to upgrade the treatment facility for Ebola and viral hemorrhagic fevers at a hospital in Sierra Leone, including increasing water storage for decontamination and enhancing the capacity and controls for medical waste.

USAID Obligated $80 Million for CDC Ebola Recovery Projects for West Africa

As of September 30, 2017, USAID's Bureau for Global Health had obligated $80 million for 15 CDC Ebola recovery projects for West Africa through an interagency

[31] Pub. L. No. 113-235, Div. J, Title IX, 128 Stat 2130, 2692 (Dec. 16, 2014).

agreement. The May 2016 interagency agreement obligated funding from the ESF account for CDC projects to build capacity to respond to infectious disease outbreaks in Guinea, Liberia, and Sierra Leone and high-risk, non-affected border countries. Specifically, USAID's interagency agreement with CDC funded such activities as strengthening disease surveillance, laboratory and emergency operations systems, workforce development, health communications and care networks, border health security, infection control, and outbreak response.

Most of the funding provided through USAID's interagency agreement with CDC funded recovery projects in the three primarily affected countries—Guinea, Liberia, and Sierra Leone. CDC funded 5 recovery projects in Guinea, 4 in Liberia, and 6 in Sierra Leone. For example, CDC funded recovery projects in Guinea that provided trainings on public health emergency preparedness, evaluated the training curriculum for laboratory professionals, and identified focal points for health information sharing among Guinea, Liberia, and Sierra Leone. In addition, CDC funded recovery projects in Liberia that provided training and guidance for laboratory operations and infection prevention control, and provided transport of specimens to laboratories. CDC also funded recovery projects in Sierra Leone that supplied hospitals with laboratory equipment and provided trainings to health-care workers on specimen management.

Appendix IV: Funding for U.S. Agency for International Development and Dept of State Ebola Response and Recovery Projects

In December 2014, Congress appropriated approximately $2.5 billion for the U.S. Agency for International Development (USAID) and Department of State (State) for necessary expenses to assist countries affected by— or at risk of being affected by—the Ebola outbreak, among other things.[32] Congress made the funds available from different accounts and subject to different periods of availability (see Table 16).

As of September 30, 2017, USAID and State had obligated approximately $1.9 billion (77 percent) of the $2.4 billion that they had allocated from the Act. Table 17 shows USAID's and State's reported allocations from the Act by appropriation account, as of September 30, 2017. As of September 30, 2017, USAID and State had obligated approximately $1.9 billion (77 percent) of the $2.4 billion that they had allocated from the Act. Table 17 shows USAID's and State's reported allocations from the Act by appropriation account, as of September 30, 2017.

[32] Pub. L. No. 113-35, Div. J., Title IX (Dec. 16, 2014). In addition, the Act appropriated funding for efforts to prevent, prepare for, and respond to the Ebola outbreak; address economic and stabilization requirements resulting from the Ebola outbreak; mitigate the risk of illicit acquisition of the Ebola virus; and promote biosecurity practices associated with Ebola outbreak response efforts.

Table 16. Fiscal Year 2015 Appropriation for USAID and State Ebola Response and Preparedness, by Account and Period of Availability (Dollars in millions)

Appropriations account	Period of availability for obligation	Dollar amount appropriated
International Disaster Assistance	Until expended	1,436.3
Economic Support Fund	Until September 30, 2016a	711.7
Global Health Programs	Until expended	312.0
Diplomatic and Consular Programs	Until September 30, 2016	36.4
USAID Operating Expenses	Until September 30, 2016	19.0
USAID Office of Inspector General	Until expended	5.6
Nonproliferation, Antiterrorism, Demining, and Related Programs	Until September 30, 2016[a]	5.3
Total		2,526.4

Source: Department of State, Foreign Operations, and Related Programs Appropriations Act, 2015. | GAO-18-350.

[a]For appropriations for the Economic Support Fund and Nonproliferation, Antiterrorism, Demining, and Related Programs accounts, funds remain available for an additional 4 years from the data on which the availability of such funds would have otherwise expired, if such funds are initially obligated before the expiration of their respective periods of availability. Pub. L. No. 113-235, Div. J, § 7011 (Dec. 16, 2014). Amount shown may not sum to total because of rounding.

Table 17. Status of USAID and State Allocations for Ebola Response and Preparedness from the Department of State, Foreign Operations, and Related Programs Appropriations Act, 2015, by Appropriation Account, as of September 30, 2017

Appropriation account	Allocations	Unobligated balances	Percentage obligated	Unliquidated obligations	Disbursements	Percentage of obligations disbursed
International Disaster Assistance[a]	1,347,281	441,230	67	65,344	840,707	93
Economic Support Fund[b]	561,675	10[c]	100	294,793	266,872[d]	48
Global Health Programs[e]	389,416	101,182	74	196,852	91,382	32
Nonproliferation, Anti-Terrorism, Demining, and Related Programs	5,300	0	100	914	4,386	83
Operating Expenses[f]	11,515	65[g]	99	4,201	7,249	63
International Narcotics Control and Law Enforcement[h]	30,000	0	100	29,612	388	1
Peacekeeping Operations[i]	2,200	0	100	0	0	0
Office of Inspector General	5,626	255	95	665	4,706	88
Diplomatic & Consular Programs	36,420	534[j]	99	0	35,886	100
Contributions to International Organizationsk	19,948	0	100	0	19,948	100

Appropriation account	Allocations	Unobligated balances	Percentage obligated	Unliquidated obligations	Disbursements	Percentage of obligations disbursed
Total	2,409,381	543,277	77	592,381	1,271,523	68

Source: GAO analysis of U.S. Agency for International Development (USAID) and Department of State (State) data. | GAO-18-350.

Notes: The calculations in this table are based on USAID's and State's most recently reported allocations, obligations, and disbursements. Disbursements differ from the data in USAID's monthly reporting, as they reflect corrections that we made, based on our analysis. State allocates Ebola funding from the Nonproliferation, Anti-Terrorism, Demining, and Related Programs, Diplomatic & Consular Programs, International Narcotics Control and Law Enforcement (INCLE), Peacekeeping Operations (PKO), and Contributions to International Organizations (CIO) accounts. USAID allocates Ebola funding from all other accounts listed in this table, with the exception of $700,000 from the Economic Support Fund (ESF) account, which State has programmed for Ebola recovery and viral hemorrhagic fever treatment in Sierra Leone. The Continuing Appropriations and Military Construction, Veterans Affairs, and Related Agencies Appropriations Act, 2017, and Zika Response and Preparedness Act (Pub. L. No. 114-223, Sept. 29, 2016) rescinded $7.5 million from the Operating Expenses account, as well as $109.5 million from bilateral economic assistance accounts, which are the International Disaster Assistance (IDA), ESF, and Global Health Programs (GHP) accounts. USAID determined the amounts rescinded from the IDA, ESF, and GHP accounts. Amounts shown may not sum to totals because of rounding.

[a]IDA account allocations are lower than the amount in the IDA appropriation for Ebola response and preparedness because USAID rescinded $69 million in response to a provision requiring a rescission from bilateral economic assistance in the Continuing Appropriations and Military Construction, Veterans Affairs, and Related Agencies Appropriations Act, 2017, and Zika Response and Preparedness Act (Pub. L. No. 114-223, Sept. 29, 2016). In addition, State transferred $19.9 million from the IDA account to the CIO account for the U.S. contribution to the United Nations Mission for Ebola Emergency Response on June 1, 2015. These allocations are listed in this table under the CIO account.

[b]ESF account allocations are lower than the amount in the ESF appropriation for Ebola response and preparedness for two reasons. First, USAID and State made three transfers of ESF funding. In July and August 2016, State notified the relevant congressional committees that it intended to transfer $2.2 million to the PKO account and $30 million to the INCLE account. On September 9, 2016, USAID notified the relevant congressional committees that it intended to transfer $106.5 million to the Global Health Programs (GHP) account. Second, rescissions as a result of the Continuing Appropriations and Military Construction, Veterans Affairs, and Related Agencies Appropriations Act, 2017, and Zika Response and Preparedness Act affected the ESF account. USAID rescinded $11.4 million from the ESF account. In addition, USAID reprogrammed a portion of its ESF Ebola funds. USAID notified the relevant congressional committees on April 8, 2016 that it intended to reprogram $295 million in ESF Ebola funds for Zika response activities and for the CDC's international Ebola response.

[c]According to USAID officials, these funds were obligated within the period of availability and remain available for obligation for an additional 4 years.

[d]Some disbursements reflected here are based on accruals from quarterly financial invoices provided by USAID's implementing partners. These data may not yet be reflected in USAID's financial system records on disbursements for Ebola response and preparedness from the Department of State, Foreign Operations, and Related Programs Appropriations Act, 2015 (Pub. L. No. 113-235, Dec. 16, 2014).

[e]GHP account allocations are $77.4 million greater than the amount in the GHP appropriation for Ebola response and preparedness because of a transfer from the ESF account and a rescission. On September 9, 2016, USAID notified the relevant congressional committees that it intended to transfer $106.5 million to the GHP account. As a result of the rescissions in the Continuing Appropriations and Military Construction, Veterans Affairs, and Related Agencies Appropriations Act, 2017, and Zika Response and Preparedness Act, USAID rescinded $29 million in GHP funding transferred from the ESF account. (Continued ...)

[f]Operating Expenses account allocations are lower than the amount in the Operating Expenses appropriation for Ebola response and preparedness because of a rescission of approximately $7.5 million in the Continuing Appropriations and Military Construction, Veterans Affairs, and Related Agencies Appropriations Act, 2017, and Zika Response and Preparedness Act (Pub. L. No. 114-223, Sept. 29, 2016).

[g]According to USAID officials, these funds have expired and are no longer available for new obligations.

[h]INCLE account funds were not appropriated for Ebola response and preparedness in the Department of State, Foreign Operations, and Related Programs Appropriations Act, 2015. Instead, State transferred ESF Ebola funding to the INCLE account in 2016, pursuant to transfer authority included in the appropriations act. On August 10, 2016, State notified the relevant congressional committees of its intent to transfer $30 million in Ebola ESF funding to the INCLE account.

[i]PKO account funds were not appropriated for Ebola response and preparedness in the Department of State, Foreign Operations, and Related Programs Appropriations Act, 2015. Instead, State transferred ESF Ebola funding to the PKO account in 2016, pursuant to transfer authority included in the appropriations act. On July 27, 2016, State notified the relevant congressional committees of its intent to transfer $30 million in Ebola ESF funding to the INCLE account.

[j]According to State officials, Diplomatic and Consular Programs account funds have expired and are no longer available for new obligations.

[k]Allocations for the CIO account are a transfer from the IDA account to the CIO account for the U.S. contribution to the United Nations Mission for Ebola Emergency Response on June 1, 2015.

Appendix V: Comments from the U.S. Agency for International Development

USAID
FROM THE AMERICAN PEOPLE

FEB 2 6 2018

David Gootnick
Director, International Affairs and Trade
United States Government Accountability Office
441 G Street, N.W.
Washington, D.C. 20548

Re: EBOLA RECOVERY: USAID Has Initiated or Completed Most Projects, but a Complete Project Inventory Is Still Needed for Evaluating Its Efforts (GAO-18-350)

Dear Mr. Gootnick:

I am pleased to provide the United States Agency for International Development's (USAID) formal response to the draft report produced by the United States Government Accountability Office (GAO) draft report entitled, *"EBOLA RECOVERY: USAID Has Initiated or Completed Most Projects, but a Complete Project Inventory Is Still Needed for Evaluating Its Efforts"* (GAO-18-350).

We are providing this letter and the enclosed USAID comments are provided for incorporation as an appendix to the GAO final report. Thank you for the opportunity to respond to your draft report and for the courtesies extended by your staff while conducting this engagement.

Sincerely,

Angelique M. Crumbly
Acting Assistant Administrator
Bureau for Management

USAID COMMENTS ON GAO DRAFT REPORT
EBOLA RECOVERY: USAID Has Initiated or Completed Most Projects, but a Complete Project Inventory Is Still Needed for Evaluating Its Efforts (GAO-18-350)

The United States Agency for International Development would like to thank the Government Accountability Office (GAO) for giving us the opportunity to respond to this draft report. We appreciate the extensive work of the audit team, which resulted in a recommendation that will help USAID enhance the management of its evaluation of Ebola recovery projects.

This report has one recommendation:

Recommendation: The Administrator of USAID should take steps to ensure that USAID's contractor compiles a complete and accurate inventory of Ebola Recovery projects prior to finalizing its analysis.

USAID agrees with GAO's recommendation that we complete a full and accurate inventory of all Ebola Pillar II programs and is working with our contractor to do so. USAID is a strong proponent of project evaluations as is set forth in section 201.3.5 of the USAID Automated Directives System. In an evaluation such as the Ebola recovery projects evaluation, it is axiomatic that all projects should be included in the universe covered by the evaluation, and USAID will ensure that the contractor compiles a complete and accurate inventory of Ebola recovery projects prior to finalizing its analysis.

USAID's operating units that have programmed Ebola recovery activities have conducted a crosswalk exercise of records from USAID Ebola recovery projects and with the contractor to identify all activities. The contractor and operating units will ensure the accuracy and completeness of the inventory used for the overarching evaluation.

In: Infectious Diseases
Editor: Philippe Georges
ISBN: 978-1-53616-401-5

Chapter 6

EBOLA OUTBREAK: DEMOCRATIC REPUBLIC OF CONGO*

Tiaji Salaam-Blyther and Alexis Arieff

For years, Congress has provided funds to prevent, detect, and respond to infectious disease threats, including those with pandemic potential like Ebola. In regular appropriations, since FY2014 Congress has annually provided $72.5 million to the U.S. Agency for International Development (USAID) for such efforts. From FY2015 to FY2017, Congress appropriated annually $55.1 million to the U.S. Centers for Disease Control and Prevention (CDC); in FY2018, it provided $108.2 million, including an authority to spend $50 million over three years for global health security efforts. In FY2015, Congress also provided over $5 billion in emergency funds for domestic and global efforts to contain the 2014-2015 West Africa Ebola outbreak (P.L. 113-235). Some of those unspent funds were used to contain a 2018 outbreak in western Democratic Republic of Congo (DRC) and are being used to fight the ongoing outbreak.

On August 1, 2018, the World Health Organization (WHO) reported a new Ebola outbreak in eastern DRC, about one week after declaring that a separate outbreak had ended in western DRC. The ongoing Ebola outbreak—the 10th to be documented in DRC—is the largest in the country's history and has continued to spread (*Figure 1*). It is occurring in North Kivu and Ituri provinces, where a protracted conflict has caused a long-running humanitarian crisis: as of mid-2018, 4.3 million people were in need of humanitarian aid. In addition to classic public health response tools (surveillance, contact tracing, isolation, and safe burials), health workers (HWs) are using an investigational

* This is an edited, reformatted and augmented version of Congressional Research Service Publication No. IF11100, dated February 6, 2019.

vaccine to counter the spread of disease. Unpredictable armed conflict and intermittent community resistance to these efforts are hindering all aspects of outbreak control.

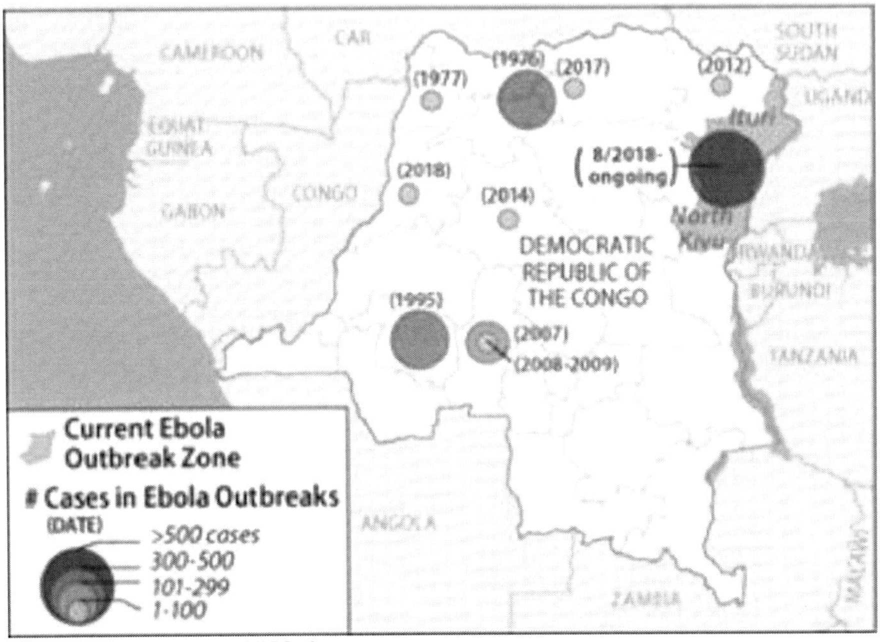

Source: CRS graphic, based on WHO data.

Figure 1. Ebola Virus Outbreaks in DRC: 1976-2019.

As of February 4, 2019, WHO reported 785 confirmed and probable Ebola cases in Ituri and North Kivu, including 484 deaths. Observers are concerned that the outbreak could spread to Goma, the capital of North Kivu, a city of over 1 million people that is also an operational hub for the United Nations (U.N.) peacekeeping mission and international relief efforts in DRC, as well as to neighboring countries. While Uganda (which borders the most affected areas in DRC) has prior experience in Ebola control, Rwanda and Burundi do not. South Sudan's current minimal state capacity and protracted armed conflict suggest a coordinated disease control response would be highly challenging.

INTERNATIONAL AND U.S. RESPONSES

Confirmed Ebola cases are being treated with experimental Ebola therapeutics in Ebola Treatment Centers (ETCs). As of January 28, 2019, six ETCs and two isolation treatment units were operational, with occupancy rates ranging from 60% to 110%, with additional ETCs being constructed. Between August 2018 and early February 2019, the DRC's Ministry of Health (MoH) and partners vaccinated roughly 73,000 Ebola cases and their contacts. In bordering countries, over 2,600 health workers (HWs) have been vaccinated in Uganda, more than 1,400 HWs in Rwanda are designated to be vaccinated (once the protocol is approved), and approximately 300 HWs have been vaccinated in South Sudan. The WHO has conducted readiness assessments in neighboring countries, and the U.N. Central Emergency Response Fund has contributed $10 million toward regional Ebola control and preparedness efforts.

When the outbreak began, USAID and CDC deployed staff to DRC and the region. In October 2018, USAID announced it had deployed a Disaster Assistance Response Team (DART) to coordinate the U.S. government response in support of the MoH, WHO, and other international partners. The United States, more broadly, is the top bilateral humanitarian donor to DRC and the top financial contributor to the U.N. peacekeeping operation there, which has provided "life-saving logistics support to the Ebola response" in North Kivu and Ituri, according to U.S. officials. U.S. support for outbreak control also includes the following:

- *USAID:* As of February 5, 2019, USAID has provided more than $33 million in FY2018-FY2019 to nongovernmental organizations (NGOs), U.N. agencies, and other partners for Ebola response in DRC and Ebola preparedness in neighboring countries. USAID funds are supporting disease surveillance, infection protection and control, risk communication and community engagement, safe and dignified burials, water and sanitation aid, and prepositioning of medical supplies.
- *CDC:* CDC personnel provide direct support to the MoH, WHO, and the DART and are supporting disease surveillance, contact tracing, data management, infection protection and control, risk communication and community engagement, laboratory strengthening, emergency management, and surveillance at points of entry. CDC staff are also supporting Ebola preparedness efforts in Rwanda, South Sudan, and Uganda.
- *U.S. Department of Defense (DOD):* DOD supplies laboratory training to Ugandan researchers and partners with them to conduct clinical trials of Ebola vaccines.

Challenges

Insecurity

Ebola cases are concentrated in Beni and Butembo districts in North Kivu, a site of armed conflict since the 1990s. Dozens of armed groups are active in the area, including the Allied Democratic Forces (ADF), a nebulous armed group implicated in attacks on U.N. peacekeepers, local military forces, and civilians. Elements of the state security forces also reportedly maintain ties with armed groups and have been implicated in serious abuses. Road travel is often dangerous, with frequent reports of militia attacks, armed robbery, and kidnappings.

Fear and misinformation have also prompted community resistance to Ebola control efforts. Health workers and facilities have been attacked, and community resistance to conducting safe burials has hindered containment efforts. Political unrest related to DRC's national elections in December 2018 has also posed challenges. The DRC government postponed voting in Beni and Butembo, citing risks of contagion (although the MoH had earlier suggested such risks would be mitigated), spurring protesters to ransack and burn down part of an ETC in Beni.

The U.S. government has placed constraints on the movement of U.S. personnel due to security threats in the east and political unrest throughout the country. In September, USAID and CDC withdrew their personnel from the outbreak zone pursuant to security concerns. The CDC Director stated to the press that the CDC's preference would have been to maintain staff in the field. U.S. personnel continue to provide technical assistance from the capital, Kinshasa, and from neighboring Rwanda and Uganda, while implementing partners (WHO and NGOs) are continuing Ebola control efforts with U.S. resources.

Health System Constraints

Low health worker density, low health spending, and prolonged conflict have weakened DRC's health system and hindered Ebola control efforts. A ratio of at least 2.3 health workers per 1,000 people is often used as a proxy for measuring minimum health delivery capacity in a given country. According to the latest available data from WHO, DRC had roughly 1.1 health workers per 1,000 people as of 2009. WHO reported that as of 2015 (latest available), health spending accounted for 5% of government spending, which would amount to roughly $3.30 per capita, one of the lowest rates in the world.

The WHO suggests that Ebola transmission may be occurring in ill-equipped, untrained, and/or understaffed health facilities. Inconsistent adherence to infection prevention and control, periodic disruptions in the personal protection equipment supply chain, and limited access to water for handwashing in some health facilities is putting health workers and patients at risk. As of February 3, 2019, 65 health workers had contracted Ebola in the current outbreak, 22 of whom died. From December 1, 2018, through January 28, 2019, 18% of confirmed Ebola cases reported having visited a health center before developing symptoms, suggesting they may have been exposed to the virus at the facility. The MoH, WHO, and other partners have identified health facilities where Ebola transmission may have occurred and are addressing lapses around triage, case detection, and infection prevention and control.

Early symptoms of Ebola and malaria are similar, and a spike in malaria cases in and around Beni City has compounded pressure on its health facilities and ETCs. A January 2019 WHO report indicated that up to 50% of people screened in ETCs had malaria. In November 2018, the DRC National Malaria Control Program, supported by WHO, the United Nations Children's Fund (UNICEF), the Global Fund, and the U.S. President's Malaria Initiative, launched a prevention and treatment campaign to curb malaria deaths and reduce pressure on the health system.

OUTLOOK

The ongoing Ebola outbreak is in its seventh month, and control efforts have shown mixed results. While the number of new cases have declined in some areas, infection rates have risen in others. Insecurity in North Kivu has disrupted response activities, raising questions about how to carry out disease control in unsafe settings. Protracted conflict in Pakistan and Afghanistan, for example, has stymied global polio eradication efforts, while political instability in Venezuela has contributed to the resurgence of malaria in the country, imperiling the rest of the region.

Political instability aside, the inability to control disease outbreaks is largely a symptom of weak domestic health systems. To address this challenge and improve countries' ability to prevent, detect, and respond to infectious disease threats, the United States and WHO co-launched the Global Health Security Agenda (GHSA) in 2014. The United States, the largest donor to this multilateral effort, pledged to support it with $1 billion from FY2015 through FY2019. Much of the emergency appropriations that have been used in support of GHSA and to control the ongoing Ebola outbreak is expected to be expended by the end of FY2019. The Trump Administration has signaled support for continuing the GHSA. Clearer signals of how the Administration proposes extending U.S. engagement may be found in the forthcoming FY2020 budget request.

In the 115th Congress, H.R. 7290, Global Health Security Act of 2018, would have codified an Obama-era executive order setting out agency roles in supporting the GHSA. In the 116th Congress, H.R. 826 would seek to facilitate research and treatment of neglected tropical diseases, including Ebola. Members may continue to debate what role, if any, the United States should play in supporting global health system strengthening efforts to bolster global health security and whether to adjust funding levels to meet ongoing and looming infectious disease threats.

In: Infectious Diseases
Editor: Philippe Georges
ISBN: 978-1-53616-401-5

Chapter 7

AFRICAN SWINE FEVER (ASF)*

Sahar Angadjivand and Joel L. Greene

Between September 2018 and May 2019, the number of African swine fever (ASF) outbreaks has rapidly increased, most notably in China, triggering economic losses in affected pork-producing countries (*Figure 1*). Since September 2018, the World Organization for Animal Health (OIE)—an intergovernmental organization coordinating, supporting, and promoting animal health and disease control—has reported that over 2.8 million hogs have been culled globally due to ASF. Many industry observers believe that the actual number of culled animals is much higher. The extent of ASF outbreaks is expected to affect international trade in pork and feedstuffs. The U.S. Department of Agriculture's (USDA) Animal and Plant Health Inspection Service (APHIS) is monitoring the global spread of ASF and has developed plans to prevent ASF introduction into the United States.

BACKGROUND

ASF is a viral disease that affects swine, including domestic pigs, feral (wild) swine, wild boar, and other exotic swine. Infected swine may exhibit symptoms including high fever, decreased appetite, and weakness. ASF leads to nearly 100% mortality rates in swine herds. There is no treatment or vaccine available for ASF. The only way to reduce the prevalence of ASF is to quarantine and depopulate (cull) all affected and exposed

* This is an edited, reformatted and augmented version of Congressional Research Service Publication No. IF11215, dated May 17, 2019.

animals. ASF does not have zoonotic potential—the infection cannot spread from animals to humans.

ASF is caused by the African swine fever virus and spreads between pigs by direct contact with an infected animal, its bodily fluids (e.g., saliva, blood, feces), or animal tissue or through indirect contact with contaminated objects. In addition, it is often introduced into a herd through the feeding of garbage. On-farm biosecurity is critical to preventing ASF from developing and spreading.

ASF Impacts on Global Pork Trade

China, the world's leader in pork production, has notified OIE of animal losses due to ASF. Between September 2018 and May 2019, China has reported over 2 million culled animals. The USDA's Foreign Agricultural Service's "Livestock and Poultry: World Markets and Trade" report for April 2019 forecasts that China's pork imports in 2019 will climb to a record high, partly due to liquidation of China's swine herd. Despite efforts to contain the disease, outbreaks continue to emerge, and it appears that China will be unable to eradicate ASF in the near term. Chinese pork imports could partially offset its lower production, and the EU, Canada, Brazil, and United States are expected to increase exports to China.

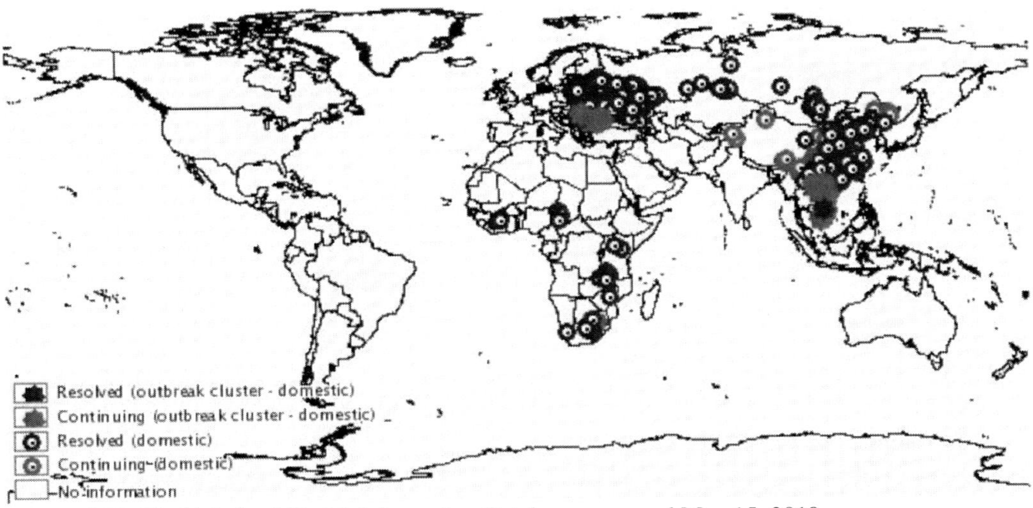

Source: OIE, World Animal Health Information Database, accessed May 15, 2019.

Figure 1. Global Distribution of ASF (January 2017-May 2019).

Because of ASF, USDA reports that U.S. pork sales to China from January to April 2019 are more than three times higher than during the same period a year ago in spite of the retaliatory tariffs China imposed on U.S. pork exports in April 2018. Higher Chinese imports will likely create an uptick in global pork trade in 2019, driving global hog prices up and leading to record sales for exporters, such as the United States.

In contrast, China is also the world's leading importer of soybeans—a source for high-protein meal used as animal feed—averaging over 90 million metric tons per year since 2016, according to USDA. A substantial decline in China's hog population could curb its soybean imports.

Potential Impacts to U.S. Pork Industry

If ASF were to be detected in the United States, the consequences to the U.S. pork industry could be severe. Upon detection of ASF in the U.S. hog population, U.S. export markets would likely impose restrictions on imports of U.S. pork. Total U.S. pork exports in 2018 reached nearly $6.4 billion (2.4 million metric tons, or 22% of production in 2018). Mexico, China, Japan, and Canada rank as the leading U.S. pork export markets.

The U.S. pork industry and USDA have both responded to the global spread of ASF. For example, out of an abundance of caution, the National Pork Producers Council cancelled the annual World Pork Expo in Des Moines, Iowa, citing a possible risk of ASF transmission. Typically, the expo draws about 20,000 domestic and foreign visitors. In another example, APHIS participated in the Canadian Food Inspection Agency's (CFIA) "African Swine Fever Forum," held April 30-May 1, 2019, to address the status, prevention, and management of ASF in North America.

APHIS's engagement with CFIA has led to the establishment of a strategy to harmonize available North American ASF diagnostic methods. According to APHIS, this collaboration resulted in estimates of resources and laboratory capacity necessary to meet the potential diagnostic demand for ASF outbreaks.

Federal ASF Management Activities

Many ASF activities are within the purview of APHIS, the lead agency for responding to animal diseases, conducting disease investigation and control activities, and overseeing zoonotic disease prevention and response. APHIS's legislative authority for this work derives mainly from the Animal Health Protection Act (7 U.S.C. §8301 *et seq.*). To carry out this work APHIS often partners with other federal agencies, including the Food and Drug Administration (FDA), the Food Safety and Inspection Service (FSIS), the Environmental Protection Agency (EPA), and Customs and Border Protection

(CBP). In addition, various agencies within individual states, such as agricultural agencies and wildlife management agencies, collaborate with APHIS.

Since the practice of feeding garbage to swine could transmit infectious diseases, APHIS is tasked with licensing and inspecting swine production facilities that feed cooked garbage to swine and to search for unlicensed facilities that may illegally feed raw garbage (9 C.F.R. Part 166). As of February 2018, APHIS reported that 22 states prohibit feeding garbage to domestic swine, while 28 states in addition to Puerto Rico and the Virgin Islands permit it.

In May 2019, APHIS announced it will enhance its ASF surveillance efforts by adding ASF testing to its existing surveillance of classical swine fever. The surveillance effort is to test samples from high-risk animals and pigs from herds that are at greater risk for disease through such factors as exposure to feral swine or garbage feeding.

APHIS and FDA Collaboration

On September 5, 2018, USDA and FDA officials met with U.S. pork industry groups to assess additional measures to prevent the spread of ASF to the United States. Following the meeting, APHIS moved to expand testing capacity for ASF within APHIS National Animal Health Laboratory Network (NAHLN) labs, and it issued the "Foreign Animal Disease Preparedness and Response Plan—Disease Response Strategy: African Swine Fever (2019)." The plan provides guidance for responding to a U.S. swine health emergency caused by ASF. It explains the protocols and the cooperative plans APHIS has with state authorities and the EPA for disposing of potentially infected carcasses.

APHIS and CBP Collaboration

APHIS has concluded that illegal entry of swine products and byproducts, such as through airline baggage and foreign mail, presents the largest potential pathway for the entry of the ASF virus. To strengthen detection, APHIS has increased the deployment of trained detector dogs, or the "Beagle Brigade." CBP enforces APHIS regulations and is responsible for confiscating illegally imported animals and animal byproducts at ports or from travelers entering the United States and for seizing such products entering the country through mail facilities. For example, in early March 2019, CBP officers stopped an attempt to smuggle over 1 million pounds of pork containing food products from China. All the products were incinerated.

APHIS AND FSIS COLLABORATION

APHIS reports to FSIS—a USDA agency that conducts official inspection of domestic, imported, and exported meat, poultry, and some egg products—when OIE receives notification of an ASF outbreak in specific regions or countries. FSIS follows established protocol to address pork and pork products from regions where ASF exists or is reasonably believed to exist (9 C.F.R. 94.8).

SWINE HEALTH FUNDING

The 116th Congress appropriated $24.8 million in the Consolidated Appropriations Act, 2019 (P.L. 116-6), for swine health, including swine surveillance, emergency preparedness, and response planning. Funds were not specific to ASF. In addition, USDA's Agricultural Research Service (ARS) received $9.6 million for research efforts on foreign animal diseases and emerging diseases. ARS is to determine how much FY2019 funding will be allocated toward ASF vaccine development. In FY2018, ARS allocated $324,000 toward ASF vaccine development. This included research using clustered regularly interspaced short palindromic repeats (or CRISPR-Cas9)—a technology that enables researchers to edit parts of genomes by altering DNA sequence—to better understand gene function toward ASF vaccine development.

The 2018 farm bill (P.L. 115-334) established the National Animal Disease Preparedness Response Program (NADPRP) and the National Animal Vaccine and Veterinary Countermeasures Bank (NAVVCB). The NADPRP is to address risks to U.S. livestock associated with the introduction of animal diseases and pests. The NAVVCB is to maintain significant quantities of vaccine and diagnostic products to respond to animal disease outbreaks. The act authorized mandatory funding of $120 million for FY2019-FY2022 and $30 million for FY2023 and for each fiscal year thereafter for the two new programs and the NAHLN. In addition, the act authorizes annual discretionary appropriations for FY2019-FY2023.

In: Infectious Diseases
Editor: Philippe Georges

ISBN: 978-1-53616-401-5

Chapter 8

GLOBAL TRENDS: TUBERCULOSIS*

Sara M. Tharakan

Tuberculosis (TB) remains a major, and evolving, health challenge in many parts of the world and a priority for the U.S. Congress and international community. The U.S. government is one of the largest donors to global TB control efforts. The 116th Congress may consider future funding needs for TB control, particularly for vaccine research and disease surveillance and detection through strengthening health care infrastructure.

TUBERCULOSIS

Transmission and Prevalence

Infectious diseases cause over 25% of deaths globally, and TB is the leading cause of death from a single infectious agent. TB is spread through the air, such as when a person inhales germs from an infected person's cough or sneeze. An estimated 23% of the global population is infected with TB bacteria, and about 10% of individuals infected with the TB bacteria will develop active TB. Latent TB becomes active and transmittable when a person's immune system is suppressed, for example due to pregnancy, chemotherapy, or HIV/AIDS. The latter represents a serious public health concern, as people with HIV are 20 to 30 times more likely to develop active TB than those without HIV.

TB is considered a disease of poverty, and the global disease burden is uneven. India, China, Indonesia, the Philippines, Pakistan, Nigeria, Bangladesh, and South

* This is an edited, reformatted and augmented version of Congressional Research Service Publication No. IF11057, Updated December 27, 2018.

Africa account for two-thirds of TB cases worldwide (see *Figure 1*). In countries without comprehensive health care infrastructure, TB control is especially difficult. The WHO estimates that 3.6 million TB cases are undetected annually, primarily because of inadequate monitoring and surveillance capacity.

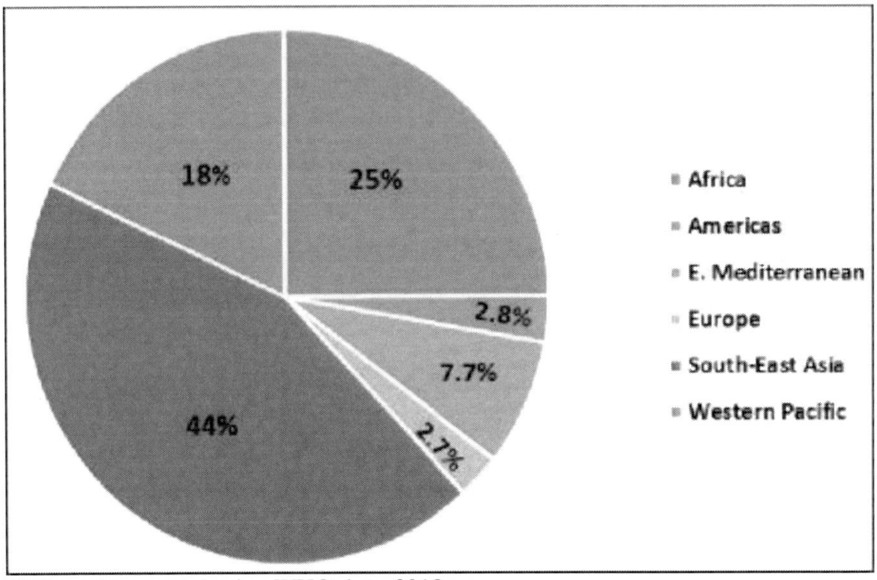

Source: CRS graphic created using WHO data, 2018.

Figure 1. Burden of New TB Cases in 2017, by WHO Region.

Diagnosis and Treatment

TB is generally diagnosed using rapid molecular tests, sputum smear microscopy, and culture-based methods. Many countries rely on the second to diagnose TB, because it is the cheapest method. However, that method detects only half of all TB cases and cannot detect Rifampicin Resistant-TB (known as RR-TB which is resistance to the first line TB drug Rifampicin), or Multi Drug Resistant (MDR)-TB.

Drug-susceptible TB is treated by a six-month course of four antimicrobial drugs. The majority of cases are curable when medicines are available and patients adhere to treatment. On average, 85% of drug-susceptible TB cases were cured in 2017. If patients do not complete the treatment regiment, they can develop MDR-TB—when TB does not respond to at least two anti-TB drugs. MDR-TB is a top concern of many global health experts because MDR-TB carriers can transmit resistant forms of TB to others. Of those who contracted MDR-TB in 2017, 55% survived.

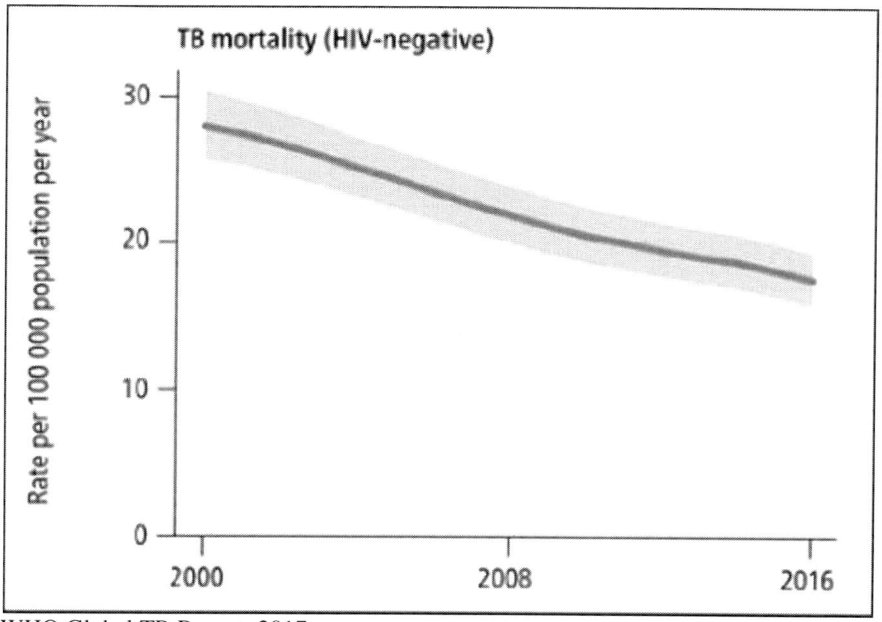

Source: WHO Global TB Report, 2017.

Figure 2. Global TB Mortality Rate, 2000-2016.

Global Developments

The international community has made significant strides in curbing TB deaths worldwide (see Figure 2); however, the disease continues to spread, mostly unabated. The international community has adopted several multiyear plans to combat TB. In 2018, reflecting a deepening global commitment to TB eradication, the WHO, the Stop TB Partnership, and the Global Fund to Fight AIDS, Tuberculosis, and Malaria (Global Fund) launched a joint initiative to scale up access to TB prevention and care. The "End TB Strategy" focuses on 30 high-burden countries to diagnose, treat and report an additional 40 million people with TB. The aim is a 95% reduction in TB deaths by 2035 and a 90% reduction in the TB incidence rate compared with 2015 levels. The strategy calls for bringing together critical interventions to ensure that all people with TB have equitable access to high-quality diagnosis, treatment and prevention services, without facing catastrophic expenditures or social repercussions.

Key TB Facts (as of 2017)

- In 2017,
  - 10 million people developed TB disease
  - TB killed 1.3 million people, about one person every 18 seconds

  - 95% of TB cases and deaths occurred in developing countries
  - Incidence (new cases per 100,000 people per year) fell by 2%
- From 1990 to 2015, TB prevalence decreased by 41%
- From 2000 to 2017, some 54 million deaths were averted through improved diagnosis and treatment adherence
- Among HIV-negative people, TB deaths fell by 29% since 2000

TB and HIV-Positive Individuals

In 2017, nearly 1 million persons living with HIV contracted TB. In 2017, TB was the leading cause of death for HIV-positive people, killing 300,000. HIV/TB co-infection remains concentrated in Africa, which accounted for 84% of all deaths due to co-infection. Overall, TB deaths among HIV-positive individuals have decreased by 44% since 2000. In 2017, 84% of people living with an HIV/TB co-infection were receiving ART treatment, compared to 36% in 2005.

2013-2017: Regional Improvements

The fastest regional declines of new cases were in the WHO Europe region (5% per year), and the Africa region (4% per year). The TB mortality rate fell by 11% per year in the WHO European region, and by 4% per year in the WHO South-East Asia region. During this period, the WHO reported notable mortality rate declines in high TB burden countries including Russia (13%), Ethiopia (12%), Sierra Leone (10%), Kenya (8%), and Vietnam (8%).

Research & Development (R&D)

Development of a vaccine is crucial to meeting WHO TB reduction targets, as an effective vaccine could protect adults from contracting TB. Twenty TB drugs and 12 TB vaccines were in clinical trials in 2018. Clinical trials conducted in Africa of the first new TB vaccine in 100 years has shown promising results.

KEY CHALLENGES

Multi-Drug Resistant-TB (MDR-TB)

MDR-TB is spreading worldwide. In 2017 nearly 600,000 people developed RR-TB compared to 425,000 cases in 2005. Overall, 75% of MDR-TB cases go undetected by health systems. Some experts indicate this reflects a need to focus on strengthening health systems to improve surveillance and detection of MDR-TB cases. The expense, complexity, and side effects of treating MDR-TB complicate treatment adherence. The development of improved treatments with shorter regiments and less severe side effects, some argue, could help control the spread of MDR-TB.

Global Funding

Global TB-related funding to 119 Low- and Middle-Income Countries (LMICs) was $6.9 billion in 2018, compared to $3.3 billion in 2006. 86% of the funding is from LMICs; however, this figure is skewed by domestic financing provided by Brazil, Russia, India, China and South Africa (BRICS). In low-income countries, international donor contributions accounted for 57% of funding.

In 2015, the WHO estimated that $9.2 billion would be needed to control TB. At the 2018 United Nations (U.N.) General Assembly High Level Meeting on TB, U.N. Members agreed that TB control would cost an additional $3 billion, in part to address the rising costs of addressing MDR-TB. Members also set goals of treating 40 million affected people and improving access to affordable treatments by 2022.

U.S. Government Response

The United States supports international efforts to address TB through bilateral programs and multilateral institutions, including the Global Fund. Bilateral efforts are coordinated by the U.S. Agency for International Development (USAID) and co-implemented with the U.S. Centers for Disease Control and Prevention (CDC), National Institutes of Health, the Department of State, and the Department of Defense.

Authorization and Funding

In December 2018, Congress enacted the PEPFAR (President's Emergency Plan for AIDS Relief) Extension Act of 2018, authorizing support for programs that combat TB, HIV/AIDS and malaria. Through the FY2018 State and Foreign Operations (SFOPS) appropriations (P.L. 115-141), Congress provided $261 million for TB prevention and treatment programs, as well as $1.35 billion for a contribution to the Global Fund. The Trump Administration proposed reducing bilateral TB funding to $178.4 million for FY 2019 (a 32% cut from FY2018), and proposed $925 million for a U.S. Global Fund contribution. Congress has not enacted FY 2019 SFOPS appropriations.

Strategy

In 2015, the Obama Administration released the "U.S. Government Global Tuberculosis Strategy" to establish policy guidance and goals for 2015-2019. It aimed to treat 13 million new positive TB cases, maintain treatment success rates for 90% of individuals with TB, diagnose and begin treating 360,000 cases of MDR-TB, and provide treatment for 100% of people diagnosed with HIV/TB co-infection. To date, the Trump Administration has not proposed a continuation of this strategy.

In: Infectious Diseases
Editor: Philippe Georges
ISBN: 978-1-53616-401-5

Chapter 9

GLOBAL MEASLES VACCINATION TRENDS*

Sara M. Tharakan

ABSTRACT

Congress has long taken an interest in infectious disease prevention and control. Measles is a highly contagious virus that is transmitted through droplets emitted from an infected person when coughing and sneezing. The virus can live for up to two hours in the airspace or on a surface where an infected person coughed or sneezed. Other people can contract the disease if they breathe contaminated air or touch their eyes, nose, or mouth after touching a contaminated surface. Up to 90% of those in the proximity of an infected person who are not immune to the disease will be infected. Symptoms usually include high fever, rash, runny nose, and ear infections. Measles can also cause hearing loss, blindness, encephalitis (an infection that causes brain swelling), severe diarrhea, and severe respiratory infections such as pneumonia. The U.S. Centers for Disease Control and Prevention (CDC) estimates that up to two of every 1,000 children infected with measles will die.

VACCINES

According to the CDC, the measles, mumps, and rubella (MMR) vaccine is 97% effective in preventing infection and related deaths, and routine MMR vaccination is recommended for all children. Figure 1 shows the estimated number of measles deaths globally, disaggregated by MMR immunization status. In countries with high case and death rates, the World Health Organization (WHO) recommends mass immunization campaigns and routine MMR vaccinations for children.

---

* This is an edited, reformatted and augmented version of Congressional Research Service, Publication No. IN11104, dated April 19, 2019.

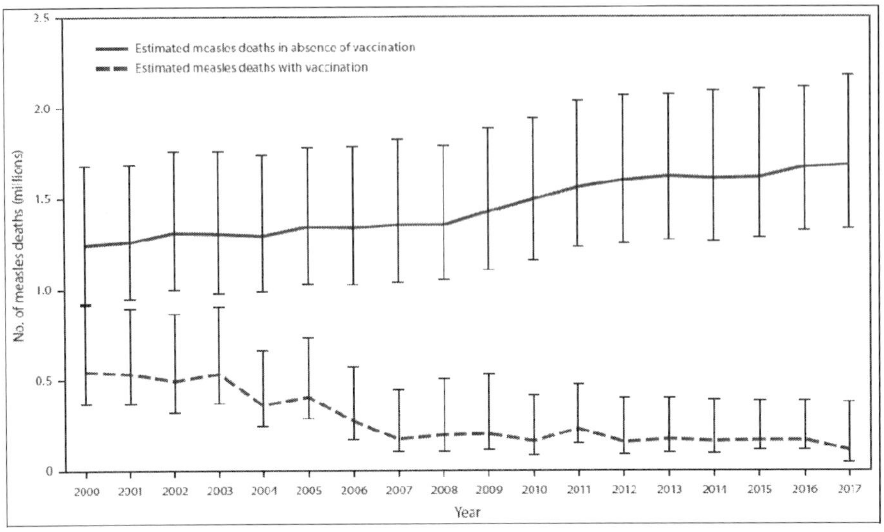

Source: Adapted by CRS from Dabbagh, A. et al., 2017.

Note: Deaths prevented by vaccination are indicated by the area between estimated deaths with vaccination and those without vaccination (cumulative total of 21.1 million deaths prevented during 2000–2017). Error bars represent upper and lower 95% confidence limits around the point estimate.

Figure 1. CDC Estimate: Annual Number of Measles Deaths, with and Without Vaccination Programs, Worldwide, 2010-2017.

In 2000 the World Health Assembly, the decisionmaking body of the WHO, endorsed the Global Vaccine Action Plan, which aimed to eliminate measles in five WHO regions by 2020. A global measles vaccination campaign ensued, and between 2000 and 2017 it resulted in an 80% drop in deaths from the disease and saved an estimated 21 million lives.

By the end of 2017, 85% of children worldwide had received one MMR dose by their second birthday, while 67% of children received the recommended two MMR doses. A 95% vaccination rate is necessary to achieve herd immunity and stop outbreak spread. Unvaccinated children and pregnant women are at the highest risk of measles and subsequent complications, including death. In 2017, there were 110,000 measles deaths globally, the majority of which were in children under five.

Regional Trends in Measles Cases

Despite the global increase in vaccination rates, measles outbreaks continue to occur. According to the WHO, one factor driving outbreaks is poverty: medical systems in many afflicted nations remain underfunded and weak, unable to vaccinate enough children to stop the virus' spread. Today, there are an estimated 21 million unvaccinated infants globally, half of whom are in five countries: Nigeria, India, Pakistan, Indonesia, and Ethiopia (see Figure 2).

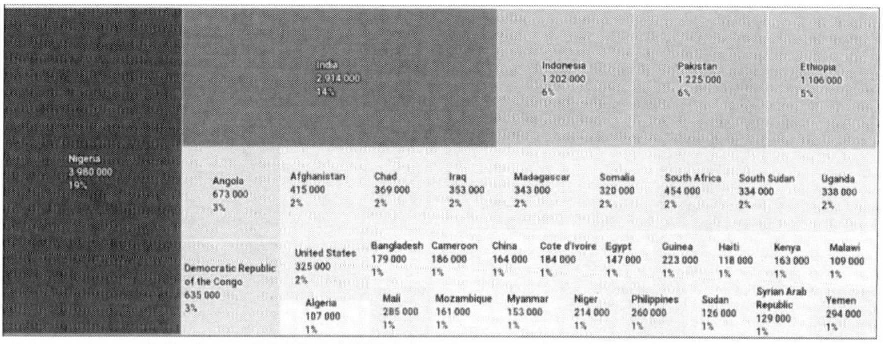

Source: Adapted by CRS from WHO/UNICEF estimates of national immunization coverage. Note: Countries comprising less than 1% of regional share of unvaccinated children are not shown.

Figure 2. Global Distribution of Children without Measles Antigen-Containing Vaccines (MCV), 2017.

Middle- and high-income countries are experiencing a resurgence of measles, due to a variety of socioeconomic, political, and cultural factors. In April 2019, the WHO reported a 300% increase in global measles cases compared to the same period in 2018. The Americas, the Middle East and Europe had the greatest upsurge in cases. Figure 3 maps out recent measles cases reported to the WHO.

In the Americas, the increase in measles cases is concentrated in three countries: the United States, Venezuela, and Brazil. In the United States, the increase in measles cases is largely because of low vaccination coverage in minority religious community pockets, and misinformation related to vaccines that has caused "vaccine hesitancy." The WHO considers vaccine hesitancy, defined as a "delay in acceptance or refusal of vaccines despite availability of vaccination services," to be one of the 10 biggest global public health threats. Venezuela, which had previously eradicated the disease, has seen a resurgence of measles cases, due in part to political and economic instability. The country's health system has collapsed, interrupting basic health services including routine vaccination campaigns. As a result, measles has returned and spread, primarily among vulnerable indigenous communities. Venezuelan refugees have caused an increase in cases throughout the region, with Brazil seeing the largest increase due to the shared Amazonian border with Venezuela.

In Europe, misinformation about vaccines and renewed interest in natural and non-GMO products have also led to vaccine hesitancy. As in the United States, experts believe that vaccine hesitancy is responsible for the increase in measles cases in Europe.

In the Middle East, the largest surge in measles cases has been in Yemen, which experts believe is due to the country's protracted conflict and humanitarian crisis.

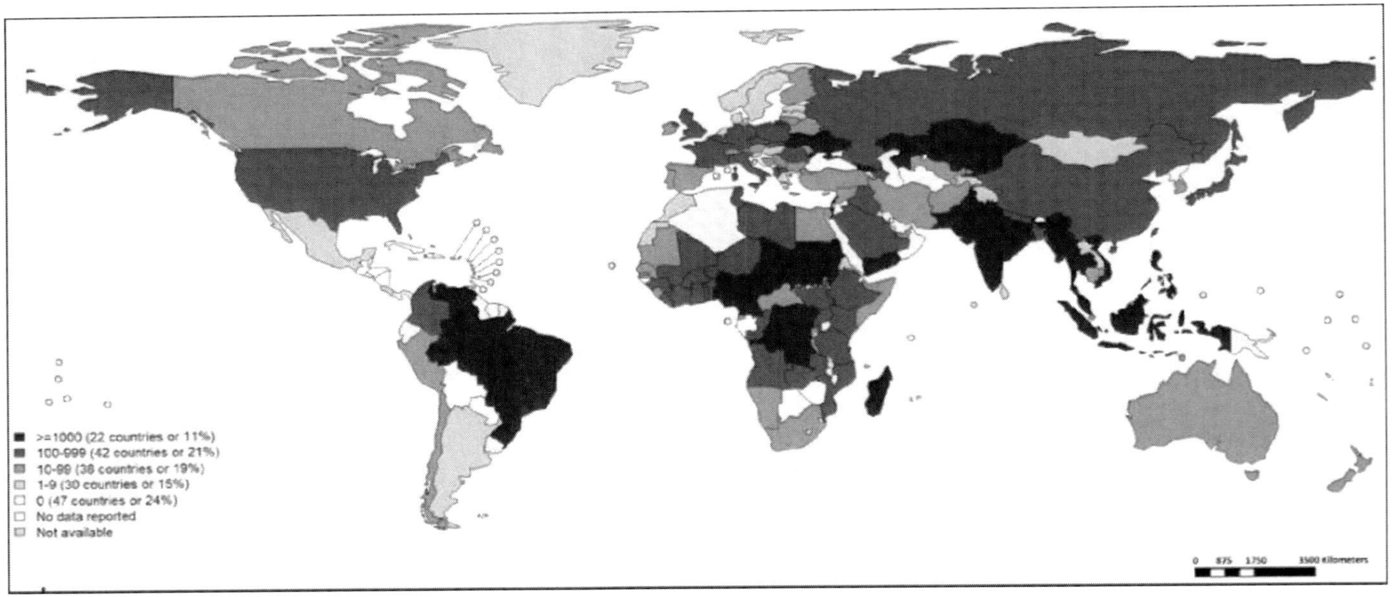

Source: World Health Organization, 2019.

Notes: Based on September 2018-February 2019 surveillance data received by the WHO in April 2019.

Figure 3. Measles Cases Reported to the WHO, September 2018-February 2019.

Relevant Agencies and U.S. Government Response

Congress has historically recognized the importance of vaccinations and immunizations. Through annual appropriations for the Department of Health and Human Services, and the Department of State, Congress funds CDC and the United States Agency for International Development (USAID) global immunization activities, as well as funding for the Global Alliance for Vaccines and Immunization (GAVI).

USAID and the CDC are the primary U.S. agencies involved in immunization provision and implementation internationally. Guided by the 2016-2020 Strategic Framework for Global Immunization, the agencies work with country governments to strengthen immunization programs through infectious disease surveillance, increasing laboratory capacity, and public health workforce capacity. They also support national routine immunization efforts through enhanced supply chain management and product procurement assistance. Related efforts are implemented bilaterally and through international partnerships with the WHO, UNICEF, the World Bank, and others.

INDEX

A

B

C

D

E

F

G

H

I

S

T

Related Nova Publications

Bacillus subtilis: Morphology, Functions and Role in Disease Management

Editor: Angelo Curtis

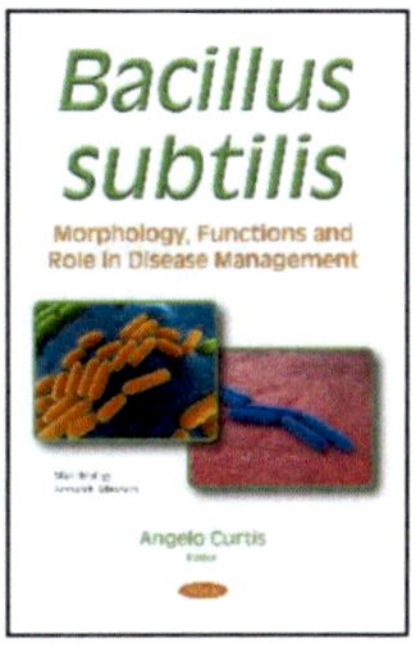

Series: Microbiology Research Advances

Book Description: In *Bacillus subtilis: Morphology, Functions and Role in Disease Management,* the authors begin by outlining the main features of chemotaxis as a behaviour, then reviewing the molecular machinery *Bacillus subtilis* uses to sense and respond to chemical cues.

Softcover ISBN: 978-1-53614-513-7
Retail Price: $95

The Role of Photosynthetic Microbes in Agriculture and Industry

Editors: Keshawanad Tripathi, Narendra Kumar, and Gerard Abraham

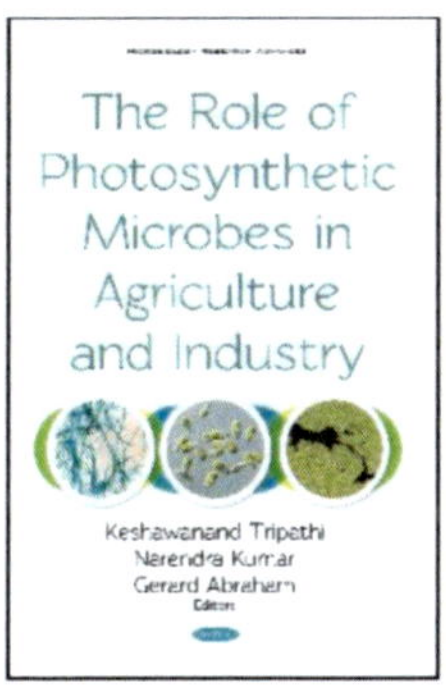

Series: Microbiology Research Advances

Book Description: This book attempts to highlight the potential and prospects of the photosynthetic microbes for the welfare of mankind in view of the anticipated population explosion and global climate change.

Hardcover ISBN: 978-1-53614-032-3
Retail Price: $195

To see a complete list of Nova publications, please visit our website at www.novapublishers.com